AF564818

Poultry Medicine

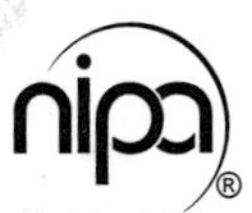

NIPA® GENX ELECTRONIC RESOURCES & SOLUTIONS P. LTD.
New Delhi-110 034

About the Editor

Dr. Tanmoy Rana obtained his Bachelor of Veterinary Sciences and Animal Husbandry degree (B.V.Sc. & A.H.) and Masters (M.V.Sc) in Veterinary Medicine, Ethics & Jurisprudence from West Bengal University of Animal and Fishery Sciences, Kolkata, India. He secured his Doctor of Philosophy (Ph.D.) in Veterinary Science from the University of Calcutta, Kolkata, India. He works currently as an Assistant Professor of the Veterinary Clinical Complex at West Bengal University of Animal and Fishery Sciences, Kolkata, India. Previously he has also worked as a Veterinary Officer, Animal Resources Development Department, Government of West Bengal, India. He is actively engaged in teaching and clinical practices in veterinary medicine and research related to animal health, production, and disease monitoring regimes. His research interests involve arsenic toxicity, molecular diagnosis, molecular toxicology and medicine, oxidative stress, immunopathology, nanoparticles, Echinococcosis, and microbes. He has published several research articles in reputed international and national journals along with review articles in international journals. He is an editorial board member (especially BMC Veterinary Research, Associate Editor of Frontier in Veterinary Science), and a reviewer of international and national journals. He is a member of many international scientific societies and organizations importantly the West Bengal Veterinary Council (WBVC), The Indian Society for Veterinary Medicine (ISVM), the Association of Public Health Veterinarians, and The Indian Science Congress Association (ISCA). He is also an associate of the West Bengal Academy of Science & Technology, West Bengal, India. He is an editor and author of so many national and international books.

Poultry Medicine

Tanmoy Rana, Ph.D.
AFWAST, FVASc., Assistant Professor
Veterinary Clinical Complex
(Veterinary Medicine, Ethics & Jurisprudence)
Department of Veterinary Clinical Complex
West Bengal University of Animal & Fishery Sciences
Kolkata-700037, West Bengal, India

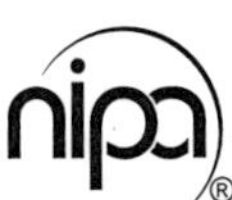

NIPA® GENX ELECTRONIC RESOURCES & SOLUTIONS P. LTD.
New Delhi-110 034

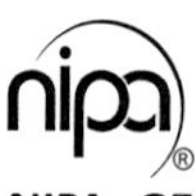

NIPA® GENX ELECTRONIC RESOURCES & SOLUTIONS P. LTD.

101,103, Vikas Surya Plaza, CU Block
L.S.C. Market, Pitam Pura, New Delhi-110 034
Ph : +91-11-43860225, Mob.: +91 9717133558, 9540816132
E-mail: newindiapublishingagency@gmail.com
Website: www.nipaersources.com

Print ISBN: 978-93-58875-12-6
ebook ISBN: 978-93-58879-26-1

Composed and Designed by NIPA®.

Preface

Poultry plays an important role in global food security as well as development economic condition by providing a readily available, affordable, and nutritious source of protein in the form of meat and eggs. It also provides income and employment opportunities, particularly in rural areas with a great contribution towards sustainable agriculture practices through the application of poultry manure as a fertilizer. In addition, poultry meat and eggs are very valuable sources of high-quality of protein that is essential for human health, Besides, poultry farming can provide a constant source of income, generation for small scale farmers in rural communities. It is well known that poultry have a relatively high feed conversion rate with a increasing demand of meat or eggs compared to other livestock. In this context, poultry health and disease and its management are well emphasized to improve productivity. The MCQ book of poultry medicine deals with both preventive and clinical medicine. The book is the valuable source of poultry medicine in which students can prepare themselves for competitive examinations like JRF/ SRF/ARS//NET, Union/State Public Service commission examination (UPSC) and Indian Forest Service's examination (IFS). This book, is well designed to markup easy understanding and easy grasping for the readership. The book is a comprehensive guidebook for the academicians to prepare question about the subject in the academic programme. The book is prepared in such a fashion that students are not feeling bored and monotonous. A brief introduction is also included in every chapter before starting of the MCQ for better understanding of the subject. The book covers more than 2000 solved multiple choice questions with their answer keys. I hope, the book will be helpful for the undergraduate and post graduates, to prepare various competitive examinations including ICAR-JRF, SRF, NET, ARS and other competitive examination. I also welcome readers to give their opinion, criticism, suggestions, and queries for bringing out the next edition for the better improvement of the readership.

Tanmoy Rana

Kolkata, India

Acknowledgement

I would like to convey my sincere gratitude to Hon'ble Vice Chancellor, West Bengal University of Animal& Fishery Sciences for providing me the opportunity to edit the book. I also express sincere thanks to all contributors who wholeheartedly helped me by sending their chapters in proper time. I am also thankful to all colleagues for their useful ideas, thoughts, and suggestions in this regard. I am also helpful to all the personnel at a publisher for helping me to edit MCQ book. I am also grateful to family members for providing great support and the time to finalize the book.

Tanmoy Rana
Kolkata, India

Contents

1

General Aspects of Poultry Preventive Medicine

K. Karthika[1], K. Jayalakshmi[2] and Tanmoy Rana[2]

[1]*Department of Veterinary Medicine, Veterinary College and Research Institute, Orathanadu, TANUVAS, Tamil Nadu*

[2]*Department of Veterinary Clinical Complex, Veterinary College and Research Institute, Orathanadu, TANUVAS, Tamil Nadu*

[2]*Department of Veterinary Clinical Complex, West Bengal University of Animal and Fishery Sciences, Kolkata*

Introduction

The Poultry industry stands as one of the most advanced sectors globally. The impact of diseases on poultry can be profoundly detrimental, affecting productivity, trade of live birds, meat and related products. Vulnerabilities in biosecurity within production sites, as well as weaknesses in disease diagnosis, pave the way for emerging pathogens to establish as persistent threats. In numerous tropical and developing nations poultry infections like viscerotropic velogenic New castle disease have become endemic, leading to disastrous losses. Many developing countries contend with a prevalence of vertically transmitted diseases among village-level flocks, including ailments like pullorum disease and mycoplasmosis. The combination of hot, humid climates fosters mycotoxicosis, compounded by prevalent immunosuppressive diseases, which in turn hinder the effectiveness of vaccination efforts. In the absence of robust quarantine measures and government – mandated control programs, disease can persist within both commercial and local flocks. The introduction of new infections further compounds the vulnerability of susceptible poultry populations.

Biosecurity, an integral part of any successful poultry production system. It involves identifying and eliminating all possible routes by which a disease could be accidentally introduced into a flock. The component of biosecurity include management, placement program, farm layout, decontamination (cleaning and disinfection), pest control, immunization directly affect productivity and profitability.

Poultry egg and meat are important sources of high quality proteins, minerals and vitamins to balance the human diet. Vaccinate all birds at one time in a house. Increase the level of antibiotics in water or feed 3-4 days before vaccination. Prevention and control of disease is an ongoing process, integrating management, nutrition, environmental control and genetics. Comprehensive disease- control strategies should be based on risk of disease and impact of disease on production cost. Disease survey should be done to ascertain the range of infections to which flocks are exposed and to define the epidemiology of diseases that are prevalent. This will facilitate development of vaccination programs of parent stock and progeny and appropriate supportive measures to prevent diseases. Vaccination programs are based on the prevalence and severity of disease agents in the area of operation and risk of introduction of disease. It is necessary to establish a balance between deleterious effect on performance following field exposure and cost associated with purchase and administration of vaccine

The major emphasis should be given for preventing disease in layer and broiler breeders to prevent the introduction of pathogen into flocks. Imported breeding stock should be free from vertically transmitted diseases like mycoplasmosis and pullorum disease and fowl typhoid. Rations should be carefully formulated to ensure free from mycotoxin. Diagnostic services should be available from the government or provided by producer. Emphasis should be placed on elimination of egg transmitted diseases and control of respiratory and immunosuppressive viral diseases.

A quarantine and depletion approach, followed by extremely through cleaning and disinfection, is considered only way to control the exotic infections, such as viscerotropic velogenic Newcastle disease, highly pathogenic avian influenza and fowl typhoid.

1. The following disease causes cyanosis of comb and swelling of wattle in poultry except
   a) Avian influenza b) Newcastle disease
   c) Avian pasteurellosis d) Infectious bronchitis
2. In-ovo vaccination is most commonly practiced for
   a) Newcastle disease b) Marek´s disease
   c) Infectious bronchitis d) Infectious bursal disease
3. Which of the following affect the T cell population in birds
   a) Chicken infectious anaemia b) Marek´s disease
   c) Avian leukosis d) Both a and b
4. When administration of vaccine in drinking water, which of the following is used to neutralize the negative effect of chlorine in the drinking water
   a) Skimmed milk powder b) Milk powder
   c) Milk d) All the above
5. Simple and cost effective method of disease prevention
   a) Biosecurity b) Vaccination
   c) Depopulation d) All the above
6. All-in all out system of rearing is effective for removal disease agents from poultry house
   a) Avian Mycoplasmosis b) Infectious coryza
   c) Avian influenza d) All the above
7. The ratio of formalin to potassium permanganate for fumigation of poultry shed
   a) 2:1 b) 1:2
   c) 1:3 d) 3:1

8. Dose of Bleaching powder for sanitation of 1000 litres of water
   a) 3g
   b) 5g
   c) 6g
   d) 8g
9. The most commonly used chemical for control of fungal diseases in poultry
   a) Copper sulphate @ 0.5%
   b) Copper sulphate @ 1.0%
   c) Chlorhexidine @ 1%
   d) Glutaraldehyde @ 2%
10. Which of the following have bactericidal, virucidal, fungicidal and sporicidal activity
   a) Sodium hypochlorite
   b) Quaternary ammonium compound
   c) Glutaraldehyde
   d) Formaldehyde
11. Rich source of IgA antibody in chicken is
   a) Respiratory tract
   b) Bile
   c) Intestinal tract
   d) Oviduct
12. Which of the following infection in chicken is predisposed to colibacillosis
   a) Mycotoxin
   b) Ranikhet disease
   c) Infectious bronchitis
   d) All the above
13. Broiler flocks affected with Chronic respiratory disease predisposed or aggravated the
   a) Colisepticemia
   b) Necrotic enteritis
   c) Fowl cholera
   d) All the above
14. Colisepticemia in chicks are controlled by
   a) Chlorination of drinking water
   b) Probiotics
   c) Wetting the litter materials
   d) All the above
15. Prevalence of *Haemophillus paragallinarum* serotypes in chicken in India
   a) Serotype A
   b) Serotype B
   c) Serotype C
   d) Both a and b
16. Necrotic enteritis in poultry is caused by
   a) *Clostridium perfringens* type B
   b) *Clostridium perfringens type C*
   c) *Clostridium septicum*
   d) *None of the above*
17. Outbreak of Coccidiosis in chicken is predisposed to
   a) Necrotic enteritis
   b) Colibacillosis
   c) Salmonellosis
   d) Newcastle disease
18. Predisposing factor for necrotic enteritis in poultry
   a) Fish meal
   b) Soya meal
   c) Bone meal
   d) None of the above

19. Casual organism for ulcerative enteritis in quail is
    a) *Clostridium perfringens*
    b) *Clostridium botulinum*
    c) *Clostridium collinum*
    d) *Clostridium sporogens*
20. The most commonly used screening test for pullorum disease in poultry
    a) Whole blood agglutination test
    b) Enzyme linked immunosorbent assay
    c) Tube agglutination test
    d) Agar gel precipitation test
21. Which of the following is vertically transmitted diseases in poultry
    a) Pullorum disease
    b) Avian mycoplasmosis
    c) Fowl typhoid
    d) All the above
22. The control of pullorum disease and fowl typhoid is achieved by
    a) Screening of breeder flock before egg laying
    b) Disinfection
    c) Water sanitation
    d) All the above
23. Drug of choice for chronic respiratory disease in chicken
    a) Tylosin
    b) Oxytetracycline
    c) Tiamulin
    d) Streptomycin
24. The first report of Newcastle disease in England
    a) 1924
    b) 1925
    c) 1926
    d) 1927
25. Which of the following disinfectant is effective against both enveloped and non enveloped virus
    a) Formalin
    b) Glutaraldehyde
    c) Quaternary ammonium compound
    d) Iodophor
26. Which of the following avian is most susceptible to aflatoxicosis
    a) Duckling
    b) Goose
    c) Turkey
    d) Chicken
27. Which of the following disease is not causes paralysis in poultry
    a) Marek´s disease
    b) Infectious bronchitis
    c) Newcastle disease
    d) Avian influenza
28. Thin shelled egg and shell-less are noticed in
    a) Infectious bronchitis
    b) Newcastle disease
    c) Egg drop syndrome
    d) All the above
29. Trickle infection in poultry is used for control of
    a) Coccidiosis
    b) Ascariasis
    c) Avian trichomoniasis
    d) Nodular taeniasis

30. Which of the following programme is followed to prevent drug resistance in poultry against coccidiosis
    a) Trickle infection
    b) Shuttle programme
    c) Step-down programme
    d) All the above
31. Identify the odd one from the following vaccine strain of infectious bronchitis
    a) Massachusetts
    b) Arkansas-99
    c) Connecticut
    d) Mukteswar
32. Watery whites are seen in
    a) Newcastle disease
    b) Infectious bronchitis
    c) EDS-76
    d) Infectious bursal disease
33. The major cause of vaccine failure in poultry
    a) Mycotoxin
    b) Improper vaccination
    c) Low potency of vaccine
    d) All the above
34. Virulence of Newcastle disease virus is assessed by
    a) Nucleotide sequencing
    b) Isolation of virus
    c) Intracerebral pathogenicity index
    d) Both a and c
35. Which of the following bacteria is transmitted from bird to human
    a) *Salmonella pullorum*
    b) Salmonella gallinarum
    c) Salmonella enteritidis
    d) Salmonella typhimurium
36. Botulism in poultry is also called as
    a) Limberneck
    b) *Lamsiektte*
    c) Western Duck Sickness
    d) Both a and c
37. Minimum lethal dose of botulinum toxin in Guineapig
    a) 0.000012 mg/Kg
    b) 0.00012 mg/Kg
    c) 0.0012 mg/Kg
    d) 0.012 mg/Kg
38. The outbreak of botulism in chicken is most commonly associated with
    a) Cl. botulinum Type A
    b) Cl. botulinum Type B
    c) Cl. botulinum Type C
    d) Cl. botulinum Type D
39. Pseudobotulism is ....
    a) Marek′s disease
    b) Newcastle disease
    c) Avian encephalomyelitis
    d) Avian influenza
40. The area enzootic for botulism, the following are prophylactically used to control the botulism in broiler farm
    a) Antibiotics
    b) Selenium
    c) Alkaline water
    d) Both a and b
41. The most susceptible species for bordetellosis
    a) Chicken
    b) Duck
    c) Turkey
    d) Quail

42. Which of the following causes upper respiratory disease in chicken except
    a) Infectious bronchitis
    b) Infectious laryngotracheitis
    c) Bordetellosis
    d) Infectious coryza
43. The most susceptible species for erysipelas
    a) Chicken
    b) Turkey
    c) Duck
    d) Guinea fowl
44. Cutaneous and muscular haemorrhage in turkey is seen in
    a) Infectious bursal disease
    b) Bordetellosis
    c) Erysipelas
    d) None of the above
45. Transmission of fowl cholera in chicken occurs through
    a) Swine and raccoons
    b) Wild birds
    c) Cannibalism & scavenging of dead birds
    d) All the above
46. Vaccine strain used in fowl cholera vaccine
    a) PM-1
    b) M-9
    c) CU
    d) All the above
47. Treatment of choice for fowl cholera in chicken
    a) Sulphaquinoxaline
    b) Tetracycline
    c) Penicillin
    d) Both a and b
48. Route of administration of fowl cholera vaccine in chicken
    a) Wing web
    b) Subcutaneous
    c) Drinking water
    d) Nasal drop
49. Age of fowl cholera vaccination in turkey
    a) 6-7th weeks
    b) 8-9th weeks
    c) 10-11th weeks
    d) 13-14th weeks
50. Repeated problem of gangrenous dermatitis in chicken is controlled by
    a) Salting the floor
    b) Use of bedding material
    c) Disinfection
    d) All the above
51. The gangrenous dermatitis is most commonly occur in the following infection
    a) Infectious bursal disease
    b) Chicken infectious anaemia
    c) Aflatoxicosis
    d) All the above
52. Wing rot in chicken is caused by
    a) *Staphylococcus aureus*
    b) Clostridium septicum
    c) *Escherchia coli*
    d) All the above
53. Diagnosis of *Mycoplasma gallisepticum* is carried out by using
    a) Haemagglutination test
    b) Enzyme linked immunosorbent assay
    c) Agar gel immunodiffusion test
    d) Both a and b

54. Which of the following used as vaccine strain in Mycoplasma vaccine
   a) F-strain
   b) TS 11 strain
   c) 6/85 strain
   d) All the above
55. Which of the following causes runting syndrome and chronic lymphoma in chicken
   a) Chicken infectious anaemia
   b) Reticuloendotheliosis
   c) Lymphoid leukosis
   d) Marek´s disease
56. Which of the following causes thymic atrophy in chicken
   a) Reticuloendotheliosis
   b) Inclusion body hepatitis
   c) Chicken infectious anaemia
   d) Both a and c
57. Duck viral enteritis is caused by
   a) Paramyxovirus
   b) Herpesvirus
   c) Circovirus
   d) Coronavirus
58. Duck viral hepatitis is caused by
   a) Enterovirus
   b) Anellovirus
   c) Herpesvirus
   d) Paramyxovirus
59. Which of the following used as vector in recombinant vaccine
   a) Fowlpox virus
   c) Adenovirus
   b) Herpesvirus of turkey
   d) All the above
60. Aflatoxicosis in poultry is most commonly caused by
   a) *Aspergillus flavus*
   b) Aspergillus fumigates
   c) *Aspergillus niger*
   d) Aspergillus tereus
61. Identify correct statement(s)
   i. Newcastle disease in chicken is caused by APMV-2&3
   ii. Inactivated vaccine was effective without initial priming with live vaccine
   iii. Diarrhoea and neurological symptoms are predominant in pigeon with ND
   iv. ND vaccine provide sterile and long term immunity
   a) (i) and (iii)
   b) (ii) and (iii)
   c) (iii) only
   d) (i), (ii), (iii) and (iv)
62. The media used for isolation of Salmonella pullorum
   a) Rappaport-vassiliadis medium
   b) Dorset egg yolk agar
   c) Eosin-methylene blue agar
   d) Stuart medium
63. Which of the following causes dermal necrosis in turkey
   a) Fowl cholera
   b) Wing rot
   c) Necrotic enteritis
   d) None of the above
64. The flock immunity is good when layers are vaccinated
   a) 50 %
   b) 60 %
   c) 70 %
   d) > 85 %

65. The most commonly used mass vaccination method in Indian condition
    a) Aerosol spray b) Drinking water
    c) Eye drop d) Nasal drop
66. Fine tremor of head and neck was observed in
    a) Newcastle disease b) Marek´s disease
    c) Avian encephalomyelitis d) Avian influenza
67. Cystic oviduct of chicken is seen in
    a) Infectious bursal disease b) Avian leukosis
    c) Infectious bronchitis d) Newcastle disease
68. Bollinger bodies in infected cells are observed in
    a) Fowlpox b) Lymphoid leukosis
    c) Marek´s disease d) Infectious laryngotracheitis
69. Epidemic tremor of chicken is caused by
    a) Astrovirus b) Anellovirus
    c) Enterovirus d) Herpesvirus
70. Emergence of new subtype of avian influenza virus arises due to
    a) Genetic reassortment b) Point mutation
    c) Conjugation d) Both a and b
71. Identify the incorrect statement(s)
    i. Pullorum disease mainly affect the adult birds
    ii. Fowl cholera mostly occur in young age
    iii. Sinusitis is most common symptoms in turkey infected with Mycoplasma gallisepticum
    iv. The birds recovered from mycoplasmosis remain lifelong carrier
    a) (i) and (ii) b) (ii) and (iii)
    c) (iii) and (iv) d) (i), (ii), (iii) and (iv)
72. Which of the following is commonly used for molecular tracking and spread of infection among the flocks
    a) PCR b) RAPD
    c) Nucleic acid probe d) LAMP
73. First outbreak of Avian influenza was reported in the world
    a) 1997 b) 2003
    c) 2004 d) 2006
74. Newcastle disease virus is classified as virulence, if the ICPI is
    a) 0.2 or above b) 0.5 or above
    c) 0.7 or above d) 0.9 or above
75. Low pathogenic Avian Influenza virus is mostly found in
    a) Migratory water fowl b) Duck
    c) Turkey d) All the above

76. Age of fowlpox vaccination
    a) 2-4th weeks
    b) 4-6th weeks
    c) 6-8th weeks
    d) 8-10th weeks
77. Take was observed in skin following vaccination against
    a) Fowlpox
    b) Fowl cholera
    c) Infectious laryngotracheitis
    d) Both a and b
78. Which of the following causes immunosuppression in chicken
    a) Marek's disease
    b) Infectious bursal disease
    c) Chicken infectious anaemia
    d) All the above
79. The permissible level of aflatoxin in poultry feed
    a) <20 ppb
    b) 50 ppb
    c) 100 ppb
    d) 200 ppb
80. Toxin binder used for aflatoxin in poultry feed
    a) HSCAS
    b) Sodium bentonite
    c) Zeolite
    d) All the above
81. Predisposing factor for candidiasis in chicken
    a) Prolonged antibiotic therapy
    b) Corticosteroids
    c) Vitamin A deficiency
    d) All the above
82. The following are treatment of choice for psittacosis except
    a) Chlortetracycline
    b) Tetracycline
    c) Doxycycline
    d) Penicillin
83. Nodular taeniasis in poultry is caused by
    a) *Raillietina echinobothrida*
    b) *Raillietina tetragona*
    c) *Raillietina cesticillus*
    d) *Daveina proglottina*
84. Age of vaccination and route administration of infectious laryngotracheitis vaccine in layers
    a) 7 weeks- eye drop
    b) 9 weeks- eye drop
    c) 10 weeks- eye drop
    d) 12 weeks-eye dop
85. Turkey towel appearance of crop was seen in
    a) Candidiasis
    b) Trichomoniasis
    c) Psittacosis
    d) Megabacteria
86. Inactivating agent used in fowl cholera vaccine
    a) Formalin
    b) Thiomersal
    c) Binary Ethyleneamine
    d) Aziridine
87. Maintenance of maternal antibody in chicks are important for prevention of
    a) Infectious bursal disease
    b) Infectious bronchitis
    c) Newcastle disease
    d) Marek's disease
88. Coarse spray vaccination is usually practiced in hatchery to control the
    a) Newcastle disease
    b) Infectious bronchitis
    c) Coccidiosis
    d) All the above

89. Optimum particle size of vaccine in coarse spray vaccination
  a) 20 μ b) 50-100 μ
  c) 100-150 μ d) 200 μ
90. The vaccine stored in liquid nitrogen is
  a) Marek´s disease vaccine b) Infectious bursal disease vaccine
  c) Mycoplasma vaccine d) Infectious bronchitis vaccine
91. Intravenous pathogenicity index of highly pathogenic avian influenza (HPAI) is
  a) 0.5 b) 0.7
  b) 1.0 d) >1.2
92. Interstitial nephritis in chicks is caused by
  a) Coronavirus b) Gumborovirus
  c) Reovirus d) Astrovirus
93. Diphtheritic lesions on mouth, oesophagus and trachea is found in
  a) Infectious laryngotracheitis b) Fowlpox
  c) Newcastle disease d) Candidiasis
94. Minimum quarantine period for importation of birds
  a) 14 days b) 21 days
  c) 28 days d) 30 days
95 Excellent choice of environmental disinfection even in the presence of organic debris
  a) Accelerated hydrogen peroxide b) Phenol
  c) Peroxymonosulfate d) Both a and c
96. Peroxymonosulfate disinfectant is effective against
  a) Bacteria including Bacterial spore b) Non- enveloped virus
  c) Cryptosporidium d) All the above
97. Big liver and spleen disease in chicken is caused by
  a) Hepatitis A virus b) Hepatitis B virus
  c) Hepatitis C virus d) Hepatitis E virus
98. The most commonly used vaccine strain for infectious bursal disease
  a) Intermediate strain b) Intermediate plus strain
  c) Delaware strain d) Classical strain
99. Oil adjuvanted inactivated vaccine is most commonly used in commercial poultry
  a) Chicks b) Growers
  c) Before egg production d) None
100. Black head in turkey is caused by
  a) *Histomonas meleagridis* *b) Heterakis gallinarum*
  c) *Salmonella gallinarum* *d) Pasteurella multocida*

101. The major source of Marek´s disease virus in commercial layers

a) Infected feather follicle
d) Faeces
b) Nasal discharge
d) Red mite

102. Shedding of avian leukosis virus in breeder flock is identified in

a) Albumin
b) Egg yolk
c) Feather follicle
d) Nasal discharge

103. The gene responsible for viral replication and triggers apoptosis in infected cell in chicken infectious anaemia

a) VP1
b) VP2
c) VP3
d) VP4

104. Tenosynovitis and arthritis in chicken is caused by

a) Reovirus
b) Astrovirus
c) Circovirus
d) None of the above

105. Prolonged clotting time was observed in birds infected with

a) Myeloid leukosis
b) Lymphoid leukosis
c) Chicken infectious anaemia
d) Reticuloendotheliosis

106. Drug of choice for tape worm infection in poultry

a) Praziquantel @ 10 mg/Kg
b) Niclosomide @ 100 mg/Kg
c) Albendazole @ 7.5 mg/Kg
d) Both a and b

107. Which of the following most frequently causes intestinal obstruction in desi chicken

a) *Ascardia galli*
b) Raillitenia cesticillus
c) *Heterakis gallinarum*
d) All the above

108. Renal coccidiosis in geese is caused by

a) *Eimeria anseris*
b) Eimeria truncata
c) *Eimeria adenoids*
d) Eimeria stediae

109. Pasteurellosis in duck is caused by

a) *Pasteurella multocida*
b) Mannheimia haemolytica
c) *Rimerella anatipestifer*
d) Biberstenia trehalosi

110. Whitish or watery diarrhoea with vent pecking is a classical symptom of

a) Infectious bursal disease
b) Newcastle disease
c) Pullorum disease
d) Fowl cholera

111. ICPI of Mesogenic Roakin strain of NDV

a) 0.4
b) 1.4
c) 1.45
d) 1.6

112. Age of occurrence of chicken infectious anaemia

a) < 3 weeks
b) 4 weeks
b) 5 weeks
d) 8 weeks

113. Drug of choice for coccidiosis
   a) Sulphadimidine b) Amprolium
   c) Ethopabate d) Monensin

114. Which of the following is used as sporulating agent
   a) 2.5% Potassium dichromate b) 2.5% Potassium chromate
   c) 5 .0% Potassium dichromate d) 5.0% Potassium chloride

115. First anticancer vaccine used in poultry
   a) HVT b) SB-1
   c) CVI988 d) None of the above

116. Identify the correct statement(s)
   i. Ornithobacterium *rhinotracheale* mainly affect the young broilers
   ii. Mushy chick disease is caused by *E.coli*
   iii. Haemorrhagic tracheitis in layer is caused by syngamus trachea
   iv. Campylobacter is a non-fastidious fast growing organism
   a) (i) only b) (i) and (ii)
   c) (i), (ii) and (iv) d) (i), (ii), (iii) and (iv)

117. Identify the correct statement(s)
   i. Swollen head syndrome in chicken is caused by Avian metapneumovirus
   ii. Infectious laryngotracheitis mainly affect the young chicken
   iii. The bird recovered from infection with mesogenic roakin strain of Newcastle disease virus has detectable hemagglutination inhibition antibodies for one year
   iv. Eye drop vaccination with Hitchner B1 results in replication of virus in harderian gland
   a) (i) and (ii) b) (i) and (iii)
   c) (i), (iii) and (iv) d) (i), (ii), (iii) and (iv)

118. Identify the incorrect statement(s)
   i. Dwarfing and curling of embryo is pathognomic lesion of infectious laryngotracheitis
   ii. Pock lesions on chorioallantoic membrane is pathognomic lesions for fowl pox
   iii. Subclinical form of IBD causes long lasting immunosuppression in chicken
   iv. Connecticut strain of infectious bronchitis virus used as vaccine strain throughout the world
   a) (i) and (ii) b) (i), (ii) and (iii)
   c) (iii) only d) (i), (ii) and (iv)

119. Identify the correct statement(s)
   i. Duck viral hepatitis (DHV) mainly affect the young duckling less than 6 weeks of age
   ii. Duck hepatitis virus causes ecchymotic haemorrhage in liver
   iii. Duckling are protected from DHV through breeder flock vaccination
   iv. Chick embryo origin of modified live DHAV-1 vaccine can be used in day old duckling
   a) (i) and (iii) b) (i) and(iv)
   c) (i), (ii) and (iii) d) (i), (ii), (iii) and (iv)

120. Identify the correct statement(s)
   i. Duck viral enteritis (DVE) mainly affect the adult ducks and causes persistent mortality
   ii. Outbreaks of DVE is frequent in duck flocks accessed to water bodies with free living waterfowl
   iii. DVEV causes damage to blood vessels result in widespread haemorrhage in body tissue
   iv. Chicken embryo-adopted modified live DVE vaccine used for vaccination of duckling
   a) (i) and (ii) b) (i), (ii) and (iii)
   c) (i), (iii) and (iv) d) (i), (ii), (iii) and (iv)

121. Identify the correct statement(s)
   i. Lentogenic virus of NDV causes serious respiratory disease in young birds
   ii. Harderian gland is the main site for IgA antibody production in chicken
   iii. Chicken and turkeys infected in lay with velogenic viruses usually have egg yolk in the abdominal cavity
   iv. Newcastle disease virus is labile in environment
   a) (i) and (ii) b) (ii), (iii) and (iv)
   c) (i), (ii) and (iii) d) (i), (ii), (iii) and (iv)

122. Identify the incorrect statement(s)
   i. Derzsy´s disease is highly contagious disease of young goosling
   ii. Goose parvovirus causes high mortality in goosling and duckling under 1 week of age
   iii. Penguin-like posture is seen in goosling with goose hepatitis
   iv. In Derzsy´s disease fibrinous pseudomembrane is observed on tongue and oral cavity
   a) (i) only b) (ii), (iii) and (iv)
   c) (i) and (iii) d) (i), (ii), (iii) and (iv)

123. Inclusion body hepatitis mainly affect the
   a) Broilers b) Layers
   c) Backyard poultry d) Quail

124. The change of vocalization in pet birds is observed in
   a) Aspergillosis   b) Tuberculosis
   c) Psittacosis   d) Mycoplasmosis

125. Screening of progeny chicks for mycoplasmosis is carried out
   a) 2 days after hatching   b) 5 days after hatching
   c) 7 days after hatching   d) 9 days after hatching

126. Recently started Animal Quarantine and Certification Services in India
   a) Delhi   b) Bangalore
   c) Mumbai   d) Chennai

127. Etiology of Brooder pneumonia in chicks
   a) *Aspergillus fumigatus*   *b) Aspergillus parasiticus*
   c) *Aspergillus flavus*   *d) Aspergillus niger*

128. Which of the followings are used for detection of elementary bodies in infected tissue of birds affected with psittacosis
   a) Macchiavello stain   b) Gimenez stain
   c) Giemsa stain   d) All the above

129. Oral canker in pigeon is caused by
   a) *Trichomonas gallinae*   *b) Candida albicans*
   b) Pigeon poxvirus   d) *Trichomonas avium*

130. Sulphur yellow droppings are seen in
   a) Histomoniasis   b) Psittacosis
   c) Pullorum disease   d) Fowl typhoid

131. Coccidial oocysts in the poultry house environment is destroyed by
   a) Heaping of manure
   b) Fumigation with NH_4OH and $KMnO_4$
   b) Application of quick lime
   d) All the above

132. Which of the following causes sudden death, acute pneumonia and weakened skull bone in young birds
   a) *Pasteurella multocida*
   b) Ornithobacterium rhinotracheale
   b) *Salmonella pullorum*
   d) Mycoplasma gallispeticum

133. White yoghurt like exudates with fibrin clots in abdominal air sacs are seen in birds infected with
   a) *Ornithobacterium rhinotracheale*   *b) Escherchia coli*
   c) *Haemophillus paragallinarum*   *d)* Both a & b

134. The most common cause of bumble foot in chicken and duck
   a) *Staphylococcus aureus*   *b) Escherchia coli*
   c) *Mycoplasma synoviae*   *d)* All the above

135. The rapid diagnostic test for tuberculosis in birds
   a) Intradermal test b) Whole blood agglutination test
   c) Enzyme linked immunosorbent assay d) Polymerase chain reaction
136. Gapes in poultry is caused by
   a) *Syngamus trachea* *b) Tetrameres mohtedai*
   c) *Ascardia galli* *d) Hymenolepsis nana*
137. Classical symptoms of Favus cups in chicken
   a) White powdery spot on comb
   b) Patchy loss of feathers
   c) Thick, crusting and hardened skin around the feather follicle
   d) All the above
138. Favus cups in chicken is also called as
   a) Avian ringworm b) Scaly leg
   b) Depluming itch d) None of the above
139. Oviduct fluke in poultry
   a) *Prosthogoniumus macrorchis* *b) Cyathocotyle bushiensis*
   c) *Sphaeridiotrema globules* *d) Philophthalmus gralli*
140. Mycotoxicosis in poultry causes
   a) Vaccination failure
   b) Impaired egg production efficiency
   c) Immunosuppression
   d) All the above
141. Sternal bursitis or breast blisters in chicken is caused by
   a) *Mycoplasma synoviae* *b) Mycoplasma gallispeticum*
   c) *Staphylococcus aureus* *d)* All the above
142. Pale, friable and swollen liver with petechial and ecchymotic haemorrhage on liver and skeletal muscle is seen in
   a) Fowl cholera b) Fowl pox
   c) Inclusion body hepatitis d) Fowl plague
143. Levinthal-cole-Lillie bodies (LCL bodies) are seen in
   a) Infectious laryngiotracheitis b) Psittacosis
   c) Fowl pox d) Lymphoid leukosis
144. The birds treated for psittacosis using chlortetracycline is kept under veterinary supervision before shipment for
   a) 14 days b) 21 days
   c) 28 days d) 45 days
145. Which of the following diseases causes more number of dead- in shells and dead chicks in the incubator
   a) Pullorum disease b) Fowl cholera
   c) Fowl typhoid d) Mycoplasmosis

146. Which of the following test is used for evaluation of antibodies in serum after vaccination of chicken against IBD
   a) ELISA b) VNT
   c) AGID d) All the above

147. Derzsy's disease is commonly called as
   a) Goosling plague b) Goose hepatitis
   c) Infectious myocarditis d) All the above

148. Pigeon malaria is caused by
   a) *Hemoproteus columbae* *b)* *Hemoproteus meleagridis*
   c) *Hemoproteus iophortyx* *d)* *Plasmodium vivax*

149. Treatment of choice for Pigeon malaria
   a) Chloroquine b) Primaquine
   c) Buparvaquone d) All the above

150. The classical signs of leucocytozoonosis in duckling and turkey poults
   a) Anaemia b) Diarrhoea with green dropping
   c) CNS symptoms d) All the above

Answer Key

1	d	2	b	3	d	4	a	5	a	6	d	7	a
8	c	9	a	10	c	11	c	12	d	13	a	14	d
15	d	16	b	17	a	18	a	19	c	20	a	21	d
22	a	23	a	24	c	25	b	26	a	27	b	28	d
29	a	30	b	31	d	32	b	33	d	34	d	35	c
36	d	37	b	38	c	39	a	40	d	41	c	42	a
43	b	44	c	45	d	46	d	47	d	48	a	49	a
50	a	51	d	52	d	53	d	54	d	55	b	56	d
57	b	58	a	59	d	60	a	61	c	62	a	63	a
64	d	65	b	66	c	67	c	68	a	69	c	70	d
71	c	72	b	73	a	74	c	75	d	76	b	77	d
78	d	79	a	80	d	81	d	82	d	83	a	84	a
85	a	86	a	87	a	88	d	89	c	90	a	91	d
92	a	93	b	94	d	95	d	96	d	97	d	98	a
99	c	100	a	101	a	102	a	103	c	104	a	105	c
106	d	107	a	108	b	109	c	110	a	111	c	112	a
113	a	114	a	115	a	116	b	117	c	118	b	119	d
120	d	121	c	122	d	123	a	124	a	125	a	126	b
127	a	128	d	129	a	130	a	131	d	132	b	133	a
134	a	135	b	136	a	137	d	138	a	139	a	140	d
141	a	142	c	143	b	144	d	145	a	146	a	147	d
148	a	149	d	150	d								

2

Viral Diseases

J.B. Kathiriya, S.H. Sindhi and K.R. Bhedi

Department of Veterinary Public Health & Epidemiology, College of Veterinary Science & A. H., Kamdhenu University, Junagadh-362001, Gujarat, India

---

1. Which of the following is not a reason for animal disease?
   a) Genetic diseases b) Deficiency diseases
   c) Environmental discomforts d) Hygiene and cleanliness
2. Which of the following steps should not be done for the prevention of infectious diseases?
   a) Proper disposal of dead infected animals
   b) Disinfection of the animal house
   c) Freedom of infected animals
   d) Vaccination of animals against major diseases
3. Which of the following virus causes Foot and Mouth disease?
   a) Coxsackievirus b) Cowpoxvirus
   c) Retrovirus d) Reovirus
4. Which of the following is not a characteristic symptom of Foot and Mouth disease?
   a) An eruption of vesicles over the lips b) Fever
   c) Increase in appetite d) Lameness
5. Cowpox is caused by cowpox virus.
   a) True b) False
6. Which of the following diseases can spread to humans while milking?
   a) Foot and Mouth disease b) Small Pox
   c) Ranikhet d) Cowpox
7. Which of the following is the highly contagious viral disease of cattle?
   a) Foot and Mouth disease b) Rinderpest
   c) Cowpox d) Ranikhet
8. Which of the following is not a method by which Rinderpest is spread amongst cattle?
   a) Contact b) Contaminated feed
   c) Flies d) Clean water

9. Which of the following is not a symptom of Rinderpest?
   a) Dysentery b) Fever
   c) Congestion d) Blueurine
10. Prophylaxis was initiated in India in 1954 and has effectively controlled rinderpest.
   a) True b) False
11. Which of the following is not a viral disease?
   a) Salmonellosis b) Ranikhetdisease
   c) Laryngotracheitis d) FowlPox
12. Which of the following is incorrect about Bird Flu?
   a) Caused by H5N1 b) Bacterialdisease
   c) Also known as Avian influenza d) Attacks poultry birds
13. Poliovirus affects which pathway during paralysis of muscles?
   a) Motor Pathway b) Sensory Pathway
   c) Inter-neuron Pathway d) Intra-neuron Pathway
14. In which of the following area the effect of Poliovirus is not fatal?
   a) Diaphragm b) Larynx
   c) Pharynx d) Limbs
15. When was Polio eradicated from India?
   a) 13 January 2011 b) 25 April 2013
   c) 27 March 2014 d) 7 August 2010
16. *Flavivirus* group causes which of the following pair of diseases?
   a) Amoebic Dysentery and Ascariasis b) Rabies and Plague
   c) Dengue and Tetanus d) Dengue and Yellow Fever
17. Which of the following is not the symptom of Classic Dengue Fever?
   a) Blood vessels become fragile b) Very high fever
   c) Pain behind the eyes d) Joints are affected
18. Chikungunya is a viral disease transmitted to humans by infected mosquitoes
   a) True b) False
19. What is the full form of SARS?
   a) Silk Associated Respiratory Syndrome
   b) Severe Acute Respiratory Syndrome
   c) Sand Acquired Respiratory Syndrome
   d) Severely Assimilated Respiratory Syndrome
20. Which of the following viruses cause Swine Flu?
   a) S1H1 virus b) X1Z1 virus
   c) H1N1 virus d) N1M1virus
21. A viral disease causing painful swelling of the parotid gland is __________
   a) Measles b) Mumps
   c) Rabies d) Influenza

22. The disease that may cause sterility due to the infection spreading to sex organs is ________

a) Mumps b) Measles

c) Swine Flu d) Chicken Pox

23. Which type of Hepatitis cannot be transferred by blood or sexual contact?

a) Hepatitis A b) Hepatitis B

c) Hepatitis C d) Hepatitis D

24. Which of the following Hepatitis virus has a different strand of genetic material?

a) Hepatitis C virus b) Hepatitis A virus

c) Hepatitis B virus d) Hepatitis D virus

25. Which vaccine is given to prevent Hepatitis B infection?

a) BCG Vaccine b) Sabin Vaccine

c) Salk Vaccine d) Recombivax HB

26. *Rhino* viruses infect the nose, respiratory passage as well as the lungs of a person suffering from cold.

a) True b) False

27. Which virus causes Small Pox disease?

a) *Variolavirus* b) *Varicellazoster*

c) *Rubeolavirus* d) *Rhabdo virus*

28. *Variola* virus has ________ as genetic material.

a) Single stranded RNA b) Double stranded RNA

c) Single stranded DNA d) Double stranded DNA

29. Small Pox vaccine is which kind of vaccine?

a) Attenuated Vaccine b) Inactivated Vaccine

c) Second Generation Vaccine d) Third Generation Vaccine

30. Who is known as the Father of Immunology?

a) Dmitry Ivanovsky b) Edward Jenner

c) Erik Acharius d) Francesco Redi

31. When was Small Pox eradicated from the world?

a) 1971 b) 1977

c) 1967 d) 1980

32. In Chicken Pox, rashes first appear on the body and then on the face.

a) True b) False

33. Which of the following is the most common late complication of Chicken Pox?

a) Fever b) Shingles

c) Small Pox d) Mumps

34. What is the full form of MMR vaccine?

a) Mumps Measles Rabies

b) Malignant Melanoma Rheumatism

c) Measles Mumps Rubella

d) Malignant-Malaria Rheumatoid

35. What is the incubation period of Rhabdo virus?
    a) 1 day-2 weeks
    b) 10-20 days
    c) 2-4 weeks
    d) 10 days-1 year
36. Which is the most important characteristic symptom of Rabies?
    a) Fear of Height
    b) Fear of Water
    c) Fear of Cats
    d) Fear of Fire
37. What is the mortality rate of humans if they contract rabies?
    a) 50% fatal
    b) 100% fatal
    c) No effects
    d) 33% fatal
38. What is the earliest sign of contracting Polio?
    a) Paralysis
    b) Inflammation of the body
    c) Inability to bend the head forward
    d) Inability to walk
39. Which of the following options is incorrect regarding the contraction of Polio?
    a) It spreads through intestinal discharges
    b) It spreads through contaminated food and water
    c) It spreads by flies
    d) It spreads through mosquito bites
40. What is the full form of OPV?
    a) Oral Polio Vaccine
    b) Oesophagus Polio Vaccine
    c) Oral Plague Vaccine
    d) Oesophagus Plague Vaccine
41. If you walked into your hen house and noticed swelling in the face and eyes and nasal discharge, which of the following diseases do your chickens most likely have?
    a) Infectious coryza
    b) Fowl typhoid
    c) Fowl cholera
    d) Chicken pox
42. Which of the following poultry diseases cannot be cured by antibiotics or a vaccine?
    a) Fowl typhoid
    b) Fowl cholera
    c) Infectious coryza
    d) Vitamin E deficiency
43. A virus's non-living property is referred to as
    a) The ability to reproduce only within the host's body
    b) The ability to go through mutation
    c) The ability to solidify or crystallise
    d) The ability to inflict sickness upon the host
44. This virus possesses both DNA and RNA sequences.
    a) The poliovirus
    b) Herpes simplex virus
    c) Cyanophage is a kind of bacteria
    d) Leuko Virus
45. The poliovirus multiplies in the part of the body known as the
    a) Muscle cells
    b) Nerve cells
    c) Intestinal cells
    d) None of the above

46. Interferons stop the infection from spreading.
   a) Fungi b) Bacteria
   c) Cancer d) None of these
47. This virus was created in the form of non-living crystals for the first time, marking a significant milestone in science.
   a) The smallpox virus b) Influenza virus
   c) Tobacco mosaic virus d) Bacteriophage
48. Causative of Chickenpox is
   a) Bacteriophage T-2 b) Varicella virus
   c) SV-40 virus d) Adenovirus
49. Tetanus germs produce a toxin. It affects
   a) Jawbones b) Involuntary muscles
   c) Voluntary muscles d) Muscles that are both voluntary and involuntary
50. This is a viral sickness that has spread throughout the worl d)
   a) Rickets b) The measles
   c) Beri-beri d) Syphilis
51. This is a contagious disease.
   a) Rabies b) Cancer
   c) Alkaptonuria d) Phenylketonuria
52. Hydrophobia, often known as rabies, is a disease that is caused by
   a) Protozoan b) Nematode
   c) Virus d) Helminth
53. What is the name of the virus that is transferred to humans by the bite of infected animals, birds, and insects?
   a) Rabies Virus b) Ebola Virus
   c) Flavivirus d) All the above
54. Identify which of the following statements concerning viruses is correct.
   a) Viruses do not contain a ribosome.
   b) Viruses can make protein.
   c) Viruses can be categorised by their shapes.
   d) Both A and C are correct
55. Disease causes a bird's health to weaken. What is a result of this weakened state?
   a) Poor productivity
   b) Reduced quality of the affected animal.
   c) Possible loss through death
   d) All of the above

56. Which of the following are indicators of birds infected with pullorum-typhiod disease?
    a) White pasty excrement (in chicks)
    b) A high death rate in the first three weeks after hatching
    c) Severe lesions on many of the internal organs
    d) All of the above are indicators, along with drowsiness, lack of appetite, drooping wings, labored breathing, swelling in joints, and a stunted or distorted body appearance.
57. Chicken Transparent-Image.png
    The primary route of transmission of pullorum-typhoid disease is by:
    a) Breathing infected particles
    b) Consumption of infected droppings
    c) Consumption of infected feed
    d) Transmission within the egg from the parent to the offspring
58. How can avian influenza be spread to a flock?
    a) Exposure of poultry to waterfowl
    b) Contaminated poultry equipment
    c) Direct bird-to-bird contact
    d) All of the above
59. Diseases that spread from one person to another are called _______.
    a) Communicable diseases
    b) Degenerative diseases
    c) Non-communicable diseases
    d) None of the above
60. Night blindness is caused due to the deficiencies of_______.
    a) Vitamin A
    b) Vitamin B
    c) Vitamin C
    d) Vitamin E
61. Which of the following diseases is an example of non-communicable diseases?
    a) Cancer
    b) Diabetes,
    c) Hypertension
    d) All of the above
62. Alzheimer's and osteoporosis are examples of _______.
    a) Communicable diseases
    b) Degenerative diseases
    c) Non-communicable diseases
    d) None of the above
63. Excessive bleeding during an injury is a deficiency of_________.
    a) vitamin A
    b) vitamin B
    c) vitamin K
    d) vitamin E
64. Goitre and the enlarged thyroid gland are mainly diagnosed in patients with deficiencies of which of the following minerals?
    a) Iron
    b) Iodine
    c) Calcium
    d) Phosphorus
65. Cystic Fibrosis and Haemophilia are examples of _______.
    a) Hereditary diseases
    b) Degenerative diseases
    c) Deficiency diseases
    d) None of the above

66. Which of the following diseases is caused by various pathogenic microorganisms?
    a) Deficiency diseases
    b) Hereditary diseases
    c) Infectious diseases
    d) Degenerative diseases
67. Which of the following diseases is caused by protein deficiency?
    a) Anaemia
    b) Kwashiorkor
    c) Hypothyroidism
    d) All of the above
68. Which of the following vitamins is also known as ascorbic acid?
    a) vitamin A
    b) vitamin B
    c) vitamin C
    d) vitamin E
69. The deficiency diseases can be prevented by ____________.
    a) Prolonged cooking
    b) Eating only fruits
    c) Eating only vegetables
    d) Eating food with good nutritional value
70. AIDS, common cold, dengue fever and influenza are examples of __________.
    a) Deficiency Disease
    b) Infectious diseases
    c) Physiological Diseases
    d) Non-infectious diseases
71. Which of the following vitamins helps in blood clotting?
    a) vitamin A
    b) vitamin C
    c) vitamin D
    d) vitamin K
72. Which of the following vitamins functions as both hormone and visual pigment?
    a) Thiamine
    b) Retinal
    c) Riboflavin
    d) Folic acid
73. Which of the following vitamin is also known as niacin and plays a vital role in many digestive tract functions?
    a) vitamin B1
    b) vitamin B2
    c) vitamin B3
    d) vitamin B12
74. The Deficiency of vitamin E leads to _______
    a) Soft Bones
    b) Bleeding in gums
    c) Weakness in muscles
    d) Neurological disorders
75. Xerophthalmia caused due to the deficiency of __________.
    a) vitamin A
    b) vitamin B
    c) vitamin C
    d) vitamin E
76. Which of the following is not an infectious disease?
    a) Dengue
    b) Scurvy
    c) Typhoid Fever
    d) Whooping cough
77. Which of the following is the main cause of blindness in children worldwide?
    a) Glaucoma
    b) Cataracts
    c) Protein deficiency
    d) vitamin A deficiency

78. Amoxicillin, Doxycycline Azithromycin, and Penicillin are some examples of ________.

a) Bacteria
b) Pathogens
c) Antibiotics
d) Vaccinations

79. Ministry of Agriculture, Govt. of India Has .... Central Poultry Development Organisations?

a) Four
b) Three
c) Two
d) Five

80. Central Poultry Development Organisation (Southern Region) Was Formerly Known As..?

a) Central Poultry Research & Training Institute
b) Southern Poultry Development Organisation
c) Central Poultry Devlopment Organisation & Training Institute
d) None of the above

81. The Directorate of Poultry Research is Located In..?

a) Lucknow
b) Hyderaba
c) Delhi
d) Bangalore

82. ALC IS a ...?

a) Viral disease
b) Bacterial disease
c) Fungal disease
d) Nutritional disorder.

83. Coryza is a..?

a) Viral disease
b) Bacterial disease
c) Fungal disease
d) Nutritional disorder

84. Coccidiosis is a..?

a) External parasite
b) Internal parasite
c) Fungal disease
d) Nutritional disorder

85. BWD is a..?

a) Summer season disease
b) Winter season disease
c) Rainy season disease
d) All of the above.

86. Death rate is highest in..?

a) Mesogenic form of disease
b) Virulent form of disease
c) Lentogenic form of diseas
d) All of the above.

87. The double wall feeder was developed by..?

a) ICAR, New Delhi
b) Department of animal husbandry, BHU, Varanasi
c) AAU, Anand
d) TNAU, Coimbatore.

88. Which is a type of brooding?

a) Natural brooding
b) Artificial brooding
c) Both a and b
d) None of the above.

89. The distance between brooder house and layer house should be atleast..?
    a) 50 m b) 75 m
    c) 100 m d) 125 m.
90. The first week temperature of brooder is..?
    a) 95 °F b) 97 °F
    c) 90 °F d) 75 °F
91. S. K. F. Is useful against..?
    a) Coccidiosis diseases b) Bacterial diseases
    c) Both a and b d) Fungal diseases.
92. Central avian research institute is located at..?
    a) Gorakhpur, UP b) Deoria, UP
    c) Azamgarh, UP d) Bareli, UP
93. Which pharmaceutical company produces lincospectin?
    a) Sun pharma b) Unichem
    c) Panacea biotec d) Novartis India
94. DIMIDON 16% is an..?
    a) External parasitic medicine b) Internal parasitic medicine
    c) Anti coccidiosis medicine d) Anti influenza medicine.
95. Multiple-Choice Questions in Poultry Diseases
    The carrier status of infection is most significant in which of the following viral diseases?
    a) Infectious bronchitis b) Infectious laryngotracheitis
    c) Newcastle disease d) Infectious bursal disease
    e) avian encephalomyelitis
96. Consolidation of one or both lungs (pneumonia) is a frequent gross lesion in turkeys affected with which of the following diseases?
    a) fowl cholera
    b) Ornithobacterium rhinotracheale infection
    c) fowl choleraand erysipelas
    d) Ornithobacterium rhinotracheale infection and bordetellosis
    e) fowl choleraand
    f) Ornithobacterium rhinotracheale infection
97. For which of the following diseases, all commercially available vaccines are only of tissueculture origin?
    a) hemorrhagic enteritis b) avian encephalomyelitis
    c) pox d) infectious laryngotracheitis
    e) infectious bronchitis
98. How many Eimeria sp. have been identified in chickens and turkeys?
    a) Sixand four, respectively b) Sevenand four, respectively
    c) Sevenand five, respectively d) Eightand six, respectively
    e) Nineand seven, respectively

99. Which of the following is NOT a known cause of false-positive reactions on the serum plateagglutination test for mycoplasmas?
   a) vaccination with inactivated oil-emulsion vaccines
   b) cross-reacting antigens shared between avian mycoplasmas and bacteria
   c) cross-reacting antigens shared between avian mycoplasmas and manyavian viruses
   d) frozen serum and/or antigen
   e) none of the above

100. Which of the following bacteria is an important cause of keratitis with perforation of thecornea in chickens and turkeys?
   a) Escherichia coli
   b) Pseudomonas aeruginosa
   c) Streptococcus fecalis
   d) Staphylococcus aureus
   e) Salmonella typhimurium

101. In chickens infected with Borrelia anserina, gross lesion is characteristically found in the
   a) Lungs
   b) Intestine
   c) Heart
   d) Spleen
   e) Liver

102. Duck hepatitis virus type 2 has been classified as
   a) Adenovirus
   b) Astrovirus
   c) Enterovirus
   d) Parvovirus
   e) Coronavirus

103. The addition of small amounts of anti-oxidants to the diet of chickens may prevent which ofthe following vitamin E/selenium-deficiency diseases?
   a) Muscular dystrophy
   b) Exudative diathesis
   c) Encephalomalacia
   d) Muscular dystrophyand exudative diathesis
   e) Exudative diathesisand encephalomalacia

104. Which of the following diseases is NOT caused by herpesvirus?
   a) Marek's disease
   b) Infectious laryngotracheitis
   c) Turkey viral hepatitis
   d) Duck virus enteritis

105. Which of the following vitamins does prevent fatty liver and kidney syndrome in chicks?
   a) Pyridoxine
   b) Vitamin B1
   c) Vitamin B12
   d) Biotin

e) Pantothenic acid

106. Sulphur-colored droppings in turkeys are associated with infection with which of thefollowing infectious agents?
   a) Astrovirus
   b) Rotavirus
   c) Eimeria gallopavonis
   d) Hexamita meleagridis
   e) Histomonas meleagridis

107. Histopathology is an important diagnostic tool for the diagnosis of which of the followingviral diseases?
   a) Infectious bursal disease
   b) Avian influenza
   c) Infectious bronchitis
   d) Newcastle disease
   e) Turkey rhinotracheitis

108. In chickens affected with infectious bronchitis, the virus can be isolated from which of thefollowing organs/tissues?
   a) Tracheas
   b) Lungs
   c) Tracheaand lungs
   d) Tracheasand cecal tonsils
   e) Tracheas, lungs, and cecal tonsils

109. Amyloidosis, particularly of the liver, most commonly occurs in which of the following typesof poultry?
   a) Quail
   b) Ostriches
   c) Ducks
   d) Geese

110. For the diagnosis of avian encephalomyelitis, a brain suspension prepared from affectedchicks is inoculated in embryonated chicken eggs via which route of inoculation?
   a) Yolk sac
   b) Allantoic cavity
   c) Amniotic cavity
   d) Chorioallantoic membrane

111. What is the most consistent and prominent gross lesion in turkeys dying oflymphoproliferative disease?
   a) Splenomegaly
   b) Hepatomegaly
   c) Thickening of peripheral nerves
   d) Tumors in the gonads
   e) Tumors in the bursa of fabricius

112. Fully productive infection with Marek's disease virus occurs only in
   a) T lymphocytes
   b) B lymphocytes
   c) Macrophages in the spleen
   d) Schwann cells of the peripheral nerves
   e) Feather follicular epithelium

113. Which of the following postures is characteristically seen in chickens affected with bilateralrupture of the gastrocnemius tendons?
   a) Lateral extension of the legs
   b) Backward extension of the legs
   c) Sitting on hock joints with the toes flexed
   d) Sitting on the back with the legs raised off the ground

114. Rodents play an important role in the epizootiology of which of the following diseases?
   a) Fowl cholera
   b) Paratyphoid
   c) Fowl choleraand necrotic enteritis
   d) Paratyphoidand necrotic enteritis
   e) Paratyphoidand fowl cholera

115. In turkeys affected with turkey viral hepatitis, prominent gross lesions occur primarily in theliver, but gross and/or microscopic lesions may also be found in the
   a) Pancreas b) Intestine
   c) Spleen d) Kidneys
   e) Myocardium

116. Extensive hemorrhages on the mucosal and serosal surfaces, parenchymatous organs,myocardium and endocardium, with free blood in the body cavities are lesionscharacteristically found in ducks and/or geese affected with which of the followingdiseases?
   a) Duck hepatitis b) Duck virus enteritis
   c) Goose parvovirus infection d) Avian influenza

117. The most common site of northern fowl mite (Ornithonyssu sylviarum) infestation in layers is
   a) Around the vent b) Under the wings
   c) The abdominal region d) The back

118. In ulcerative enteritis, gross lesions are characteristically found in the intestine and, in mostcases, in the
   a) Spleen b) Proventriculus
   c) Liver d) Spleenand liver

119. A large cystic growth in the kidneys of a chicken is a characteristic feature for which of the following tumors?
   a) Myeloblastoma b) Renal cell carcinoma
   c) Nephroblastoma d) Marek's disease tumor

120. Irregular thickening of the bones of legs in chickens refers to as
   a) Osteopetrosis b) Osteoporosis
   c) Osteochondrosis d) Osteomalacia

121. Which of the following tests is used to confirm that an isolated virus is type A influenzavirus?
   a) Hemagglutination test b) Hemagglutination-inhibition test
   c) Agar-gel immunodiffusion test d) Virus-neutralization test

122. In histomoniasis, flagellated Histomonas meleagridis can be demonstrated in wet smearsprepared from the
   a) Liver b) Cecal lumen
   c) Cecal mucosaand liver d) Cecal lumenand liver

123. Intranuclear inclusion bodies in the myocardium may be seen in goslings and/or ducklingsaffected with which of the following diseases?
   a) Duck hepatitis b) Duck virus enteritis
   c) Derzy's disease d) Avian influenza

124. The highest rate of mortality due to spontaneous cardiomyopathy in turkeys occurs duringwhat week of life?
   a) First week b) Second week
   c) Forth week d) Fifth week

125. High dietary levels of which of the following minerals may lead to metabolic acidosis, whichcould interfere with renal vitamin D3 metabolism and result in increased incidence of tibialdyschondroplasia?

a) Phosphorusand chloride
b) Sodiumand potassium
c) Chlorideand potassium
d) Phosphorusand sodium

126. Which of the following gross lesions is characteristically seen in pheasants infected withgroup avian adenovirus?

a) Enlargement and mottling of the spleenand congestion of the lungs
b) Enlargement and mottling of the spleenand hemorrhagic enteritis
c) Petechial hemorrhages in the liverand congestion of the lung
d) Petechial hemorrhages in the liverand hemorrhagic enteritis

127. Staphylococcus was isolated from swollen joints of turkeys. Which of the followingbiochemical tests would confirm that the isolate is not *Staphylococcus epidermidis.*

a) Catalase test
b) Oxidase test
c) Coagulase test
d) Indole test

128. Avian leukosis/sarcoma viruses that occur in chickens have been divided into how manysubgroups?

a) 4
b) 5
c) 6
d) 7

129. Derzy's disease in goslings is caused by

a) Adenovirus
b) Herpesvirus
c) Astrovirus
d) Parvovirus

130. Small submucosal nodules in the oesophagus are suggestive of which of the followingconditions?

a) Intoxication with the T-2 mycotoxin
b) Vitamin A deficiency
c) Candidiasis
d) Trichomoniasis

131. Which of the following infectious agents is known to induce hemorrhagic tracheitis inchickens?

a) Infectious laryngotracheitis virus
b) Velogenic newcastle disease virus
c) Infectious laryngotracheitis, velogenic newcastle disease virus, and avian influenzavirus
d) Infectious laryngotracheitis virus, velogenic newcastle disease virus, and infectiousbronchitis virus

132. If you observe nervous signs and turbidity or opacity of the eyes in many 7-day-old turkeypoults, infection with which of the following bacteria would be first on your list of rule-outs?

a) Escherichia coli
b) Salmonella arizonae
c) Pseudomonas aeruginosa
d) Streptococcus faecalis

133. Which of the following live vaccines can be administered by the wing-web stab method?
   a) Avian encephalomyelitis vaccine
   b) Avian encephalomyelitisand fowl cholera vaccines
   c) Avian encephalomyelitisand viral arthritis vaccines
   d) Fowl choleraand viral arthritis vaccines

134. Which of the following neoplasm-induce viruses is egg-transmitted?
   a) Marek's disease virus
   b) Lymphoid leukosis virus
   c) Marek's disease virusand lymphoid leukosis virus
   d) Lymphoid leukosis virusand reticuloendotheliosis virus

135. The main clinical manifestation of acute ionophore toxicity in chickens and turkeys is
   a) Blindness
   b) Leg weakness
   c) Respiratory signs
   d) Diarrhoea

136. Two-week-old chicks had subcutaneous edema, ascites, and hydropericardium. Toxicitywith which of the following salts would be on your list of rule-outs?
   a) Copper sulphate
   b) Calcium carbonate
   c) Nitrate and nitrite salts
   d) Sodium chloride

137. Cytological examination of touch preparations from visceral tumors of Marek's diseasereveals that the predominant cells are
   a) Lymphocytes
   b) Lymphoblasts
   c) Myelocytes
   d) Myeloblasts

138. Which of the following is the most common lesion induced by *Staphylococcus aureu* inchickens and turkeys?
   a) Encephalitis
   b) Panophthalmitis
   c) Salpingitis
   d) Arthritis/osteomyelitis

139. In chickens infected with the chicken infectious anemia virus, there is a decrease innumbers of which blood cells?
   a) Leukocytes
   b) Erythrocytes
   c) Leukocytesand thrombocytes
   d) Leukocytes, erythrocytes, and thrombocytes

140. Which of the following avian viruses does express hemagglutination activity followingtreatment with the enzyme neuraminidase?
   a) Infectious bursal disease virus
   b) Infectious bronchitis virus
   c) Infectious laryngotracheitis virus
   d) Avian encephalomyelitis virus

141. Which of the following avian viruses does cause pocks on the chorioallantoic membrane ofembryonated chicken eggs?
   a) Poxvirusand infectious laryngotracheitis virus
   b) Poxvirusand viral arthritis virus
   c) Infectious laryngotracheitis virusand viral arthritis virus
   d) Poxvirus, infectious laryngotracheitis virus, and viral arthritis virus

142. The double immunodiffusion test is used to define the type of influenza virus. Thisserological test identifies which of the following antigens of influenza virus?
   a) Matrix antigens
   b) Nucleocapsid antigen
   c) Hemagglutinin antigen
   d) Matrixand nucleocapsid antigens

143. Which of the following supplements is commonly used in the culture media used for theisolation of avian mycoplasmas?
   a) Swine serum
   b) Yeast extractand sodium chloride
   c) Swine serumand glucose
   d) Swine serum, yeast extract, and glucose

144. Central chromatolysis of neurons in the brain and spinal cord is a histopathologic lesion ofdiagnostic significance in which of the following diseases?
   a) Marek's disease
   b) Avian encephalomyelitis
   c) Eastern equine encephalitis
   d) Newcastle disease

145. In chronic stages of Mycoplasma synoviae infection, it has been indicated that which of thefollowing organs/tissues may be more reliable for the isolation of the mycoplasma?
   a) Foot pads
   b) Tendons
   c) Tracheas
   d) Ovaries

146. The etiology of hemorrhagic enteritis in turkeys is
   a) Adenovirus
   b) Paramyxovirus
   c) Rotavirus
   d) Enterovirus

147. Which of the following lesions is NOT found in pigeons acutely infected with Chlamydia psittaci?
   a) Hepatomegaly
   b) Splenomegaly
   c) Diffuse hemorrhages ın the proventriculus
   d) Pericarditisand perihepatitis

148. MacConkey's agar can be used for the isolation of all of the following bacteria EXCEPT
   a) Escherichia coli
   b) Bordetella avium
   c) Pasteurella multocida
   d) Pseudomonas aeruginosa

149. Egg transmission occurs with which of the three groups of avian adenoviruses?
   a) Group I
   b) Groups I and II
   c) Group I and III
   d) Group II and III

150. Migratory waterfowl are considered as an important source of infection of poultry with whichof the following viral diseases?
 a) Avian influenza b) Newcastle disease
 c) Avian encephalomyelitis d) Infectious bronchitis
151. The presence of a caseous mass in the pharyngeal region of a pigeon arouses suspicion ofwhich of the following diseases?
 a) Wet pox b) Chlamydiosis
 c) Trichomoniasis d) Candidiasis
152. Which of the following vitamins must be hydroxylated in the liver and kidneys in order tobecome metabolically active?
 a) Vitamin A b) Vitamin C
 c) Vitamin D d) Vitamin E
153. Nodules in the mucosal surface of the ceca in a pheasant is a characteristic lesion forinfection with
 a) Salmonella typhimurium b) Histomonas meleagridis
 c) Eimeria colchici d) Heterakis isolonche
154. Spondylolisthesis in chickens results from subluxation of the
 a) Fourth thoracic vertebra b) Notarium
 c) Synsacrum d) Third caudal vertebra
155. Which of the following bacteria does typically induce liver granulomas in turkeys?
 a) Clostridium septicum *b) Eubacterium tortuosum*
 c) Streptobacillus moniliformis *d) Staphylococcus aureus*
156. What are the predominant clinical signs of paramyxovirus serotype 1 infection in pigeons?
 a) Respiratoryand neurologic signs b) Neurologic signsand diarrhea
 c) Respiratory signsand diarrhea d) Respiratory signs, neurologic signs, and diarrhea
157. Which of the following anticoccidials is an ionophore?
 a) Zoalene b) Narasin
 c) Diclazuril d) Halofuginone
158. During the life cycle of Eimeria spp. in the intestine, the schizonts produce
 a) Sporozoites b) Merozoites
 c) Microgametes d) Macrogametes
159. Coligranulomas occur in which of the following organs?
 a) Liverand spleen b) Intestineand mesentery
 c) Liver , intestine, and mesentry d) Spleen, intestineand mesentry
160. Knemidocoptes mutans
 a) Induces which of the following lesions in chickens?
 b) Crusty lesion under the wings
 c) Scabby lesion around the vent
 d) Scaly lesion on the legs
 e) Small subcutaneous nodules

Answer Key

1	d	2	c	3	a	4	c	5	a	6	d	7	b
8	d	9	d	10	a	11	a	12	b	13	a	14	d
15	c	16	d	17	a	18	a	19	b	20	c	21	b
22	a	23	a	24	c	25		26	b	27	a	28	d
29	a	30	b	31	d	32	a	33	b	34	c	35	d
36	b	37	b	38	c	39	d	40	a	41		42	
43	c	44	d	45	c	46	d	47	c	48	b	49	c
50	b	51	a	52	c	53	d	54	d	55	d	56	d
57	d	58	d	59	a	60	a	61	d	62	b	63	c
64	b	65	a	66	c	67	b	68	c	69	d	70	b
71	d	72	b	73	c	74	c	75	a	76	b	77	d
78	c	79		80		81		82	a	83	b	84	
85	c	86		87		88		89		90		91	
92	d	93	b	94	d	95	d	96	b	97	c	98	c
99	d	100	c	101	a	102	b	103	a	104	d	105	b
106	e	107	a	108	e	109	c	110	a	111	a	112	e
113	c	114	e	115	a	116	b	117	a	118	d	119	c
120	a	121	c	122	b	123	c	124	b	125	a	126	a
127	c	128	c	129	d	130	b	131	c	132	b	133	b
134	d	135	b	136	d	137	a	138	d	139	d	140	b
141	d	142	d	143	d	144	b	145	c	146	a	147	c
148	c	149	c	150	a	151	c	152	c	153	d	154	a
155	b	156	b	157	b	158	b	159	c	160	d		

3

Bacterial Diseases

Karthik Itherni, Amita Dubey, Yamini Verma and Amita Tiwari

College of Veterinary Science and Animal Husbandry Jabalpur, NDVSU

1. How does the toxin of Clostridium botulinum affect the nervous system?
   a) Blocks inhibitory transmitter substance
   b) Stimulates macrophages
   c) Causes haemolysis and tissue destruction
   d) Induces systemic shock and death
2. What is the specific effect of the toxin produced by Clostridium perfringens on host cells?
   a) Blocks inhibitory transmitter substance b) Induces systemic shock
   c) Causes ribosomal dysfunction d) Disrupts plasma membranes
3. Which bacterium produces a toxin that blocks cholinergic neurotransmitters and causes paralysis?
   a) Clostridium perfringens b) Clostridium botulinum
   c) Vibrio cholerae d) Corynebacterium diphtheriae
4. How does airborne transmission of bacterial diseases primarily occur?
   a) Ingestion b) Inhalation
   c) Mucosal contamination d) Cutaneous contamination
5. What is the typical diameter of droplet nuclei involved in airborne infection?
   a) 10-100 μm b) 0.15 pm
   c) 0.1-5 μm d) 1-10 μm
6. Which bacterial structures play a crucial role in the attachment and entry into epithelial cells?
   a) Flagella
   b) Capsules
   c) Fimbrial proteins and lipoteichoic acids
   d) Toxins
7. What is the function of lipoteichoic acids in Streptococcus and some other Gram-positive cocci?
   a) Bind to fibronectin b) Cause urinary infections
   c) Compose fibrillae on the bacterial surface d) Inhibit attachment

8. In Escherichia coli, which type of pili is associated with causing urinary infections by binding to mannose (host receptor)?
   a) Type I proteins
   b) Type P proteins
   c) Type S proteins
   d) Flagellar proteins
9. What is the term for the defense mechanism where normal commensal flora inhibits bacterial colonization by excreting toxic metabolites and bacteriocins?
   a) Antibody defense
   b) Mucosal defense
   c) Colonization resistance
   d) Bacterial tropism
10. Besides mucosal antibodies, what are the other antibacterial substances that contribute to colonization resistance?
   a) Fimbriae
   b) Lactoferrin
   c) Lipoteichoic acids
   d) Flagella
11. What is the primary role of arthropods in the transmission of bacterial pathogens?
   a) Production of toxins
   b) Mechanical carriers
   c) Attachment to host cells
   d) Formation of fibrils on the bacterial surface
12. Which Clostridium species is associated with Botulism (limberneck) in chickens?
   a) *C. chauvoei*
   b) *C. botulinum*
   c) *C. colinum*
   d) *C. difficile*
13. What disease does *C. colinum* cause in chickens, quail, pigeons, and other birds?
   a) Black quarter (blackleg)
   b) Pseudomembranous colitis
   c) Ulcerative enteritis
   d) Gangrenous dermatitis
14. Which Clostridium species is responsible for Necrotic enteritis and Gangrenous dermatitis in chickens and turkeys?
   a) C. septicum
   b) C. perfringens
   c) C. botulinum
   d) C. colinum
15. Which toxin type is primarily responsible for outbreaks of Botulism in poultry?
   a) Type A
   b) Type C-alpha
   c) Type E
   d) Type G
16. What is the main pathogenesis of Botulism caused by Type C in broiler chickens?
   a) Inhalation of spores
   b) Consumption of preformed toxin
   c) Toxico-infection in the gut
   d) Direct bacterial invasion
17. What are the main clinical signs of Botulism in chickens?
   a) Respiratory distress and coughing
   b) Firm paralysis of muscles
   c) Aggressive behavior and pecking
   d) Flaccid paralysis of legs, wings, neck, and eyelids

18. What is required for the definitive diagnosis of Botulism in chickens?
    a) Necropsy examination
    b) Detection of bacterial DNA
    c) Presence of maggots in the crop
    d) Detection of toxin in serum, crop, or gastrointestinal washings
19. What is the causative agent of Ulcerative Enteritis (UE) in chickens and turkeys?
    a) Clostridium botulinum
    b) Clostridium colinum
    c) Clostridium difficile
    d) Clostridium perfringens
20. What was the original name for Ulcerative Enteritis due to its prevalence in quail?
    a) Avian Influenza
    b) Quail Fever
    c) Quail Disease
    d) Feather Drop Syndrome
21. What are considered predisposing factors for Ulcerative Enteritis?
    a) Bacterial contamination
    b) Fungal infections
    c) Coccidiosis, infectious bursal disease, and stress conditions
    d) Viral invasions
22. Which organ shows yellowish to grey necrotic lesions in Ulcerative Enteritis?
    a) Kidney
    b) Spleen
    c) Liver
    d) Heart
23. What is the usual age range of birds affected by Necrotic Enteritis (NE)?
    a) Less than 2 weeks
    b) 2-4 weeks
    c) 4 weeks or older
    d) Adults only
24. Which bacterium is responsible for causing Necrotic Enteritis in chickens and turkeys?
    a) Clostridium difficile
    b) Clostridium botulinum
    c) Clostridium perfringens
    d) Clostridium colinum
25. What toxins are believed to be responsible for intestinal mucosal necrosis in Necrotic Enteritis?
    a) Alpha toxin produced by C. perfringens type A and C
    b) Beta toxin produced by C. perfringens type C
    c) Both a and b
    d) Gamma toxin
26. Where are C. perfringens types A and C found before migrating to the small intestine in Necrotic Enteritis?
    a) Small intestine
    b) Lungs
    c) Large intestine and caeca
    d) Liver
27. What are considered predisposing factors for Necrotic Enteritis?
    a) High humidity
    b) Outbreaks of avian influenza
    c) Changes in diet and inadequate cleaning
    d) Viral invasions

28. What is the characteristic lesion of Necrotic Enteritis in the small intestine?
    a) Ulcers with hemorrhagic borders
    b) Extensive necrosis with deeply fissured and often congested mucosa
    c) Abscess formation
    d) Thickening of the intestinal walls
29. Which two clostridia are commonly involved in Gangrenous Dermatitis (GD)?
    a) Clostridium difficile and C. perfringens type A
    b) Clostridium septicum and C. perfringens type A
    c) Clostridium botulinum and C. difficile
    d) Clostridium tetani and C. novyi
30. What is the main age group affected by Gangrenous Dermatitis (GD)?
    a) Chicks under 2 weeks old
    b) Broilers over 4 weeks of age
    c) Turkeys of any age
    d) Layers during egg-laying period
31. What is the underlying predisposing factor that allows GD to occur?
    a) High humidity
    b) Genetic mutations
    c) Compromised (damaged) immune system
    d) Excessive heat
32. What condition, often associated with avian retroviruses, predisposes chickens to Gangrenous Dermatitis?
    a) Blue Wing Disease (BWD)
    b) Infectious Coryza
    c) Fowl Cholera
    d) Avian Encephalomyelitis
33. What is the causative agent of Avian Listeriosis in poultry?
    a) Clostridium perfringens
    b) Salmonella enteritidis
    c) Listeria monocytogenes
    d) Escherichia coli
34. In the encephalitic form of Avian Listeriosis, what neurological signs may be observed?
    a) Limb weakness
    b) Ataxia (muscular incoordination) and torticollis (stiff neck)
    c) Seizures
    d) Wing drooping
35. Which poultry conditions are commonly associated with Staphylococcus aureus infections?
    a) Avian influenza and Newcastle disease
    b) Coccidiosis and Marek's disease
    c) Arthritis and tenosynovitis, gangrenous dermatitis, subdermal abscesses, spondylitis, and osteomyelitis
    d) Infectious bronchitis and infectious bursal disease

36. Where is Staphylococcus aureus often found in apparently normal chickens?
    a) Gastrointestinal tract
    b) Respiratory system
    c) Skin, nares, beak, and foot
    d) Bloodstream
37. What can predispose poultry to Staphylococcosis?
    a) High humidity conditions
    b) Adequate sanitation practices
    c) Injury to the skin or mucous membrane, fowl-pox, and unhealed navel in chicks
    d) Proper vaccination protocols
38. Which disease is characterized by swollen and painful joints, often affecting the hock and feet regions?
    a) Gangrenous Dermatitis (GD)
    b) Subdermal Abscesses
    c) Arthritis and Tenosynovitis
    d) Spondylitis and Osteomyelitis
39. In which condition may subdermal staphylococcal plantar abscesses ("bumble foot") occur?
    a) Gangrenous Dermatitis (GD)
    b) Subdermal Abscesses
    c) Arthritis and Tenosynovitis
    d) Staphylococcal Septicaemia
40. What is the usual site of lesion in Gangrenous Dermatitis (GD) in broiler chickens?
    a) Wing tips and dorsal pelvic region
    b) Feet and sternal bursa
    c) Thoracic vertebrae and spinal cord
    d) Head of femur and tibiotarsus
41. Which bones may be affected by osteomyelitis in Staphylococcosis?
    a) Beak and skull
    b) Femur, tibiotarsus, and sometimes other bones
    c) Radius and ulna
    d) Pelvic girdle bones
42. What is the main consequence of Colisepticaemia in poultry?
    a) Gangrenous Dermatitis
    b) Airsacculitis and respiratory disease
    c) Ulcerative Enteritis
    d) Botulism
43. What factors can predispose chickens to Colisepticaemia?
    a) Adequate ventilation and clean water
    b) Viral infections, coccidiosis, nutritional deficiencies, and Ranikhet disease
    c) Dry, dusty conditions and overcrowding
    d) High humidity and proper sanitation practices
44. How does E. coli typically spread to other chickens during hatch?
    a) Through direct contact with infected birds
    b) Via contaminated feed
    c) Through contaminated well water
    d) Faecal contamination of the eggs

45. What is a characteristic sign of Colisepticaemia in affected birds?
    a) Bright and active behavior
    b) Dropping of wings
    c) Limb paralysis
    d) Making short sharp sounds ("snicking")
46. Which age group of chickens is usually affected by Colisepticaemia?
    a) Chicks under 4 weeks
    b) Birds between 4 and 12 weeks
    c) Laying hens
    d) Roosters
47. Which condition may result from an ascending infection from the cloaca in Colisepticaemia?
    a) Gangrenous Dermatitis
    b) Yolk sac infection
    c) Necrotic Enteritis
    d) Infectious Bursal Disease (IBD)
48. What is the characteristic finding in the peritoneal cavity in cases of peritonitis due to Colisepticaemia?
    a) Fibrin and free yolk
    b) Dark and congested liver
    c) White and caseous deposits in airsacs
    d) Thickened pericardial sac
49. What microscopic changes are observed in the trachea during Colisepticaemia?
    a) Accumulation of necrotic heterophils
    b) Fibroblast proliferation
    c) Replacement of ciliated cells by immature non-ciliated cells
    d) Thickened and opaque airsacs
50. What are the reproductive disorders encompassed by the term "egg peritonitis" in poultry?
    a) Cannibalism and vent pecking
    b) Peritonitis, salpingitis, and impaction of the oviduct
    c) Yolk sac infection and omphalitis
    d) Overcrowding and huddling
51. What may be observed in the abdominal cavity during the postmortem examination of birds affected by egg peritonitis?
    a) Milky fluid and distorted ovaries
    b) Distended abdomens and inspissated yolk
    c) Yellow inspissated yolk sac and inflamed navel
    d) Rupture of the oviduct wall and inflamed intestines
52. What is another term for yolk sac infection in chicks?
    a) Vent pecking
    b) Omphalitis
    c) Mushy chick disease
    d) Inspissated inflammatory debris
53. What bacterium is commonly involved in yolk sac infection, either as the primary causal agent or a secondary opportunist?
    a) Clostridium
    b) Staphylococcus aureus
    c) Escherichia coli (E. coli)
    d) Pseudomonas

54. What is a common sign of yolk sac infection in chicks?
   a) Distended abdomens and a tendency to huddle
   b) Cannibalism and vent pecking
   c) Engorged and dilated blood vessels in the yolk sac
   d) Insipid yolk and inflamed navel

55. What is the primary finding during the postmortem examination of chicks affected by yolk sac infection?
   a) Thickened and necrotic navel
   b) Engorged blood vessels in the yolk sac
   c) Fetid (foul-smelling) yolk sac with abnormal color and consistency
   d) Ruptured intestines with haemorrhages

56. What is a characteristic feature observed during postmortem examination in birds affected by Coligranuloma (Hjarre's Disease)?
   a) Soft, reddish nodules in the liver
   b) Yellow nodular granulomas in the mesentery and intestinal wall
   c) Enlarged spleen with dark discoloration
   d) Fluid-filled air sacs

57. Which organ is occasionally affected in birds with Coligranuloma, presenting as hard, discolored, and swollen?
   a) Lungs
   b) Spleen
   c) Kidneys
   d) Liver

58. What is the causative agent of Infectious Coryza (Fowl Coryza)?
   a) Escherichia coli
   b) Mycoplasma gallisepticum
   c) Haemophilus paragallinarum
   d) Salmonella enterica

59. How does Infectious Coryza primarily spread among chickens?
   a) Airborne transmission over long distances
   b) Contaminated drinking water
   c) Vertical transmission from parent to offspring
   d) Via bites from infected mosquitoes

60. What plays an important role in the colonization of the upper respiratory tract by Haemophilus paragallinarum?
   a) Feathers
   b) Capsule and hemagglutination antigen
   c) Ovaries
   d) Airsacs

61. What is a characteristic sign of severe Infectious Coryza in chickens?
   a) Increased feed consumption
   b) Normal ocular discharge
   c) Marked conjunctivitis with closed eyes
   d) Decreased water consumption

62. What is a common gross lesion observed in chickens affected by Infectious Coryza?
    a) Enlarged liver
    b) Swollen wattles
    c) Hypertrophied muscles
    d) Thickened eggshells
63. Microscopically, what is a characteristic finding in the upper respiratory tract of chickens with Infectious Coryza?
    a) Presence of feathers
    b) Proliferation of ciliated cells
    c) Accumulation of caseous material
    d) Atrophy of the lungs
64. Which of the following is a common microscopic lesion associated with Haemophilus paragallinarum infection in the lower respiratory tract?
    a) Hypertrophied air sacs
    b) Necrotic liver tissue
    c) Thickened oviduct walls
    d) Accumulation of necrotic heterophils in caseous exudate
65. Which organ is often affected by Haemophilus paragallinarum, presenting a hard, discolored, and swollen appearance?
    a) Kidneys
    b) Liver
    c) Heart
    d) Spleen
66. What microscopic changes are associated with chronic Infectious Coryza in the upper respiratory tract?
    a) Proliferation of ciliated cells
    b) Accumulation of fibrinous material
    c) Atrophy of the oviduct
    d) Hyperplasia of the lungs
67. In severe forms of the disease, what might be observed grossly in the eyes of chickens affected by Infectious Coryza?
    a) Normal appearance
    b) Marked conjunctivitis with closed eyes
    c) Hypertrophied corneas
    d) Enlarged tear ducts
68. What is the primary causative agent of Fowl Cholera?
    a) Escherichia coli
    b) Mycoplasma gallisepticum
    c) Pasteurella multocida
    d) Salmonella enterica
69. Which form of Fowl Cholera is characterized by birds found dead without warning signs?
    a) Acute
    b) Chronic
    c) Peracute
    d) Localized
70. What contributes to the virulence of Pasteurella multocida in causing Fowl Cholera?
    a) Physical presence of the capsule
    b) Presence of feathers
    c) Specific hemagglutination antigen
    d) Chemical substance associated with the capsule

71. What are the signs of the acute form of Fowl Cholera?
    a) Lameness and torticollis
    b) Cyanosis and fetid diarrhea
    c) Depression and anorexia
    d) Swelling of the wattles

72. What type of lesions are commonly seen in the lungs of turkeys with Fowl Cholera?
    a) Petechiation
    b) Oedema
    c) Necrotic foci
    d) Pneumonia

73. What is a characteristic gross lesion observed in the peracute form of Fowl Cholera?
    a) Caseous arthritis
    b) Oedema of the lungs
    c) Multiple petechiation throughout the viscera
    d) Swollen wattles

74. What is a common microscopic finding in the lungs of turkeys affected by Fowl Cholera?
    a) Necrotic foci
    b) Fibrous tissue proliferation
    c) Caseous exudate
    d) Engorged blood vessels

75. What is the primary etiological agent responsible for pullorum disease in poultry?
    a) Salmonella arizonae
    b) Salmonella gallinarum
    c) Salmonella pullorum
    d) Paratyphoid salmonellae

76. Which Salmonella serotype is associated with fowl typhoid in mature birds?
    a) Salmonella arizonae
    b) Salmonella gallinarum
    c) Salmonella pullorum
    d) Paratyphoid salmonellae

77. What is the primary mode of transmission for Salmonella pullorum from hens to chicks?
    a) Vertical transmission
    b) Airborne transmission
    c) Waterborne transmission
    d) Direct contact transmission

78. Which age group of chicks is mainly affected by pullorum disease, showing signs such as excessive dead-in-shell chicks and respiratory distress?
    a) Under 1 week
    b) 1-2 weeks
    c) 2-3 weeks
    d) 3-4 weeks

79. What is a common characteristic lesion in chicks that die soon after hatching due to pullorum disease?
    a) Distended caeca
    b) Enlarged hock joints
    c) Inflamed, unabsorbed yolk sac
    d) Necrotic foci in the liver

80. Which Salmonella serotype is primarily associated with arizonosis in turkeys?
    a) Salmonella arizonae
    b) Salmonella gallinarum
    c) Salmonella pullorum
    d) Paratyphoid salmonellae

81. What is the primary source of economic losses associated with salmonellae infections in poultry?
    a) Decreased hatchability
    b) Reduced egg production
    c) Lameness in growing birds
    d) Cyanosis in mature birds

82. Which type of test is commonly used to detect Salmonella pullorum antibodies in blood samples?
   a) PCR (Polymerase Chain Reaction)
   b) Rapid slide agglutination test
   c) ELISA (Enzyme-Linked Immunosorbent Assay)
   d) Western Blot
83. What is a common characteristic lesion in older birds affected by pullorum disease?
   a) Distended caeca b) Enlarged hock joints
   c) Abnormal ovary d) Necrotic foci in the liver
84. What is the primary causative agent of Fowl Typhoid (FT)?
   a) Salmonella arizonae b) Salmonella pullorum
   c) Salmonella gallinarum d) Paratyphoid salmonellae
85. Which age group of birds is primarily affected by Fowl Typhoid, leading to increased mortality and a drop in egg production?
   a) Chicks under 1 week b) 1-2 weeks
   c) 2-3 weeks d) Growers or adult birds
86. What is a common characteristic clinical sign of Fowl Typhoid in affected birds?
   a) Cyanosis b) White viscous droppings
   c) Swollen hock joints d) Distended caeca
87. How is Fowl Typhoid primarily spread among birds?
   a) Airborne transmission
   b) Vertical transmission
   c) Waterborne transmission
   d) Lateral spread through contaminated food or water
88. What is a consistent finding in the gross lesions of birds affected by Fowl Typhoid in the acute phase?
   a) Enlarged spleen b) Swollen friable liver
   c) Necrotic foci in the lungs d) Yellow fluid in the pericardial sac
89. Which of the following is a characteristic feature of Fowl Typhoid in young chicks?
   a) Enlarged hock joints
   b) Discrete necrotic foci in the gizzard
   c) Coppery bronze sheen on the liver surface
   d) Retained yolks
90. What is a feature of chronic Fowl Typhoid in laying birds?
   a) Catarrhal enteritis b) Retained yolks leading to rupture
   c) Fibrin attached to the heart surface d) Dark brown bone marrow
91. Which Salmonella serotype has the same antigenic structure as S. gallinarum, allowing the use of a common test for detection?
   a) Salmonella arizonae b) Salmonella pullorum
   c) Salmonella enteritidis d) Salmonella typhimurium

2. What is the primary causative agent of Arizonosis?
   a) Salmonella gallinarum
   b) Salmonella arizonae
   c) Salmonella pullorum
   d) Salmonella typhimurium

93. How does Arizonosis primarily spread among young turkey poults?
   a) Vertical transmission through eggs
   b) Airborne transmission
   c) Lateral transmission through contaminated food and water
   d) Contact with infected adult turkeys

94. What is a common feature of Arizonosis signs in affected poults compared to chicks with salmonellosis?
   a) Respiratory distress
   b) Huddling tendency
   c) Cyanosis
   d) Swollen hock joints

95. What is a characteristic finding in the lesions of birds affected by Arizonosis?
   a) Enlarged spleen
   b) Discrete necrotic foci in the liver
   c) Typhlitis with white caseous casts
   d) Swollen airsacs with yellow deposits

96. What is the primary causative agent of Avian Spirochaetosis?
   a) Treponema gallinarum
   b) Borrelia anserina
   c) Salmonella gallinarum
   d) Spirochaeta pullorum

97. How is Avian Spirochaetosis primarily transmitted among birds?
   a) Mosquito bites
   b) Soft tick (Argas persicus) bites
   c) Direct contact with infected birds
   d) Contaminated water ingestion

98. What is a characteristic sign of Avian Spirochaetosis in affected birds?
   a) Cyanosis or pallor
   b) Swollen hock joints
   c) Paresis (partial paralysis)
   d) Conjunctivitis

99. Which organ exhibits marked enlargement and mottling, making it a characteristic lesion in Avian Spirochaetosis?
   a) Liver
   b) Kidneys
   c) Spleen
   d) Intestine

100. What is the preferred diagnostic method for detecting spirochaetes during Avian Spirochaetosis?
   a) Culture in nutrient media
   b) Serological tests
   c) Microscopic examination of silver-stained tissue sections
   d) Polymerase chain reaction (PCR)

101. Which tick species is the primary vector responsible for transmitting Borrelia anserina in Avian Spirochaetosis?
   a) Ixodes ricinus
   b) Rhipicephalus sanguineus
   c) Amblyomma americanum
   d) Argas persicus

102. Which clinical sign is NOT commonly associated with Avian Spirochaetosis?
   a) Anorexi b) Paralysis
   c) Cyanosis d) Swollen wattles
103. What is the preferred temperature range for ticks of the genus Argas, the main reservoirs of Borrelia anserina?
   a) 0-10°C b) 10-20°C
   c) 20-30°C d) 30-40°C
104. What is the main diagnostic advantage of dark-field microscopy in Avian Spirochaetosis?
   a) It stains the spirochaetes
   b) It reveals lesions in tissue sections
   c) It allows observation of live, unstained spirochaetes
   d) It enhances antigen-antibody reactions
105. What is the primary cause of mortality in birds affected by Avian Spirochaetosis?
   a) Respiratory failure b) Nervous system damage
   c) Septicemia d) Liver failure
106. Which tissue section staining technique is commonly used to demonstrate spirochaetes in Avian Spirochaetosis?
   a) Hematoxylin and eosin (H&E) b) Gram staining
   c) Periodic acid-Schiff (PAS) d) Silver Impregnation
107. Avian tuberculosis is caused by which bacterium?
   a) Mycobacterium tuberculosis b) Mycobacterium avium
   c) Salmonella gallinarum d) Borrelia anserina
108. What is the characteristic feature of Mycobacterium avium when stained by the Ziehl-Neelsen method?
   a) Gram-positive b) Acid-fast
   c) Capsulated d) Spore-forming
109. How does avian tuberculosis primarily spread among birds?
   a) Respiratory droplets b) Contaminated eggs
   c) Infected faeces d) Direct contact with carriers
110. What is a common source of virulent Mycobacterium avium in the environment?
   a) Water b) Air
   c) Soil d) Plant material
111. Unthriftiness, decreased egg production, and finally death are characteristic signs of avian tuberculosis in birds. What is a less common clinical sign?
   a) Cyanosis b) Polydipsia
   c) Polyphagia d) Tachypnea
112. Gross lesions in avian tuberculosis are usually observed in which organs?
   a) Heart and lungs b) Kidneys and intestines
   c) Liver and spleen d) Brain and muscles

113. What is the characteristic appearance of tubercles in the spleen?
a) Smooth b) Nodular
c) Knobby d) Pustular

114. In the histopathological examination, what is the central zone of the tubercle primarily characterized by?
a) Proliferation of lymphocytes b) Coagulative necrosis
c) Vascularization d) Amyloid deposition

115. What is the primary method used for the definitive diagnosis of avian tuberculosis?
a) Clinical signs observation b) Tuberculin test
c) ELISA d) Cultural examination

116. Which immunological test involves injecting avian tuberculin into one wattle to determine the presence of avian tuberculosis?
a) Agglutination test b) ELISA
c) Tuberculin test d) Western blot

117. What does a positive reaction in the tuberculin test indicate?
a) Absence of avian tuberculosis b) Presence of antibodies
c) Hot, soft, oedematous swelling d) Negative reaction

118. The egg is considered a minor source of spread for avian tuberculosis. What is the primary material for transmission?
a) Contaminated feed b) Infected faeces
c) Airborne particles d) Blood transmission

119. In addition to chickens, which avian species is relatively uncommonly affected by avian tuberculosis?
a) Ducks b) Geese
c) Turkeys d) Parrots

120. Which bacterial serotypes of Mycobacterium avium are most virulent and responsible for avian tuberculosis?
a) Serotype 4, 5, 6 b) Serotype 1, 2, 3
c) Serotype A, B, C d) Serotype X, Y, Z

121. Where are gross lesions typically observed in avian tuberculosis?
a) Heart and lungs
b) Kidneys and bladder
c) Liver, spleen, intestines, and bone marrow
d) Brain and nervous system

122. Which organ, when affected, can give the spleen an "irregular, knobbly" appearance?
a) Kidney b) Lungs
c) Spleen d) Heart

123. What is the characteristic feature of tuberculosis in the chicken regarding bone marrow?
a) Presence of hemorrhages b) Pale yellow tubercular nodules
c) Swollen and congested appearance d) Lack of lesions

124. In which region can tubercular nodules be best observed in the long bones of the legs?
  a) Femoro-tibiotarsal
  b) Tibiotarsal-tarsometatarsal
  c) Femoro-fibular
  d) Tibiotibial

125. Which avian species is commonly affected by tuberculosis in the lungs?
  a) Chickens
  b) Turkeys
  c) Ducks
  d) Waterfowl, mainly ducks

126. What condition, caused by staphylococcal infection, is sometimes mistaken for tuberculosis?
  a) Leukosis
  b) Arthritis
  c) Bumble foot
  d) Osteoporosis

127. What are the derived cells that phagocytose tubercle bacilli early in the tubercle formation process?
  a) Fibrocytes
  b) Lymphocytes
  c) Histiocytes
  d) Eosinophils

128. What is the necrotic change resembling coagulative necrosis in the central zone of the tubercle caused by?
  a) Vascularization
  b) Avascularity of the cellular mass
  c) Presence of lymphocytes
  d) Proliferation of fibrocytes

129. What is the appearance of the cellular mass in the central zone after necrobiotic changes occur?
  a) Stains lightly with eosin
  b) Fused & stains deeply with eosin
  c) Becomes transparent
  d) Develops a granular texture

130. In what formation are giant cells arranged in the tubercle?
  a) Circular
  b) Scattered
  c) Palisade
  d) Clumped

131. What is a rare occurrence in fowl regarding the tubercular lesion?
  a) Calcification
  b) Amyloid-like degeneration
  c) Proliferation of lymphocytes
  d) Rapid cellular degeneration

Answer Key

1	a	2	d	3	b	4	b	5	b	6	c	7	c
8	a	9	c	10	b	11	b	12	b	13	c	14	b
15	b	16	c	17	d	18	d	19	b	20	c	21	c
22	c	23	c	24	c	25	c	26	c	27	c	28	b
29	b	30	b	31	c	32	a	33	c	34	b	35	c
36	c	37	c	38	c	39	b	40	a	41	b	42	b
43	b	44	d	45	d	46	b	47	b	48	a	49	c
50	b	51	a	52	c	53	c	54	a	55	c	56	b
57	d	58	c	59	a	60	b	61	c	62	b	63	c
64	a	65	b	66	a	67	b	68	c	69	c	70	d
71	b	72	b	73	c	74	a	75	c	76	b	77	a
78	b	79	b	80	a	81	b	82	b	83	c	84	c
85	d	86	b	87	d	88	b	89	b	90	b	91	b
92	b	93	a	94	c	95	c	96	b	97	b	98	a
99	c	100	c	101	d	102	d	103	c	104	c	105	c
106	d	107	d	108	b	109	c	110	c	111	a	112	c
113	c	114	b	115	b	116	c	117	c	118	b	119	c
120		121	c	122	c	123	b	124	b	125	d	126	c
127	c	128	b	129	b	130	c	131	a				

4

Fungal Diseases

Karthik Itherni, Amita Dubey, Maneesh Jatav and Y. Verma

College of Veterinary Science and Animal Husbandry, Jabalpur, Madhya Pradesh

1. What is a characteristic feature of fungal cell walls?
   a) Peptidoglycans
   b) Ergosterol and polysaccharides
   c) Antiphagocytic capsules
   d) Fruiting bodies
2. How do fungi reproduce in tissues?
   a) Binary fission
   b) Budding
   c) Simple division of round, yeast-like forms or slender, tubular hyphae
   d) Spore formation
3. What is a mycelium?
   a) A type of fungal cell
   b) A bacterial pathology
   c) A collection of hyphae
   d) A form of fungal reproduction
4. Which structure is rarely visible in body fluids or exudates?
   a) Mycelium
   b) Conidia
   c) Sporangia
   d) Fruiting bodies
5. 8. What is a characteristic feature of dimorphic fungi?
   a) Rapid growth on media
   b) Formation of antiphagocytic capsules
   c) Non-communicable tissue forms
   d) Production of infective spores in nature
6. 10. Why are leukopenic patients as vulnerable to fungi as to bacteria?
   a) Lack of antiphagocytic capsules
   b) Presence of mycotoxins
   c) Dimorphic nature of fungi
   d) Impaired phagocytic competence
7. What are synonyms for pulmonary aspergillosis in avian species?
   a) Brooder pneumonia and mycotic pneumonia
   b) Avian influenza and bronchitis
   c) Infectious bronchitis and laryngotracheitis
   d) Ranikhet disease and conjunctivitis

8. Which species of fungus is a major cause of aspergillosis in poultry?
   a) Candida albicans
   b) Aspergillus fumigatus and Aspergillus flavus
   c) Rhizopus stolonifer
   d) Cryptococcus neoformans
9. What is the primary mode of transmission for avian aspergillosis?
   a) Ingestion of contaminated feed
   b) Direct contact between infected birds
   c) Inhalation of fungal spores
   d) Sexual transmission
10. What is the characteristic clinical sign observed in chicks infected within the first 3-5 days after hatching?
   a) Gurgling and rattling noises
   b) Dyspnoea and polypnea
   c) Lethargy and stunted growth
   d) Blindness and torticollis
11. How are granulomas in avian aspergillosis usually observed grossly?
   a) As green to black lesions
   b) As separate white plaques or caseous nodules
   c) As pinkish-red spots on the skin
   d) As fluid-filled cysts
12. What is the characteristic feature of the ocular form of aspergillosis?
   a) Lethargy and stunted growth
   b) Blindness and torticollis
   c) Keratoconjunctivitis
   d) Chronic pulmonary insufficiency
13. What staining method may be required for the microscopic identification of Aspergillus hyphae in lesions?
   a) Hematoxylin and eosin (H&E)
   b) Gram staining
   c) Periodic Acid-Schiff (PAS)
   d) Giemsa staining
14. What is a characteristic gross manifestation of avian aspergillosis in the lungs or airsacs?
   a) Hemorrhagic lesions
   b) White caseous nodules
   c) Enlarged spleen
   d) Yellow discoloration
15. Which tissues are commonly affected by the haematogenous spread of Aspergillus spores in avian aspergillosis?
   a) Gastrointestinal tract
   b) Liver and gallbladder
   c) Brain, pericardium, bone marrow, and kidney
   d) Muscular system
16. In chronic cases of avian aspergillosis, what respiratory difficulty may be produced by the aspergillosis-induced exudate?
   a) Asthma
   b) Wheezing
   c) Acute respiratory distress
   d) Blockage of the trachea or syrinx

17. Which medium is commonly used for culturing granulomas or plaques in avian aspergillosis?
    a) Blood agar
    b) Sabouraud dextrose agar with antibiotics
    c) MacConkey agar
    d) Chocolate agar
18. What is another name for thrush in birds, specifically referring to oral, oesophageal, or crop candidiasis?
    a) Sour crop b) Mycosis of the digestive tract
    c) Candidiasis d) Moniliasis
19. What is the most common causative agent of crop mycosis in birds?
    a) Candida krusei b) Oidium pullorum
    c) Candida albicans d) Aspergillus fumigatus
20. Under what conditions does candidial overgrowth leading to crop mycosis often occur?
    a) Low environmental humidity
    b) High bacterial flora
    c) Prolonged administration of antibiotics
    d) High nutritional intake
21. What age group of birds is more susceptible to crop mycosis?
    a) Over 3 weeks of age b) Under 1 week of age
    c) Between 1 and 2 weeks of age d) Between 2 and 3 weeks of age
22. What is the primary reason for mortality directly due to candidiasis in birds?
    a) Neurological symptoms b) Renal failure
    c) Reduced feed intake d) Gastrointestinal disease
23. What is a characteristic gross appearance of lesions in the crop due to candidiasis?
    a) Hemorrhagic nodules
    b) Multifocal to confluent layers of white cheesy material
    c) Black discoloration
    d) Green pus accumulation
24. Pseudomembranes and diphtheritic membranes in the crop, oesophagus, and mouth are highly suggestive of which disease?
    a) Avian influenza b) Candidiasis
    c) Trichomoniasis d) Newcastle disease
25. What is another name for Thrush in birds?
    a) Sour crop b) Oidiomycosis
    c) Moniliasis d) All of the above
26. Which fungus is usually responsible for causing Crop Mycosis in birds?
    a) Candida albicans b) Trichophyton megninii
    c) Dactylaria gallopava d) Oidium pullorum

27. What is the primary clinical sign of Thrush in severely affected birds?
    a) Weight gain
    b) Neurological abnormalities
    c) Open-mouthed breathing
    d) Gurgling and rattling noises
28. What is the primary site of lesions in Favus?
    a) Feather follicles
    b) Lungs
    c) Intestines
    d) Kidneys
29. What are the depressions around follicles in feathered skin known as in Favus?
    a) Scabs
    b) Cups
    c) Holes
    d) Nodules
30. What is the main fungal species causing Favus?
    a) Candida albicans
    b) Trichophyton megninii
    c) Dactylaria gallopava
    d) Oidium pullorum
31. What is the primary symptom of Dactylariosis in chickens and turkey poults?
    a) Open-mouthed breathing
    b) Torticollis and incoordination
    c) Weight loss
    d) Gurgling noises
32. How does Dactylariosis differ from mycotic encephalitis of aspergillosis?
    a) Lesser malacia and hemorrhage
    b) Greater number of giant cells
    c) No ocular lesions
    d) Lower mortality rate
33. What part of the nervous system is primarily affected in Dactylariosis?
    a) Peripheral nerves
    b) Spinal cord
    c) Cerebellum
    d) Brain
34. What distinguishes Dactylariosis from mycotic encephalitis of aspergillosis?
    a) Lower mortality rate
    b) Presence of ocular lesions
    c) Greater malacia and hemorrhage
    d) Fewer giant cells
35. Which fungus is responsible for causing Histoplasmosis in poultry?
    a) Trichophyton megninii
    b) Candida albicans
    c) Dactylaria gallopava
    d) Histoplasma capsulatum
36. What is the primary public health concern associated with Histoplasmosis?
    a) Airborne transmission
    b) Contaminated water sources
    c) Person-to-person contact
    d) Consumption of infected poultry products
37. What is the primary causative fungus of Cryptococcosis?
    a) Candida albicans
    b) Trichophyton megninii
    c) Cryptococcus neoformans =
    d) Histoplasma capsulatum
38. In poultry, where are sporadic cases of Cryptococcosis often reported?
    a) Commercial farms
    b) Backyard flocks
    c) Hatcheries
    d) Broiler houses

39. What is the primary causative fungus of aflatoxicosis in poultry?
   a) Trichophyton megninii
   b) Candida albicans
   c) Aspergillus flavus
   d) Histoplasma capsulatum

40. Where is aflatoxin commonly found in feed grains?
   a) Temperate regions
   b) Arctic regions
   c) Tropics or subtropics
   d) Mediterranean regions

41. Which aflatoxin is usually present in the highest concentration and is the most toxic?
   a) Aflatoxin B1
   b) Aflatoxin B2
   c) Aflatoxin G1
   d) Aflatoxin G2

42. How does aflatoxin affect the liver in chickens?
   a) Causes liver enlargement
   b) Leads to liver discoloration
   c) Increases liver lipid content
   d) All of the above

43. At what level of aflatoxin concentration is aflatoxicosis economically significant in growing birds?
   a) > 0.5 ppm
   b) > 1.0 ppm
   c) > 2.0 ppm
   d) > 10.0 ppm

44. In which environmental conditions is aflatoxin production most likely to occur?
   a) Cold and dry
   b) Warm and humid
   c) Temperate and rainy
   d) Subzero temperatures

45. Which part of the avian body is most prominently affected by aflatoxicosis?
   a) Kidneys
   b) Gastrointestinal tract
   c) Liver
   d) Lungs

46. What is a characteristic gross lesion associated with aflatoxicosis in the liver?
   a) Green discoloration
   b) Enlargement and friability
   c) Hemorrhagic nodules
   d) Keratinized plaques

47. Which of the following is a microscopic lesion observed in aflatoxicosis?
   a) Oidium pullorum
   b) Clear vacuoles in hepatocytes
   c) Pseudomembrane formation
   d) Favus cups

48. What is the primary source of aflatoxin contamination in poultry feed?
   a) Fresh vegetables
   b) Clean water
   c) Mouldy grains
   d) Commercial vitamin supplements

49. Which histopathological feature is characteristic of the liver in chickens affected by aflatoxicosis?
   a) Fibrous encapsulation
   b) Lymphoid hyperplasia
   c) Multifocal hemorrhages and proliferation of bile ductules
   d) Epithelial hyperplasia

50. Which hematopoietic response is triggered in the liver due to aflatoxin-induced anemia?**
   a) Thrombocytosis
   b) Erythropoiesis
   c) Extramedullary hematopoiesis
   d) Leukocytosis
51. What effect does aflatoxin have on the bile ducts in the liver?
   a) Fibrosis
   b) Necrosis
   c) Proliferation
   d) Lymphocytic infiltration
52. Which immune organ exhibits atrophy in chickens affected by aflatoxicosis, contributing to immunosuppression?
   a) Thymus
   b) Spleen
   c) Bursa of Fabricius
   d) Bone marrow
53. What is a characteristic microscopic lesion in the cerebellum associated with aflatoxicosis?
   a) Cyst formation
   b) Gliosis
   c) Meningeal and encephalitic necrosis
   d) Neuronal hyperplasia
54. Which cellular response is significantly increased in aflatoxicosis compared to aspergillosis in the brain?
   a) Neutrophil infiltration
   b) Lymphocytic aggregation
   c) Giant cell formation
   d) Eosinophilic infiltration
55. Which cellular component in the liver is affected by aflatoxin-induced toxicity in late-stage embryos?
   a) Hepatocytes
   b) Kupffer cells
   c) B lymphocytes
   d) Macrophages
56. Which fungi are primarily responsible for producing ochratoxins in poultry feed?
   a) Candida albicans and Aspergillus flavus
   b) Penicillium veridicatum and Aspergillus ochraceus
   c) Trichophyton megninii and Dactylaria gallopava
   d) Histoplasma capsulatum and Cryptococcus neoformans
57. What is the most toxic and prevalent ochratoxin in poultry?
   a) Ochratoxin B
   b) Ochratoxin C
   c) Ochratoxin D
   d) Ochratoxin A
58. What is the primary target organ affected by ochratoxin A in acute lethal mycotoxicosis in chickens?
   a) Heart
   b) Liver
   c) Kidneys
   d) Pancreas
59. What is the primary manifestation of acute ochratoxicosis in poultry kidneys, leading to mortality?
   a) Hyperuricemia
   b) Urate deposits
   c) Acute proximal tubular epithelial necrosis
   d) Dehydration

60. What is the main microscopic lesion observed in the kidneys during acute ochratoxicosis?
   a) Interstitial inflammation
   b) Vacuolar change in hepatocytes
   c) Acute tubular necrosis
   d) Fibrosis

61. Which species is most sensitive to ochratoxin ingestion, with ducks being seven times more susceptible than chickens?
   a) Broilers
   b) Turkeys
   c) Ducks
   d) Layers

62. What are the clinical signs of ochratoxicosis in poultry survivors, indicating chronic exposure?
   a) Depression and dehydration
   b) Stunted growth and poor feathering
   c) Increased clotting time, anaemia, and immunosuppression
   d) Polyuria and acute renal failure

63. What is the primary clinical sign of trichothecene mycotoxicosis in chickens?
   a) Ulcers in the esophagus
   b) Poor feathering
   c) Swollen kidneys
   d) Enlarged liver

64. Where do chickens suffering from trichothecene mycotoxicosis develop ulcers?
   a) Dorsal surface of the tongue
   b) Hard palate,
   c) Mouth commissures
   d) All the above

65. Which of the following is a microscopic feature of ulcerative stomatitis in trichothecene mycotoxicosis?
   a) Increased epithelial layers
   b) Hypochromatic erythrocytes
   c) Inflammatory cell infiltration in ulcerated areas
   d) Enlarged liver cells

66. What is the predominant effect on the blood in chickens affected by trichothecene mycotoxicosis?
   a) Increased red blood cell count
   b) Polychromatic erythrocytes
   c) Decreased red blood cell count
   d) Hyperchromatic erythrocytes

67. Which mycotoxin is nephrotoxic and produced by Penicillium citrinum, mainly in maize and rice?
   a) Ochratoxin A
   b) Citrinin
   c) Fumonisin B1
   d) Moniliformin

68. What is the primary effect of Oosporein ingestion in chicks?
   a) Dermatitis
   b) Acute renal failure
   c) Cardiotoxicity
   d) Leg deformities

69. Which Fusarium mycotoxin is associated with equine leukoencephalomalacia and porcine pulmonary edema syndrome, but shows resistance in chickens compared to turkeys?
    a) Fumonisin B1
    b) Moniliformin
    c) Fusarochromanone
    d) Zearalenone
70. Which mycotoxin, produced by Fusarium moniliforme, is known to be cardiotoxic in poultry and has been linked to acute myocardial necrosis in ducks, chickens, and turkey poults?
    a) Zearalenone
    b) Moniliformin
    c) Fusarochromanone
    d) Ergotism
71. What is the primary effect of Fusarochromanone (TDP-1) in chicks?
    a) Nephrotoxicity
    b) Dermatitis
    c) Cardiotoxicity
    d) Leg deformities and tibial dyschondroplasia
72. Ergotism, caused by Claviceps sp., is associated with necrosis of which parts in poultry?
    a) Liver, kidneys, and spleen
    b) Beak, comb, and toes
    c) Skin, comb, and wattles
    d) Intestines and cecum
73. Which mycotoxin is produced by Gibberella zeae (Fusarium graminearum) and exhibits estrogenic activity?
    a) Zearalenone
    b) Fumonisin B1
    c) Ochratoxin A
    d) Citrinin
74. What is the characteristic effect of Fusarium-produced mycotoxins known as Trichothecenes on chickens suffering from mycotoxicosis?
    a) Yellow discoloration of the liver
    b) Ulcers at the commissures of the mouth and on the hard palate
    c) Nephrotoxicity and polyuria
    d) Dermatitis and vesicular lesions
75. Which mycotoxin is linked to vesicular dermatitis (sore throat disease) in Leghorn birds, causing vesicles and crusts on the comb, wattles, face, and eyelids?
    a) Ergotism
    b) Fusarochromanone
    c) Zearalenone
    d) Oosporein
76. Which statement about ochratoxicosis in poultry is correct?
    a) Ducks are more sensitive than chickens.
    b) Ochratoxin A has no nephrotoxic effects.
    c) It mainly affects adult hen testicular weights.
    d) Acute renal failure is not associated with ochratoxicosis.

77. What is the primary gross lesion associated with aflatoxicosis in chickens?
    a) White foci on the liver
    b) Ulcers in the mouth and palate
    c) Swollen, hard kidneys with white urate deposits
    d) Yellow discoloration of the liver

78. Which mycotoxin is characterized by its stable nature and is not destroyed during normal milling and storage processes?
    a) Fumonisin B1 b) Aflatoxin
    c) Ochratoxin A d) Citrinin

79. In young poultry, which organ shows atrophy due to aflatoxicosis?
    a) Liver b) Spleen
    c) Thymus d) Kidneys

80. What is the most commonly seen mycotoxicosis in poultry, both in terms of prevalence and economic importance?
    a) Ochratoxicosis b) Trichothecene mycotoxicosis
    c) Aflatoxicosis d) Ergotism

81. Which technique is commonly used for the isolation and identification of specific toxins in the definitive diagnosis of mycotoxicosis?
    a) ELISA b) PCR
    c) Feeding trials d) Vaccination

82. What is the primary purpose of conducting feeding trials in the diagnosis of mycotoxicosis?
    a) Identifying gross lesions
    b) Confirming the presence of mycotoxins
    c) Analyzing feed composition
    d) Evaluating vaccination efficacy

83. Which analytical technique involves the use of antibodies to detect and identify specific mycotoxins in poultry rations?
    a) Thin layer chromatography
    b) High-performance liquid chromatography
    c) Monoclonal antibody-based technology
    d) Mass spectrometry

Answer Key

1	b	2	c	3	c	4	a	5	d	6	d	7	a
8	b	9	c	10	b	11	b	12	c	13	c	14	b
15	c	16	d	17	b	18	d	19	c	20	c	21	b
22	c	23	b	24	b	25	d	26	a	27	c	28	a
29	b	30	b	31	b	32	b	33	d	34	c	35	d
36	a	37	c	38	b	39	c	40	c	41	a	42	d

43	b	44	b	45	c	46	b	47	b	48	c	49	c
50	c	51	c	52	c	53	c	54	c	55	c	56	b
57	d	58	c	59	c	60	c	61	c	62	c	63	a
64	d	65	c	66	c	67	b	68	b	69	a	70	b
71	d	72	c	73	a	74	b	75	a	76	a	77	d
78	b	79	c	80	c	81	c	82	b	83	c		

5

Mycoplasma Diseases

Ganesh K. Sawale

Department of Veterinary Pathology, Mumbai Veterinary College, Parel, Mumbai

Introduction

Avian mycoplasmosis is caused by several pathogenic mycoplasma of which mycoplasmosis due to *Mycoplasma gallisepticum* (Mg), *Mycoplasma synoviae* (MS) and *Mycoplasma meleagridis* are important. The mycoplasma are group of bacteria that lack cell wall due to which the shape of bacteria is pleomorphic. Due to lack of cell wal, mycoplasma are resistant to those drug which act on cell wall and includes Penicillin and its derivatives. Mycoplasma primarily affects respiratory system and joints in birds and respiratory and urogenital system in humans. The avian mycoplasma are mainly transmitted by vertical route (egg transmission), but can also transmitted by horizontal route. *Mycoplasma gallisepticum* (Mg) causes chronic respiratory disease (CRD) in chicken, turkeys and game birds. *Mycoplasma synoviae (Ms)* causes infectious synovitis in chicken and turkeys whereas *Mycoplasma meleagridis* cause disease in turkey. The Mg and Ms belongs to class of Mollicutes (Molecutis: soft tissue), order Mycoplasmatales and family Mycoplasmataceae. The CRD caused by Mg affects respiratory system and air sac in presence of other respiratory pathogen/ stress or immunosuppression. Clinically, CRD affected birds show respiratory rales, gasping, nasal discharge, and rhinitis with mortality due to complication with other respiratory viral pathogens or *E. coli infection.* The Ms has affinity for tendon and ligaments of joint causing severe lameness due to tenosynovitis with mild lesions in respiratory system and air sac. The Ms affected birds show lameness, breast blister and increased culling of male breeder birds. The Mg and Ms causes significant losses in poultry industry due to decreased egg production, condemnation and downgrading of carcass and decreased hatchability. *Mycoplasma meleagridis* in turkey associated with air sacculitis and drop in egg production.

Ureaplasma is another genus under order Mycoplasmatales. Ureaplasma hydrolyses urea whereas mycoplasma cannot. Ureaplasma generally affects urogenital tract of humans. The *Ureaplasma urealyticum, Ureaplasma diversum* are important pathogens associated with genital infection in human beings.

The mycoplasma often called as PPLO (pleuropneumonia like organism) and the media used for isolation as PPLO broth or PPLO agar. The most common drug used for treatment of Mycoplasma infection in birds includes Tylosin, Tiamutin, Tilmicosin. Mycoplasma infections can also be treated with Quinolone and Tetracycline.

1. Which of the following is incorrect match.

   a) Diene's stain: Mycoplasma b) Fontana stain: Spirochaetes

   c) Machiavello stain: Chlamydia d) Acid fast stain: Staphylococci

2. Mycoplasma organisms are pleomorphic in nature due to
   a) Absence of cell wall
   b) Due to rigid cell wall
   c) Small in size
   d) All of these
3. *Mycoplasma spp.* are closely related to
   a) Gram positive bacteria
   b) Gram negative bacteria
   c) Acid fast bacteria
   d) None of these
4. *Mycoplasma gallisepticum* attaches to host cell through
   a) Fimbriae
   b) Adhesins molecule
   c) Pili
   d) All of these
5. The genome of Mycoplasmas ranges from
   a) 0.1–0.5 Mb
   b) 0.58–1.38 Mb
   c) b. 1.4–3 Mb
   d) 3–5 Mb
6. The size of Mycoplasmas ranges from
   a) 0.05–0.1 μm
   b) 0.2–0.3 μm
   c) 0.4–0.5 μm
   d) 0.5–1 μm
7. The chronic respiratory disease in chicken is caused by
   a) *Ureaplasma urealyticum*
   b) Mycoplasma gallisepticum
   c) *Mycoplasma synoviae*
   d) All of these
8. Chronic respiratory disease is generally more severe in
   a) Chicken
   b) Turkeys
   c) Duck
   d) Quails
9. The infectious synovitis in chicken is caused by
   a) *Ureaplasma urealyticum*
   b) *Mycoplasma gallisepticum*
   c) Mycoplasma synoviae
   d) All of these
10. The infectious sinusitis in turkey is name given to disease caused by
   a) *Ureaplasma urealyticum*
   b) Mycoplasma gallisepticum
   c) *Mycoplasma synoviae*
   d) None of these
11. The *Mycoplasma gallisepticum* in chicken is transmitted by
   a) Direct contact (Horizontal route)
   b) Through egg (Vertical route)
   c) Carrier birds
   d) All of these
12. The *Mycoplasma gallisepticum* mainly affects
   a) Respiratory system
   b) Air sac
   c) Both a and b
   d) None of these
13. The chronic respiratory disease in chicken show signs of
   a) Respiratory rales
   b Gurgling throat sound
   c) Joint swelling & lameness
   d) Only a and b
14. The chronic respiratory disease in adult chicken show signs of
   a) Respiratory rales
   b) Decreased egg production
   c) Decreased weight gain
   d) All of these

15. The exaggerated signs of chronic respiratory disease are more commonly seen in
    a) Male birds b) Female birds
    c) Both a and b d) None of these
16. In broiler chicken, CRD is most commonly seen in
    a) Below 2 week age b) 2-3 week age
    c) 4-8 week age d) Adult age
17. The gross lesions in CRD includes
    a) Air sacculitis b) Exudate in trachea & bronchi
    c) Pneumonia d) All of these
18. The gross lesions in CRD includes following Except
    a) Air sacculitis b) Exudate in trachea & bronchi
    c) Joint swelling d) Pneumonia
19. One of the most common sign of CRD in turkey is
    a) Lameness b) Swelling of joints
    c) Swelling of Infraorbital sinuses d) Pneumonia
20. Uncomplicated CRD in chicken generally causes
    a) High morbidity and low mortality b) High mortality
    c) High morbidity and high mortality d) None of these
21. The CRD is most commonly complicated with
    a) Salmonella spp b) E. coli
    c) Pasteurella multocida d) All of these
22. The complication of CRD is seen with following diseases except
    a) Ranikhet disease b) Colisepticemia
    c) Avian coccidiosis d) Bird flu
23. The CRD can be complicated with
    a) Ranikhet disease b) Infectious bronchitis
    c) Bird flu d) All of these
24. The postmortem lesions of air sacculitis and cheesy content in air sac is most commonly seen in one of the following disease
    a) Histomoniasis b) Avian coccidiosis
    c) Chronic respiratory disease d) None of these
25. The following are the vertically transmitted diseases of poultry except
    a) CRD b) Infectious synovitis
    c) Mycoplasma meleagridis infection d) Histomoniasis
26. Polyserositis is one of characteristic gross lesion seen in
    a) *CRD* b) *Colisepticemia*
    c) Both a and b d) None of these
27. The diagnosis of Mycoplasma gallisepticum is done with following test except
    a) Gram stain b) Indirect FAT
    c) Indirect Immunoperoxidase test d) Growth inhibition test

28. The following are the medicine used for treatment of CRD except
    a) Tylosin b) Tiamulin
    c) Tetracycline d) Penicillin
29. The amoxicillin and penicillin don not kill mycoplasma as it lacks
    a) Nucleus b) Mytochondria
    c) Cell wall d) Golgi bodies
30. Mycoplasmas are resistant to one of the following drug
    a) Tylosin b) Tiamulin
    c) Beta-lactams d) Tetracycline
31. Diagnosis of Mycoplasma gallisepticum is carried out using
    a) Nurient agar b) Blood agar
    c) PPLO agar d) Cell culture
32. Diagnosis of Mycoplasma gallisepticum is carried out using all except
    a) PCR b) MG-ELISA
    c) Plate/tube agglutination test d) Grams stain
33. One of the important component of PPLO broth which support growth of *Mycoplasma* is
    a) 1-2 % agar b) 5-10 % sheep blood
    c) 5-10 % dextrose d) 10-15 % serum
34. *Mycoplasma gallisepticum* show characteristic colonies on PPLO agar as
    a) Medusa head colonies b) Swarming growth
    c) Fried egg colony d) None of these
35. Chronic respiratory disease must be differentiated from following disease except
    a) 1-2 % agar b) 5-10 % sheep blood
    c) 5-10 % dextrose d) 10-15 % serum
36. The live vaccine used for control of Mycoplasma gallisepticum include(s)
    a) The F strain b) ts-11
    c) 6/85 stain vaccine d) All of these
37. For control of Mycoplasma gallisepticum , the preferred route of vaccination for F- strain is
    a) Intranasal/ Eye drop method b) Fine spray
    c) Intramuscular route route d) None of these
38. For control of Mycoplasma gallisepticum , the preferred route of vaccination for ts-11 strain is
    a) Intranasal method b) Eye drop method
    c) Intramuscular route route d) None of these
39. For control of Mycoplasma gallisepticum , the preferred route of vaccination for 6/85 strain is
    a) Fine spray b) Drinking water
    c) Intramuscular route route d) None of these

40. The method of choice for prevention of CRD on farm is
  a) MG free breeding stock
  b) Treatment of affected flock
  c) Vaccination with live strain of MG
  d) None of these
41. Prevention of *Mycoplasma gallisepticum* (MG) in farm can be achieved by
  a) Procuring breeder birds free from MG
  b) Strict biosecirity
  c) Egg dipping with macrolide before hatching
  d) All of these
42. The *Mycoplasma meleagridis* infection is mainly seen in
  a) Chicken b) Turkeys
  c) Quails d) Ducks
43. The *Mycoplasma meleagridis* infection is usually in apparent infection in all except
  a) Recently hatched poults b) Adult turkey
  c) Grower turkey d) None of these
44. The Mycoplasma meleagridis infection is in turkey show signs of
  a) Respiratory rales b) Sinusitis
  c) Crooked neck (Wry necks) d) All of these
45. The *Mycoplasma meleagridis* in turkey spread by
  a) Horizontal route via aerosols b) Vertical route through eggs
  c) Infected semen d) All of these
46. The skeletal abnormality in Mycoplasma meleagridis infection in turkey include all except
  a) Leg deformities b) Crooked neck (Wry necks)
  c) Shortening of the tarso-metatarsal bone d) All of these
47. Immunosuppression is one of the important feature of
  a) Mycoplasma meleagridis *b)* *Mycoplasma gallisepticum*
  c) *Mycoplasma synoviae* *d)* None of these
48. The lesions of Mycoplasma meleagridis infection in poult include(s)
  a) Airsacculitis b) Crooked neck (Wry necks)
  c) Osteomylitis d) All of these
49. The lesions of Mycoplasma meleagridis infection in adult breeder include(s)
  a) Airsacculitis b) Sinusitis
  c) Synovitis d) All of these
50. Avian skeletal disorder historically known as turkey syndrome 65 (TS 65) is given for one of the following disease
  a) *Mycoplasma gallisepticum* infection b) *E. Coli* infection
  c) Mycoplasma meleagridis infection d) *Mycoplasma synoviae* infection

51. The infection due to *Mycoplasma synoviae* (MS) in chicken is commonly called as
    a) Infectious sinusitis b) Infectious synovitis
    c) CRD d) None of these
52. The exaggerated clinical signs of Infectious synivitis are more commonly seen in
    a) Male birds b) Female birds
    c) Both a and b d) None of these
53. The following is one of the test in which cross reactivity of MG with MS do not occur
    a) Plate agglutination test b) Tube agglutination test
    c) Haemagglutination inhibition d) None of these
54. The following is one of the test in which cross reactivity of MG with MS do not occur
    b) Plate agglutination test b) Tube agglutination test
    c) ELISA d) None of these
55. Infectious synovitis in chicken is spread by
    a) Horizontal route b) Vertical route
    c) Both a and b d) None of these
56. The following are the pathogenic strains of Mycoplasma synoviae except
    a) WVU1853 b) K1968
    c) K1858 d) ts-304
57. The most important route of transmission of infectious synovitis is
    a) Aerosal b) Vertical
    c) Flies d) None of these
58. The primary target organ of Mycoplasma synoviae in birds is
    a) Intestine b) Joints
    c) Liver d) Kidney
59. The main clinical signs of Mycoplasma synoviae infection in include(s)
    a) Watery diarrhoea b) Severe respiratory rales
    c) Lameness d) All of the these
60. The clinical signs of Mycoplasma synoviae infection in include(s)
    a) Anaemia b) Lameness
    c) Swelling of hock & foot pad joint d) All of the these
61. The Mycoplasma synoviae infection in chicken generally causes mortality of
    a) less than 10 percent b) 10-20 percent
    c) 20-30 percent d) 30-50 percent
62. The gross lesions of Mycoplasma synoviae infection in chicken includes
    a) Caseous exudate in joint b) Sternal bursitis
    c) Swollen & edematous tendons d) All of these

63. Infectious synovitis in chicken must be differentiated from
    a) Viral arthititis
    b) Fowl typhoid
    c) Pullorum disease
    d) All of the these

Answer Key

1	d	2	a	3	a	4	b	5	b	6	b	7	b
8	b	9	c	10	b	11	d	12	c	13	d	14	d
15	a	16	c	17	d	18	c	19		20	a	21	b
22	c	23	d	24	c	25	d	26	c	27	a	28	d
29	c	30	c	31	c	32	d	33	d	34	c	35	d
36	d	37	a	38	b	39	a	40	a	41	d	42	b
43	a	44		45	d	46	d	47	a	48	d	49	d
50	c	51	c	52	a	53	c	54	c	55	c	56	d
57	b	58	c	59	c	60	d	61	a	62	d	63	d

6

Ectoparasitic Infestation

Manaswini Dehuri

Department of Veterinary Parasitology, College of Veterinary Sciences and Animal Husbandry, OUAT, Bhubaneswar-751003

Flea of Brds

Ceratophyllus gallinae – commonest flea of domestic poultry may be responsible for irritation, restlessness and even anaemia Feeds readily on humans and domestic pets and its often acquired in the handling of poultry and from injured and wild birds brought into houses could migrate into rooms from nests under adjacent caves.

Echidnophaga gallinacea -'stick tight' flea-seen on the skin of the fowl (usually comb and wattles). Absence of genal and pronotal comb. Fleas established in a poultry house - Remove and burn all litter them spray the poultry house with an insectide.

Mites of Birds

Cnemidocoptes (Knemidocoptes)-only burrowing genus of domestic birds.

Hosts: Poultry and cage birds

C. mutan - "scaly leg"

C. gallianae -"depluming itch"

C. pilae cage bird -"scaly face", "tassel foot"

Morphology- Circular body and short, stubby legs and the avain hsot are sufficient for generic diagnosis.

In *C. gallinae*, mites burrow into shaft of the feather leading to inflammation and itching which in turn lead to pecking.Affected birds swallow falling feathers, egg production falls, infection is by contact.

C. mutans burrow into epidermal scales from tibiotarsal downward and as far as downs of the toes leading to inflammation. Scales are displaced from normal position with progress of the infection, a dry crust accumulates under the scale, and gland of pedipalp secretes irritant materials which stimulates exudation of serum which contributes to scaly nature of the legs. Vesicles can be found ,covered and filled with tissue fluids. The flexion of joints become difficult because of crust and the bird become lame. Birds peck the crust due to irritation, egg production reduces in laying birds and in advanced stages death occur dueto starvation and thirst.This is common in poorly kept birds.

C. pilae is most often seen in budgerigars because of their popularity, but other psittacines (e.g. parrot, parakeet, cokatrel)

It attacks bare and lightly feathered areas including the beak, head, neck, inside of the wings, legs and feet.The mites are deep in the skin, but cause little pruritus lesion develop slowly, over a number of months.Changes are first seen on the head with scales at the angle of the beak which spreads over the face ("scaly face')affecting the core and horny tissue of the beak. Beak may become distorted due to the mites burrowing in the matrix andcrossbeak may develop.

When the limbs are affected an extreme from of scaly leg may develop and toes may slough off in severely affected birds.

Ornithonyssus syviarium (Northern Mite of Poultry)

- 1mm, elongate to oval mite usually found on birds, it also may be found on nests or within poultry houses. Legs relatively long can be seen with naked eyes. Color may vary from red to black depending on recent feeding.

- Feeds intermittently on birds, produces irritation, weight loss, decrease egg pox, anaemia and even death.

- Known to bite humans.

- Anus on the anterior half of the ventral anal plate.

May help in the spred of NewCastleDisease and chlamydiosis.

Dermanyssus gallinae (Red mite of poultry)

- Similar in appearance to Ornithonyssus syviarium.1mm in length, elongate to oval whitish grayish/black and feeds onbirds.

- Has distinct red colour when it has recently fed on its host's blood (red mite of poultry).

- Lays eggs in the cracks in the wall of poultry houses.

- Nymphal stage and adults are periodic parasites hiding in cracks and crevices of the poultry houses and making frequent visits to the host to feed.

- Because of their blood-feeding activity, these mites may produce significant anaemia and much irritation to the host.

- Birds are listless, decrease egg production . Loss of blood may results in death.

- Anus of D. gallinae is on the posterior half of the ventral anal plate.

* Vector of Borrelia anserina (avian spirochaetosis).

Biting Lice of Birds

Menopon gallinae -shaft louse of poultry Hosts: fowl, ducks and pigeons

Pale yellow in color The thoracic and abdominal segmentseach have one dorsal row of bristles. It moves about rapidly. Lay eggs in cluster on feathers.

Holomenopon leucoxanthum

Host: Ducks

Causes "wet feather". Soiled and tattered plumage that they preen continuously. If large body areas are affected plumage no longer repel water and birds become chilled and may die from pneumonia.

Menacanthus stramineus- Yellow " body louse" of poultry. Host:fowl, turkey, peacock.

Seen in parts of body with dense feathering like breast, thighs, and around the anus.

Cuclotogaster heterographus- Head louse' of poultry

Host: fowl and patridges.

Site: skin and feathers the head and neck

Lipeurus caponis-“Wing louse” of poultry . Host: Fowl and pheasants .slender elongate louse seen on the under-side of the large wing feathers and moves about very little.

Gonniocotes gallinae- Fluff louse” Hosts: Fowls, pheasants the pigeons

fluff seen at the base of the feathers

Multiple Choice Question

1. Which of the following is shaft louse of poultry:
   a) Menopon gallinae b) *Heterodoxus spinigerum*
   c) *Menacanthus stramineus* d) *Holomenopon leucoxanthum*
2. The eggs of which louse in poultry have filaments
   a) shaft louse b) body louse
   c) wing louse d) fluff louse
3. Wet feather of ducks is due to infestation by
   a) *Menopon gallinae* b) *Heterodoxus spinigerum*
   c) *Menacanthus stramineus* d) *Holomenopon leucoxanthum*
4. Lice infestation in poultry birds is mostly due to
   a) biting lice b) sucking lice
   c) both d) none
5. Lice infestation in poultry causes
   a) anaemia b) restlessness
   c) both d) none
6. Which is the most economically important lice in intensive poultry farm
   a) *Menopon gallinae* b) *Heterodoxus spinigerum*
   c) Menacanthus stramine***us*** d) *Holomenopon leucoxanthum*
7. The lice with one row of dorsal bristle on thorax and abdomen segment
   a) Menopon gallinae b) *Heterodoxus spinigerum*
   c) *Menacanthus stramineus* d) *Holomenopon leucoxanthum*
8. The lice with one row of dorsal bristle on thorax and abdomen segment
   a) *Menopon gallinae* b) *Heterodoxus spinigerum*
   c) Menacanthus stramineus d) *Holomenopon leucoxanthum*
9. *Lipeurus caponis* is commonly known as
   a) shaft louse b) head louse
   c) wing louse d) fluff louse
10. *Cuclogaster heterographus* is commonly known as
    a) shaft louse b) head louse
    c) wing louse d) fluff louse
11. Sucking lice belongs to the order
    a) Siphunculata b) Hemiptera
    c) Mallophaga d) Siphonaptera

12. Which is known as roost mite of poultry
    a) *Ornithonysus sylvarium* b) *Ornithonyssus bursa*
    c) *Megninia ginglymura* d) *Dermanyssus gallinae*
13. Which is not true for lice infestation
    a) depluming b) reduced egg production
    c) hair ball formation d) secondary bacteria infection
14. Maggots of blow flies are an example of _________ association with host
    a) Obligatory b) Facultative
    c) Accidental d) None
15. *Goniocotes gallinae* is commonly known as
    a) shaft louse b) head louse
    c) wing louse d) fluff louse
16. Which of the following flea affects poultry birds
    a) *Ceratophyllus gallinae* b) *Echidnophaga gallinacea*
    c) Both d) None
17. *Echidnophaga gallinacea* has the following features
    a) pronotal comb b) genal comb
    c) both d) none
18. *Ceratophyllus gallinae* has the following features
    a) pronotal comb b) genal comb
    c) both d) none
19. *Echidnophaga gallinacea* attaches to which part of the body
    a) comb b) wattle
    c) eyes d) all of the above
20. The insecticide commonly used in control of poultry fleas
    a) carbaryl b) malathion
    c) pyrethroids d) All of the above
21. Which is known as poultry tick
    a) *Ornithodorus sp* b) Argas sp
    c) *Otobius sp* d) All of them
22. Fowl tick act as vector of
    a) *Agyeptionella pullorum* b) *Borrelia anserina*
    c) Both d) None
23. Which is known as tropical fowl mite
    a) *Ornithonysus sylvarium* b) Ornithonyssus bursa
    c) *Megninia ginglymura* d) *Dermanyssus gallinae*
24. *Goniocotes gallinae* is commonly known as
    a) shaft louse b) head louse
    c) wing louse d) fluff louse

25. Large chicken louse is a common name for
    a) *Goniocotes dissimilis* b) Goniocotes gigas
    c) both a & b d) *Goniocotes gallinae*
26. Chewing louse of swan is common name for
    a) *Chelopistes meleagridis* b) *Anatoecus dentatus*
    c) Trinoton anseinum d) None
27. Which is not a clinical sign of blue bug infestation
    a) loss in egg production b) irritation
    c) anemia d) None
28. Which is known as northern fowl mite
    a) Ornithonysus sylvarium b) *Ornithonyssus bursa*
    c) *Megninia ginglymura* d) *Dermanyssus gallinae*
29. The biting fly that transmits *Hymenolepis carioca*
    a) *Hypoderma* b) Stomoxys
    c) *Chrysomyia* d) *Oestrus ovis*
30. ________ act as vectors for transmission of *Leucocytozoon* to chickens
    a) Anopheles b) Cullicoides
    c) Simulium d) Culex
31. Which is not a feature of red mite of poultry
    a) grayish white in colour b) long chelicerae
    c) 3 anal setae d) no anal shield
32. Which is known as feather mite of poultry
    a) *Ornithonysus sylvarium* b) *Ornithonyssus bursa*
    c) Megninia ginglymura d) *Dermanyssus gallinae*
33. *Dermanyssus* sp transmits
    a) RMSF b) CCHF
    c) Buttonese fever d) Avian spirochetosis
34. Red mite of poultry shows which effect on host
    a) sub acute anemia b) neutrophilia
    c) lymphocytosis d) None
35. Which poultry mite is a nocturnal feeder
    a) feather mite b) Tropical mite
    c) Red mite d) All
36. Which poultry mite causes dermatitis in human beings
    a) red fowl mite b) Tropical fowl mite
    c) northern fowl mite d) All
37. Which of the following is not used in treating fowl mites
    a) Carbamates b) Macrolides
    c) Pyrethroids d) Organophosphates

38. *Salmonella gallinarum* can be transmitted by
   a) red fowl mite b) Tropical fowl mite
   c) northern fowl mite d) All
39. ________ act as vectors for transmission of *Haemoproteus* to ducks and geese
   a) Anopheles b) Cullicoides
   c) Pseudolynchia d) Culex
40. Tasel foot mite is the common name for
   a) *C. pilae* b) C. *gallinae*
   c) *C. mutans* d) C. both a & c
41. Which mite has chitinised transverse and longitudinal bars below head
   a) *Laminosioptes cysticola* b) *Cnemidocoptes sp*
   c) *Cytodites nudus* d) *Chelopistes sp*
42. Which of the fly transmit leucocytozoonosis to ducks, turkeys, and other birds
   a) Anopheles b) Cullicoides
   c) Simulium d) Culex
43. *Pseudolynchia canariensis* transmit the blood parasites
   a) Trypanosoma b) Haemoproteus
   c) Both d) None
44. Which of the following is not a bottle fly
   a) Calliphora b) Lucilia
   c) Hypoderma d) Chrysomia
45. *Plasmodium gallinaceum* (chicken malaria) is transmitted by
   a) *Culex sp* *b)* *Anopheles sp*
   c*)* *Aedes sp* *d)* Both a & b
46. Little house flies that can develop on poultry farms belongs to
   a) Musca sp b) *Fannia* sp.
   c) Lucilia sp d) None
47. Lice is transmitted in poultry farms by
   a) contact b) egg crates
   c) both d) none
48. Transmission of lice by phoresy occurs in case of
   a) *Menopon gallinae* *b)* *Heterodoxus spinigerum*
   c) *Musca domestica* *d)* *Pseudolynchia canariensis*
49. Common louse of turkey is common name for
   a) *Chelopistes meleagridis* b) *Anatoecus dentatus*
   c) *Trinoton anseinum* d) None
50. Head louse of duck is common name for
   a) *Chelopistes meleagridis* b) *Anatoecus dentatus*
   c) *Trinoton anseinum* d) None

51. Rounded head with two large bristles in head is found in which louse
    a) *Menopon sp* b) *Heterodoxus sp*
    c) *Gonoides sp* d) *Chelopistes sp*
52. Which of the following belongs to order Amblycera
    a) *Menopon sp* b) *Heterodoxus sp*
    c) *Gonoides sp* d) *Chelopistes sp*
53. Which of the following belongs to order Ischnocera
    a) *Menopon sp* b) *Menacanthus sp*
    c) *Lipeurus sp* d) *Chelopistes sp*
54. Crest flea of birds is a common name for
    a) *Ceratophyllus gallinae* b) *Echidnophaga gallinacea*
    c) Both d) None
55. Stick tight flea of poultry does not produce
    a) blindness b) anemia
    c) irritation d) none
56. Eggs produced by Echidnophaga gallinacea is
    a) sticky b) dry
    c) both d) none
57. Stick tight flea can attach to which part of poultry
    a) comb b) eyes
    c) both d) none
58. Foreshortened thorax are found in which flea
    a) *Ctenocephalides sp* b) *Pulex sp*
    c) *Xenopsylla sp* d) *Echidophaga sp*
59. Which of the following mite has the ability to attack human beings
    a) red fowl mite b) Tropical fowl mite
    c) northern fowl mite d) All of the above
60. Which is commonly called air sac mite of birds
    a) *Laminosioptes cysticola* b) both a &c
    c) *Cytodites nudus* d) *Chelopistes sp*
61. Mite that forms small nodules in muscle tissue of neck, breast, flanks & vents
    a) *Laminosioptes cysticola* b) *Mycoptes sp*
    c) *Cytodites nudus* d) *Chelopistes sp*
62. Mite that attacks the legs of fowl
    a) *C. pilae* b) *C. gallinae*
    c) *C. mutans* d) both a & c
63. Depluming itch is the common name for
    a) *C. pilae* b) *C. gallinae*
    c) *C. mutans* d) both a & c

64. Scaly face mite is the common name for
   a) *C. pilae* b) *C. gallinae*
   c) *C. mutans* d) both a & c
65. Which of the following is a burrowing mite
   a) *Laminosioptes cysticola* b) *Cnemidocoptes sp*
   c) *Cytodites nudus* d) *Chelopistes sp*
66. Copulatory suckers in mites of fowl are absent in
   a) male b) female
   c) Both d) None
67. Absence of spines and scales in dorsal surface of mite with faint striations
   a) *Laminosioptes cysticola* b) *Chelopistes sp*
   c) *Cytodites nudus* d) *Cnemidocoptes sp*
68. Lameness,distortion of feet and claws is due to which mite
   a) *C. pilae* b) *C. gallinae*
   c) *C. mutans* d) both a & c
69. Anti platelet enzyme present in flea saliva
   a) hyaluronidase b) apyrase
   c) serpin d) none
70. Flea have which type of mouthparts
   a) piercing and sucking b) sucking and lapping
   c) both d) none
71. Dorsal plate gradually tapers to a blunt point with a small setae
   a) *D. gallinae* b) *O.bacoti*
   c) *O.sylvarium* d) O.bursa
72. The following arthropod is nocturnal in habit
   a) Anopheles b) Sand fly
   c) both a & b d) Aedes
73. Anus present in posterior half of anal plate in case of
   a) *D. gallinae* b) *O.bacoti*
   c) *O.sylvarium* d) *O.bursa*
74. Which is not correct for Musca fly
   a) no mandibles b) retractile proboscis
   c) preudocracheal tubes present d) None
75. Trumpets are seen in the pupa of
   a) *Anopheles sp* b) *Aedes sp*
   c) *Culex sp* d) All of these
76. The type of metamorphosis in housefly is
   a) Ametabolous b) Holometabolous
   c) Hemimetabolous d) All of these

77. An example of insect growth regulator is
    a) Cyromazine b) Dichlorphon
    c) Dichlorvos d) None of these
78. Which of the following louse has tarsi ending in two claws
    a) *Menopon gallinae* b) both a & c
    c) *Menacanthus stramineus* d) None
79. The pathogenesis of body louse includes
    a) anemia b) death
    c) inflammation d) all of above
80. Which is not a feature of head louse
    a) tarsi ending in three claws b) rounded head
    c) three bristles on head d) none of above
81. Dark brown lateral tergal plate is present in which louse
    a) shaft louse b) body louse
    c) head louse d) fluff louse
82. Brown chicken louse is common name for
    a) *Goniocotes dissimilis* b) *Goniocotes gigas*
    c) both a & b d) *Goniocotes gallinae*
83. Which is found in tail feather of birds
    a) Lipeurus caponis b) *Goniocotes gigas*
    c) *Menopon gallinae* d) *Menacanthus stramineus*
84. A triangular head armed with spine & 4 segmented antenna is found in
    a) *Lipeurus caponis* b) *Goniocotes gigas*
    c) *Menopon gallinae* d) *Menacanthus stramineus*
85. The most common and destructive louse of domestic chicken is
    a) *Menacanthus stramineus* b) *Goniocotes gigas*
    c) *Menopon gallinae* d) *Lipeurus caponis*
86. The life cycle of red mite can be completed in a minimum of
    a) 1 month b) 1 week
    c) 1 year d) none of the above
87. Northen fowl mite can transmit
    a) Equine encephalitis b) *Newcastle disease*
    c) both a & b d) none of the above
88. Which is mostly found in temperate areas
    a) *D. gallinae* b) *O.bacoti*
    c) *O.sylvarium* d) *O.bursa*
89. Which female fowl mite is ovoviviparous
    a) *D. gallinae* b) *C. gallinae*
    c) *O.sylvarium* d) *O.bursa*

90. Which mite may cause feather pulling activity in pullets
    a) *Megninia ginglymura* b) *Cnemidocoptes mutans*
    c) Both a & b d) *Ornithonyssus bursa*
91. The life cycle of lice can be completed in a minimum of
    a) 1 month b) 1 week
    c) 1 year d) none of the above
92. Which of the following is pale yellow louse of poultry:
    a) *Menopon gallinae* b) *Heterodoxus spinigerum*
    c) *Menacanthus stramineus* d) *Holomenopon leucoxanthum*
93. Which is not true about head louse of poultry
    a) Maxillary palp absent b) five segmented antenna
    c) one row of abdominal spine d) none
94. Small head with well developed occipital lobe is seen in which flea
    a) chicken flea b) stick tight flea
    c) both a & b d) rat flea
95. Which is not true about stick tight flea
    a) 2 occular bristles b) genal comb absent
    c) pronotal comb present d) both a & c
96. The smallest louse infesting poultry
    a) shaft louse b) body louse
    c) wing louse d) fluff louse
97. The dorsal shield tapers to become tongue like in case of
    a) D. *gallinae* b) *O.bacoti*
    c) *O.sylvarium* d) *O.bursa*
98. Eggs of fowl mites are laid in
    a) cracks and crevices b) host
    b) litter d) all of these.
99. Which is not a mite infesting poultry
    a) D. *gallinae* b) *O.bacoti*
    c) *O.sylvarium* d) *O.bursa*
100. The most common fly in poultry house
    a) house fly b) blue bottle fly
    c) green bottle fly *d)* flesh fly

Answer Key

1	a	2	b	3	d	4	a	5	c	6	c	7	a
8	c	9	c	10	b	11	a	12	d	13	c	14	b
15	d	16	c	17	d	18	a	19	d	20	d	21	b
22	c	23	b	24	d	25	b	26	c	27	d	28	a
29	b	30	b	31	d	32	c	33	d	34	a	35	c
36	d	37	b	38	a	39	b	40	a	41	b	42	c
43	b	44	c	45	a	46	b	47	c	48	d	49	a
50	b	51	c	52	a	53	c	54	b	55	d	56	b
57	c	58	d	59	d	60	c	61	a	62	d	63	b
64	a	65	b	66	a	67	d	68	c	69	b	70	a
71	d	72	c	73	a	74	d	75	d	76	b	77	a
78	b	79	d	80	a	81	c	82	a	83	a	84	d
85	a	86	b	87	c	88	c	89	b	90	a	91	a
92	a	93	b	94	c	95	c	96	d	97	c	98	d
99	b	100	a										

7

Endo Parasites of Poultry

***Banothu Dasmabai*[1] *and Lunavat Gopala*[2]**

[1]Department of Veterinary Parasitology, CVSc, Rajendranagar, PVNRTVU Hyderabad, Telangana-500030

[2]Department of Veterinary Microbiology, CVSc, Rajendranagar, PVNRTVU Hyderabad, Telangana-500030

---

1. Prosthogonimus pellucidus is found in
   a) Fowl b) Duck
   c) Both d) None
2. Heterakis gallinarum is found in
   a) Fowl b) Pea fowl
   c) Guinea fowl d) All
3. Ascaridia galli occurs in
   a) Fowl b) Guinea fowl
   c) Goose d) All
4. Subulura spp. occurs in
   a) Fowl b) Guinea fowl
   c) Turkey d) All
5. Syngamus trachea are found in
   a) Fowl b) Guinea fowl
   c) Phesant d) All
6. Histomonas meleagridis are found in
   a) Fowl b) Guinea fowl
   c) Phesant d) All
7. Hammer shaped hooks in the rostellum is found in which of the following tapeworms
   a) Raillietina cesticillus b) Moniezia expansa
   c) Davainea proglottina d) None
8. Which of the following morphological feature is related to Syngamus trachea
   a) Pin shaped spicule
   b) Male & female remain permanently copulated
   c) Both
   d) None

9. The common predilection site of Heterakis gallinarum is
   a) Stomach b) Small intestine
   c) Large intestine d) All
10. The common predilection site of Histomonas meleagridis is
   a) Caecum b) Liver
   c) Both d) None
11. The common predilection site of Eimeria sps is
   a) G.I tract b) Genital tract
   c) Both d) None
12. Tetrameres sps are
   a) Facultative parasites b) Heteroxenous parasites
   c) Monoxenous parasites d) Stenoxenous parasites
13. Histomonas sps are
   a) Monoxenous parasites b) Temporary parasites
   c) Heteroxenous parasites d) Stenoxenous parasites
14. Caecal cocceidiosis is caused by
   a) E. nicatrix b) E. tenella
   c) E. brunetti d) None
15. Rectal coccidiosis is caused by-
   a) E. nicatrix b) E. tenella
   c) E. brunette d) None
16. Prosthogonimus is a bird fluke present in
   a) Bursa fabricius b) Oviduct
   c) Posterior part of Intestine d) All
17. Which one acts as II intermediate host of Prosthognimus
   a) Sand fly b) Warble fly
   c) Black fly d) Dragon fly
18. Tapeworm of which order are found in poultry
   a) *Dilepididea* b) *Davaineidea*
   c) *Thysanosomidae* d) *Hymcholepidea*
19. Which one is the commonest tapeworm of domestic fowl
   a) Davainea b) Raillietina
   c) Cotugnia d) None
20. Which tapeworm is found in both mammals & poultry
   a) Davainea b) Dipylidium
   c) Choanotaenea d) Hymenolepis
21. Which one is known as Dwarf Tapeworm?
   a) Dipylidium b) Moneizia
   c) Hymenolepis d) All

22. Intermediate host for Hymenolepis nana
    a) Floor beettle b) Rat flea
    c) Dung beettle d) All
23. Intermediate host for Hymenolepis diminuta
    a) Floor beetle b) Rat flea
    c) dung beettle d) All
24. IH for Hymenolepis carioca
    a) Floor beettle b) Rat flea
    c) Dung beettle d) All
25. Life cycle of Hymenolepis is
    a) Direct b) Indirect
    c) Both d) May be direct or indirect
26. Which one is the smallest tapeworm of poultry
    a) Davainea b) Rallietina
    c) Cotugnia d) None
27. Davainea in poultry is found in
    a) Crop b) Liver
    c) Duodenum d) Caecum
28. Intermediate host for davainea is
    a) Snail b) Fish
    c) Crab d) Oribated mites
29. Intermediate host for Raileitina is-
    a) Snail b) Fish
    c) Crab d) Ant
30. Heterakis gallinarum is commonly known as
    a) Pinworm of Poultry b) Hook worm of poultry
    c) Caecal worm of poultry d) Faecal worm of poultry
31. *Heterakis gallinarum* acts as carrier for a protozoan parasite called-
    a) *Hestromonas meleagridis* b) *Cryptosporiduim baileyi*
    c) Haemoproteus d) Leucocytozoon
32. *Histomonas meleagridis* leads to which disease in turkey
    a) Black head of turkey b) Infectious enterohepatitus
    c) Both d) None
33. Which one is the true ascarid worm of poultry
    a) *Heterakis gallinarum* b) *Ascaredia galli*
    c) *Amoeba taenia* d) *Ascaridia columbae*
34. Largest Nematode found in poultry is
    a) *Heterakis gallinarum* b) *Ascaredia galli*
    c) *Amoeba taenia* d) *Ascaridia columbae*

35. The predilection site of *H. gallinarum* of birds
   a) *Small intestine* b) *Caeca*
   c) Crop d) *Proventriculus*
36. Which helminth is found in the small intestine of domestic birds
   a) *Cherlospirura spp.* b) *Capillaria caudinflata*
   c) *Tetrameres spp.* d) *Strongyloides ovium*
37. Which helminth is found in the large intestine of domestic birds
   a) *Filicollis spp.* b) *Hartertia spp.*
   c) *Heteraksi isolonche* d) *Polymorphus spp*
38. Which helminth is found in the lungs of domestic birds
   a) *Syngamus trachea* b) *Histiocephalus spp.*
   c) *Davainea proglottina* d) *Amidostomum anseris*
39 . Which helminth is not found in the Oesophagus of domestic birds?
   a) *Capllaria controta*
   b) *Ornithostrongylus quadriradiatus*
   c) *Gongylonema ingluvicola*
   d) *Tetrameres spp.*
40. Which helminth is not found in the Proventriculus of domestic birds?
   a) *Dispharynz spp.* b) *Trichostrongylus tenuis*
   c) *Echinuria spp.* d) *Tetrameres spp.*
41. Which helminth is not found in the Gizzard of domestic birds
   a) *Amidostomum anseris* b) *Histocephalus spp.*
   c) *Syngamus trachea* d) *Streptocara spp.*
42. Which helminth is not found in the small intestine of domestic birds
   a) *Gongylonema ingluvicola* b) *Ascaridia galli*
   c) *Polymorphus spp.* d) *Strongyloides avium*
43. Which helminth is not found in the large intestine of domestic birds?
   a) *Heterakis gallinarum* b) *Heterakis isolonche*
   c) *Tricholstongylus tenuis* d) *Davainea proglottina*
44. In domestic birds, *Amoebotaenia spheoides* is found in the
   a) Large Intestine b) Small Intestine
   c) Lungs d) Gizzard
45. In domestic birds, *Ornithostrongylus quadriradiatus* is found in the
   a) Oesophagus b) Proventriculus
   c) Gizzard d) Lungs
46. White crust formation in bunches in intestinal lumen is characteristic of which infection -
   a) Coccidiosis b) Giardiosis
   c) Besnoitiosis d) All

47. Nodular tapeworm disease of fowl is caused by -
    a) Raillietina b) Daveinea
    c) Echinobothridia d) None
48. Life cycle of which of the following tape worm is direct
    a) *Ascaridia galli* b) *Taenia solium*
    c) *Hymenolepis nana* d) All
49. Naiads of Dragon fly act as II intermediate host in case of
    a) Echinostoma b) Dicrocoelium
    c) Prosthogonimus d) All
50 Snail may act as both I & II intermediate host in case of
    a) *Echinostoma revolutum* b) Echinochasmus
    c) Prosthogonimus d) Notocolylus
51. Nodules in intestine of poultry may be due to
    a) Paracooperia b) Coccidea
    c) *Ascaridia galli* d) Raillietina
52. Circumscribed necrotic areas on liver on poultry indicate which infection -
    a) Hemonchus b) Coccidia
    c) Histomonas d) Oxyspirura
53. Typhlitis in poultry can be associated with -
    a) Coccidia b) Histomonas
    c) Both d) None
54. Carcinoma of liver & pancreas can be associated with-
    a) Prosthogonimus b) Heterophyes
    c) Eurytrema d) Dicrocoelium
55. Egg production is hampered due to which of the following parasite-
    a) Dicrocoelium b) Eurytrema
    c) Heterophyes d) Prosthogonimus
56. Human beings get the infection of Hymenolepis nana by
    a) Ingestion of eggs b) Auto infection
    c) Both d) None
57. The infective stage of Echinophasmus sps is
    a) Cysticercoid b) Cysticercus
    c) Stribilocercus d) Metacercaria
58. The infective stage of Raillietina sps is
    a) Cysticercoid b) Cysticercus
    c) Procercoid d) Pleurocercoid
59. The infective stage of Eimeria sps is
    a) Sporulated oocyst b) Unsporulated oocyst
    c) Both d) None

60. *Davainea proglottina* causes
   a) Haemorrhagic enteritis b) Haemorrhagic gastritis
   c) Both d) None
61. Site of predilection in Eimeria tenella is
   a) Caecum b) Small intestine
   c) Rctum d) Colon
62. Site of predliction in Eimeria necatrix is
   a) caecum b) small intestine
   c) rectum d) colon
63. Site of predliction in Eimeria brunetti is
   a) Caecum b) Small intestine
   c) Rectum d) Colon
64. Site of predliction in Eimeria acervulina is
   a) Caecum b) Small intestine
   c) Rectum d) Colon
65. Doubled pored tapeworm of poultry is
   a) Rallietina cysticellus b) R.echinobothrida
   c) Cotugnia diagnophora d) None
66 IH of Davainea proglottina is
   a) Slug b) Limax
   c) Arion d) All
67. Rostellum armed with spanner shaped hooks seen in
   a) Hymenolepis nana b) Hymenolepis carioca
   c) Railletina d) None
68. Saw shaped segment seen in
   a) Amoebotaenia cuneata b) Railletina tetragona
   c) Davienia proglottina d) None
69. Hammer shaped hooks seen in
   a) Amoebotaenia cuneate b) Railletina cysticellus
   c) Davienia proglottina d) None
70. Regularly alternating genital pore seen in
   a) Amoebotaenia cuneate b) Railletina
   c) Davienia progllotina d) None
71. Oesophagus has a strong posterior bulb,12 pairs of caudal papillae seen in a
   a) Heterakis b) Ascardia galli
   c) Oxyuris d) None
72. Posterior bulb in Oesophagus is absent ,10 pairs of caudal papillae seen in
   a) Heterakis b) Ascardia galli
   c) Oxyuris d) None

73. Adult male & female remain in permanent copulation
    a) Heterakis b) Ascardia galli
    c) Oxyuris d) Syngamu
74. Female nematode is globular in
    a) Heterakis b) Ascardia galli
    c) Tetramere sps d) Syngamus
75. Aseptic peritonitis is caused by
    a) Prosthogonimus pellucidus b) Heterakis
    c) Ascardia galli d) Tetramere sps
76. Black head in Turkey is caused by
    a) Histomonas meleagridis b) Heterakis
    c) Ascardia galli d) Tetramere sps
77. Salt and Pepper appearance of Intestine Shown by
    a) Eimeria acervulina b) Eimeria tenella
    c) Eimeria truncate d) Eimeria brunetti
78. Oviduct fluke is
    a) Prosthogonmus ovatus b) Paragonimus westermanii
    c) Fasciola hepatica d) None
79. 4 sporocysts each with 2 sporozoite seen in
    a) Eimeria b) Isospora
    c) Tyzzenia d) Wenyonela
80. Ballooning of intestine seen in
    a) E.tenella b) E. necatrix
    c) E.acervulina d) None
81. Ladder likelesions in intestine seen in
    a) E.tenella b) E. necatrix
    c) E.acervulina d) None
82. Administartion of vaccine in eimeria vaccine in poultry is
    a) Oral route b) Allantoic route
    c) Intra ocular d) All
83. The suckers of Raillietina cesticellus are
    a) Circular b) Oval
    c) Both d) None
84. The suckers of Raillietina cesticellus are
    a) Armed b) Unarmed
    c) Both d) None
85. The shape of Amoebotaenia cuneate is
    a) Triangular b) Rectangular
    c) Both d) None

86. Eimeria sps are
    a) Facultative parasite
    b) Heteroxenous parasites
    c) Monoxenous endoparasites
    d) Stenoxenous parasites
87. Which of the following show indirect life cycle
    a) Davainea
    b) Raillietina sps
    c) Amoebotaenia
    d) all
88. Common name of *Capillaria annulata* ?
    a) Hair worms
    b) Thread worms
    c) Both a &b
    d) Only a
89. Prediliction site of Capillaria annulata?
    a) Oesophagus
    b) Crop
    c) Small Intestine
    d) Both a &b
90. Intermediate host for Capillaria annulata?
    a) Beetles
    b) Earthworms
    c) Cockroaches
    d) Housefly
91. Common name of Trichimonas gallinae ?
    a) Canker
    b) Frounce
    c) Roup
    d) All of the Above
92. The Axostyle of Trichomonas gallinae ?
    a) Protrudes beyond the body
    b) Reaches half the length of the body
    c) Equal to the body length
    d) Absence pf axostyle
93. Reproduction of Trichimod as
    a) Horizontal binary fission
    b) Longitudinal binary fission
    c) Both a & b
    d) Only a
94. The circumscribed disk-shaped lesions are often described as 'yellow buttons' is characteristic of which infection
    a) *Trichomonas gallinae*
    b) *Capillaria annulata*
    c) *Gongylonema ingluvicola*
    d) *Tetrameres Americana*
95. Which of the following is called Gullet worm
    a) *Trichomonas gallinae*
    b) *Capillaria annulata*
    c) *Gongylonema ingluvicola*
    d) *Tetrameres Americana*
96. Which of the following is called Globular roundworm
    a) *Trichomonas gallinae*
    b) *Capillaria annulata*
    c) *Gongylonema ingluvicola*
    d) *Tetrameres americana*

97. The males are pale white, slender and the females are bright red and almost spherical,

a) *Trichomonas gallinae* b) *Capillaria annulata*

c) *Gongylonema ingluvicola* d) *Tetrameres Americana*

98. Intermediate hosts for *Tetrameres Americana*

a) Cockroaches b) Grasshoppers

c) Beetles d) All of the Above

99. Common name of Dispharynx nasuta

a) Spiral stomach worm b) Globular worm

c) Gullet worm d) Thread worm

100. The cuticle is ornamented with four wavy cordons that recurve anteriorly and do not fuse is characteristic morphology of

a) *Tetrameres Americana* b) *Dispharynx nasuta*

c) *Tetrameres Crami* d) *Capillaria annulata*

101. Intermediate hosts for *Dispharynx nasuta*

a) Copepods b) Isopods

c) Fishes d) Bettles

102. Gizzard worm is common name of

a) *Amidostomum skrjabini* b) *Epomidiostomum anatinum*

c) *Epomidiostomum orispinum* d) All of the Above

103. Location of *Ascardia galli*

a) Crop b) Oesophagus

c) Small intestine d) Large intestine

104. Largest nematode of poultry

a) Ascarids b) Tetramers

c) Gongylonema d) Capillaria

105. Earthworms acts as transport host for

a) *Ascardia galli* b) *Heterakis gallinarum*

c) *Dispharnyx nasuta* d) *Capillaria annulata*

106. Smallest tapeworm of poultry

a) *Daevinea proglottina* b) *Raillientina cesticillus*

c) *Raillietina tetragona* d) *Cotugnia digonopora*

107. Double pored tapeworm of poultry

a) *Daevinea proglottina* b) *Raillientina cesticillus*

c) *Raillietina tetragona* d) *Cotugnia digonopora*

108. Largest tapeworm of poultry

a) *Daevinea proglottina* b) *Raillientina cesticillus*

c) *Raillietina tetragona* d) *Cotugnia digonopora*

109. Nodular tapeworm of poultry
   a) *Raillientina echinobothridia*   b) *Raillientina cesticillus*
   c) *Raillietina tetragona*   d) *Cotugnia digonopora*
110. *Eimeria acervulina* predilection site
   a) Caecum   b) Jejunum
   c) Duodenum   d) Ileum
111. Caecal coccidiosis is caused by
   a) *Eimeria acervulina*   b) *E. tenella*
   c) *E. brunetti*   d) *E. necatrix*
112. Rectal coccidiosis is caused by
   a) *Eimeria acervulina*   b) *E. tenella*
   c) *E. brunetti*   d) *E. necatrix*
113. Intestinal coccidiosis is caused by
   a) *Eimeria acervulina*   b) *E. tenella*
   c) *E. brunetti*   d) *E. necatrix*
114. Typical ladder-like lesions appear in the middle part of the intestine is characteristic of
   a) *Eimeria acervulina*   b) *E. tenella*
   c) *E. brunetti*   d) *E. necatrix*
115. Caecal worm of poultry
   a) *Ascardia galli*   b) *Heterakis gallinarum*
   c) *Tetrameres Crami*   d) *Capillaria annulata*
116. Worms are permanently in copula forming a Y shape, they are the only parasites found in the trachea of domestic birds
   a) *Ascardia galli*   b) *Heterakis gallinarum*
   c) *Tetrameres Crami*   d) *Syngamus trachea*
117. What is the Gapeworm of poultry
   a) *Ascardia galli*   b) *Capillaria hepatica*
   c) *Tetrameres Crami*   d) *Syngamus trachea*
118. Infective stage of *Syngamus trachea*
   a) L_1 b) L_2
   c) L_3 d) L_4
119. What is Air sac mite of poultry?
   a) Sarcoptes   b) Psoroptes
   c) Cytodites   d) Otodectes
120. Infectious enterohepatitis is caused by
   a) *Ascardia galli*   b) *Capillaria hepatica*
   c) *Tetrameres Crami*   d) *Histomonas meleagridis*

Answer Key

1	c	2	d	3	d	4	d	5	d	6	d	7	a
8	b	9	b	10	c	11	a	12	b	13	a	14	b
15	c	16	d	17	d	18	b	19	a	20	d	21	c
22	a	23	b	24	c	25	d	26	a	27	c	28	a
29	d	30	c	31	a	32	c	33	b	34	b	35	b
36	b	37	c	38	a	39	d	40	b	41	c	42	a
43	a	44	b	45	a	46	a	47	c	48	c	49	c
50	a	51	d	52	c	53	c	54	a	55	d	56	c
57	d	58	a	59	a	60	a	61	a	62	b	63	c
64	b	65	c	66	d	67	b	68	a	69	c	70	c
71	a	72	b	73	d	74	c	75	a	76	a	77	a
78	a	79	a	80	b	81	c	82	d	83	a	84	b
85	a	86	c	87	d	88	c	89	d	90	b	91	d
92	a	93	b	94	a	95	c	96	d	97	d	98	d
99	a	100	b	101	b	102	a	103	c	104	a	105	a
106	a	107	d	108	c	109	a	110	c	111	b	112	c
113	c	114	a	115	b	116	d	117	d	118	c	119	c
120	d												

8

Rickettisial Diseases

Ganesh K. Sawale[1] and G.P. Bharkad[2]

[1]*Department of Veterinary Pathology, Mumbai Veterinary College, Parel, Mumbai*

[2]*Department of Veterinary Parasitology, College of Veterinary & Animal Sciences Udgir, Maharashtr, India*

Introduction

Rickettsial diseases in poultry are caused by various species of bacteria belonging to the genus Rickettsia. These diseases can have significant economic implications for the poultry industry due to decreased production, increased mortality, and trade restrictions. Rickettsial diseases affecting poultry are relatively uncommon compared to other pathogens but can still occur. Rickettsial organisms are tiny, pleomorphic, weakly gram-negative bacilli that multiply by binary fission. The Rickettsia requires an arthropod for transmission and to complete its life cycle. The organisms are non-motile and non-capsulated and possess both DNA and RNA. Some of the rickettsial diseases affecting poultry include:

1. **Rocky Mountain spotted fever:** Chickens can be infected with various species of Rickettsia, including *Rickettsia rickettsia*, which causes Rocky Mountain spotted fever in humans. In chickens, rickettsial infections can lead to symptoms such as fever, lethargy, decreased egg production, respiratory distress, and neurological signs.
2. **Typhus:** Avian typhus, caused by *Rickettsia typhi*, can affect poultry, causing symptoms such as weakness, ruffled feathers, decreased egg production, and mortality. It can be transmitted to humans through contact with infected birds or feces.
3. **Aegyptianellosis:** Aegyptianellosis is a rickettsial disease of chicken and other birds caused by *Aegyptianellapullorum* affecting erythrocytes and the liver, thus causing anaemia and hepatitis. Parasite produces an endocytoplasmic inclusion body of 0.3 by 4μm with 26 bodies. Inclusion bodies are polymorphic and can be round, oval, ring, or horseshoe-shaped and detected by Giemsa or Pappenheim stain. The arthropod, mainly ticks (*Argus persicus*) transmits the infection to chicken.
4. **Q. Fever:** Although primarily a zoonotic disease affecting various mammals, including livestock. It is caused by *Coxiellaburnetii.* Q. fever, in addition to humans, can also infect birds, including poultry. Infected birds may show symptoms such as lethargy, decreased egg production, and reproductive disorders. Q. fever can be transmitted to humans through contact with contaminated dust, urine, feces, or aerosols from infected birds (Walker, 1996).

Preventing rickettsial diseases and other infections in poultry involves implementing strict biosecurity measures, including proper sanitation, control of vectors such as ticks and mites, and isolation of sick birds. Additionally, consulting with a veterinarian for proper diagnosis and treatment is essential if poultry show signs of illness.

1. On the basis of cause of disease, the genus Rickettsiae consist of
   a) Typhus fever group b) Spotted fever
   c) Chlamydial group d) Both a and b
2. Rickettsia are considered as a
   a) Mycoplasma b) Bacteria
   c) Virus d) Fungus
3. In Gram's staining,*Rickettsia* stain
   a) Gram positive b) Gram negative
   c) Acid fast d) None of these
4. Rickettsia are considered to be
   a) Pleomorphic b) Cocco-bacilli
   c) Spiral d) Both a and b
5. The Rickettsial organism size ranges from
   a) 0.1–0.2μmby 0.58–1.38 μm b) 3μm by 5μm
   c) 0.3-0.6μm by 0.8-2μm d) All of these
6. The special stain used to demonstrate Rickettsial inclusion is/are
   a) Machiavello stain b) Acid fast stain
   c) Silver Fontana stain d) All of these
7. The special stain used to demonstrate Rickettsial inclusion is/are
   a) Acid fast stain b) Gimenez
   c) Leishman stain d) All of these
8. The special stain used to demonstrate Rickettsial inclusions is/are
   a) Giemsa stain b) Castaneda stain
   c) Machiavello stain d) All of these
9. In Machiavello stain, the Rickettsial inclusions take
   a) Deep blue colour b) Deep red colour
   c) Bluish purple colour d) All of these
10. In Gimenez stain, the Rickettsial inclusions take
   a) Deep red colour b) Deep bluecolour
   c) Bluish purple colour d) All of these
11. In Giemsa stain, the Rickettsial inclusions take
   a) Deep red colour b) Deep golden yellow colour
   c) Bluish purple colour d) All of these
12. In Castaneda stain, the Rickettsial inclusions take
   a) Deep red colour b) Deep golden yellow colour
   c) Bluish purple colour d) All of these

13. The following are the special stain used to demonstrate rickettsial inclusions except
    a) Machiavello stain
    b) Castaneda stain
    c) Grams's stain
    d) Giemsa stain
14. The given below statement(s) is/ are true for Rickettsia
    a) They grow in cell culture
    b) They grow on cell free media
    c) They grow on blood agar media
    d) Both b and c
15. The given below statement(s) is/ are true forRickettsia
    a) They are obligate intracellular parasite
    b) They are obligate extracellular parasite
    c) They are strictly anaerobic organism
    d) They facultative anaerobic organism
16. The given below statement(s) is/ are true forRickettsia
    a) They grow in cell culture
    b) They grow in embryonated eggs
    c) Theygrow in susceptible animals
    d) All of these
17. The optimum temperature required for growth of Rickettsia in cell culture is
    a) 20-30 ^{0}C
    b) 32-35 ^{0}C
    c) 40-45 ^{0}C
    d) 45 -50^{0}C
18. The preferred route/method of cultivation of Rickettsia in embryonated egg is
    a) Amniotic sac inoculation
    b) Yolk sac inoculation
    c) Allantoic sac inoculation
    d) Chorioallantoicmembraneinoculation
19. The cultivation of Rickettsia is carried out in
    a) HeLa cell line
    b) Detriot 6
    c) Mouse fibroblast cell culture
    d) All of these
20. The cultivation of Rickettsia is carried out in
    a) Hep-2 cell line
    b) Sheep Blood agar
    c) Nutrient broth
    d) All of these
21. The preferred laboratory animal used for isolation of rickettsia is/ are
    a) Rat
    b) Guinea pig
    c) Horse
    d) Only a and b
22. The Rickettsial micro-organism grow by
    a) Sporulation
    b) Binary fission
    c) Production of offspring within cytoplasm
    d) All of these
23. The following statements are true for Rickettsia except
    a) Rickettsia contain both DNA and RNA
    b) Rickettsia has cell wall
    c) Rickettsia is bigger than virus and smaller than bacteria
    d) Rickettsia are grow on agar based cultural media

24. The following statements are true for Rickettsia except
 a) Transmitted by direct contact b) Transmitted by ticks
 c) Transmitted by mites d) Transmitted by lice and flea
25. The following statements are true for Rickettsia except
 a) Transmitted by direct contact b) Transmitted by ticks
 c) Transmitted by mites d) Transmitted by lice and flea
26. Rickettsial organism are generally transmitted by
 a) Direct contact b) Aerosal route
 c) Venereal route d) Hematophagus arthropod vectors
27. Rickettsial organism possess how many antigens
 a) One b) Two
 c) Three d) Four
28. Rickettsial organism surface antigens include all except
 a) Group specific soluble antigen b) Flaggelar (H) antigen
 c) Species specific antigen d) An alkali stable polysaccharide
29. Weil- Felix reaction used in diagnosis of
 a) Rickettsia b) Mycoplasma
 c) Viruses d) Acid fast bacteria
30. One of the test used for diagnosis ofRickettsial infection include(s)
 a) Coombs test
 b) Isolation of organism on nutrient agar and broth
 c) Weil- Felix reaction
 d) All of these
31. Weil- Felix reaction involves sharing of antigen of rickettsia with
 a) Pseudomonas b) Proteus
 c) Streptococcus d) Staphyllococcus
32. Rickettsia are considered as an obligate..
 a) Intracellular parasite b) Extracellular parasite
 c) Both a and b d) None of these
33. The etiological agent of rocky mounted spotted fever..
 a) *Rickettsia rickettsii* b) *Coxiellaburnetii*
 c) *Aegyptianellapullorum* d) All of these
34. The Rocky mounted spotted fever is transmitted by
 a) Inhalation b) Venereal route
 c) Ticks d) All of these
35. The main reservoir host of rocky mounted spotted fever includes all except
 a) Cattle b) Dog
 c) Opossum d) Birds

36. The pathogenicityof *Rickettsia rickettsii* include all except
    a) Induces toxin like action which damages endothelium cell
    b) Induces increased capillary permeability
    c) Infect all cells except red blood cell and endothelial cells
    d) Causes haemoconcentration
37. In addition to dog and cat, the reservoir host for *Rickettsia rickettsii* is.
    a) Cattle b) Buffaloes
    c) Elephant d) Birds
38. The causative agent of Avian typhus is
    a) *Rickettsia rickettsii* b) *Rickettsia typhi*
    c) *Coxiellaburnetii* d) None of these
39. The natural reservoir host for *Rickettsia typhi*is
    a) Rats b) Rabbits
    c) Cattle d) Buffalo
40. The *Rickettsia typhi*, a causative agent of avian typhus is transmitted by
    a) Tick (*Argus percicus*) b) Fleas (*Xenopsyllacheopis*)
    c) Mites (*Dermanyssusgallinae*) d) By direct contact
41. The clinical signs of avian typhus include all except
    a) Weakness b) Decreased egg production
    c) Nasal discharge with respiratory distress d) Ruffled feathers
42. The avian typhus is transmitted from infected birds to human by
    a) Contact b) Faeces
    c) Bites of tick d) Both a and b
43. The diagnosis of avian typhus is done by the following method/ test except
    a) Neil Mooser or Tunica reaction b) IFA
    c) Isolation of organism on nutrient agar d) ELISA
44. The test used to differentiate *Rickettsia typhi*, infection and *Rickettsia prowazekii*is
    a) Neil Mooser or Tunica reaction b) IFA using polyclonal antibodies
    c) Isolation of organism on nutrient agar d) ELISA
45. In Neil Mooser or Tunica reaction test, the male guinea pigs are inoculated intraperitonally with blood of patient infected with*Rickettsia typhi*develop signs of
    a) Severe diarhoea and mortality b) Fever and scrotal swelling
    c) Maculopaular rashes on whole skin d) All of these
46. In Neil Mooser or Tunica reaction testis used to diagnose disease caused by
    a) *Rickettsia prowazekii* b) *Rickettsia typhi*
    c) *Mycoplasma spp.* d) All of these
47. Laboratory animal used for diagnosis of Avian typhus by Neil Mooser or Tunica reaction testis
    a) Rat b) Mice
    c) Guinea pigs d) Hamster

48. In Neil Mooser or Tunica reaction is useful testused to differentiate between
   a) *Rickettsia prowazekii*and *Rickettsia typhi*
   b) *Rickettsia Rickettsii*and *Rickettsia burnettii*
   c) *Mycoplasma synovia and Mycoplasma gallisepticum*
   d) *Rickettsia Rickettsii*and *Rickettsia typhi*
49. Aegyptianellosis in chicken is caused by
   a) *Rickettsia typhi* b) *Aegyptianellapullorum*
   c) *Anaplasmamarginale* d) *Rickettsia Rickettsii*
50. The *Aegyptianellapullorum* causing Aegyptianellosis in chicken primarily affects
   a) Red blood cell b) White blood cell
   c) Platelets d) All of these
51. The primary target organs for Aegyptianellosis in chicken is
   a) White blood cell and spleen b) Red blood cell and liver
   c) Platelets and bone marrow d) All of these
52. The Aegyptianellosis in chicken ismainly transmitted by
   a) Inhalation b) Bite of tick
   c) Bite of mite d) All of these
53. The tick responsible for transmission of Aegyptianellosis to chicken is
   a) *Rhipicephalus bursa* b) *Boophilusmicroplus*.
   c) *Argus persicus* d) All of these
54. The clinical signs of Aegyptianellosis in chicken is / are
   a) Nasal discharge and respiratory distress b) Anaemia and hepititis
   c) Bloody diarrhoea and dehydration d) All of these
55. The *Aegyptianellapullorum* in chicken produces inclusion body (morula)in
   a) Erythrocytes b) Enterocytes
   c) Platelets d) All of these
56. The shape of inclusion body (morula) of *Aegyptianellapullorum* is
   a) Polymorphic b) Round
   c) Horse-shoe d) All of these
57. The most common stain used to demonstrate inclusion body (morula) of *Aegyptianellapullorum* is
   a) Acid fast stain b) Giemsa stain
   c) Methylene blue stain d) All of these
58. Theinclusion body (morula) of *Aegyptianellapullorum* in erythrocyte is
   a) 0.3 by 4µm b) 1 by 6 µm
   c) 2 by 8µm d) All of these
59. Among the birds, Aegyptianellosis infection is seen in
   a) Parrot b) Chicken
   c) Quails d) All of these

60. The drug of choice for treatment of Aegyptianellosis in chicken is
 a) Enrofloxacin b) Penicillin
 c) Doxycyeline d) All of these
61. Aegyptianellosis in chicken can be treated by
 a) Enrofloxacin b) Tetracycline
 c) Penicillin d) All of these
62. Q fever in poultryis caused by
 a) *Rickettsia typhi* b) *Aegyptianellapullorum*
 c) *Anaplasmamarginale* d) *Rickettsia Rickettsii*
63. The clinical signs of Q fever in chicken include(s) all except
 a) Lethargy b) Anaemia and hepititis
 c) Decreased egg production d) Reproductive disorders
64. The Q fever can be transmitted from chicken to human through
 a) Faeces b) Urine
 c) Aerosal d) All of these
65. The spotted fever Rickettsia was first discovered by
 a) Rudolf Virchow b) Havard Taylor Ricketts
 c) Julius Cohnheim d) None of these
66. The Havard Taylor Ricketts discovered spotted fever Rickettsia in year
 a) 1885 b) 1906
 c) 1932 d) 1953
67. The family Rickettsiaceaewas named after the Scientist
 a) Rudolf Virchow b) Havard Taylor Ricketts
 c) Julius Cohnheim d) None of these
68. The etiological agent of Scrub typhus
 a) *Rickettsia typhi* b) *Aegyptianellapullorum*
 c) *Orientiatsutsugamushi* d) *Rickettsia Rickettsii*
69. The reservoir host for *Orientiatsutsugamushi* causing Scrub typhus is
 a) Man b) Dog
 c) Migratory birds d) All of these
70. The *Orientiatsutsugamushi* causing Scrub typhus in migratory bird is transmitted by
 a) Tick b) Mite
 c) Direct contact d) All of these

References

Walker DH.Rickettsiae.In: Baron S, editor. Medical Microbiology.4th edition Galveston (TX): University of Texas Medical Branch at Galveston; 1996 Chapter 38. Available from: https://www.ncbi.nlm.nih.gov/books/NBK7624

Answer Key

1	b	2	b	3	b	4	d	5	c	6	a	7	b
8	d	9	b	10	a	11	c	12	c	13	c	14	a
15	a	16	d	17	b	18	b	19	d	20	a	21	d
22	b	23	d	24	a	25	a	26	d	27	c	28	b
29	a	30	c	31	b	32	a	33	a	34	c	35	a
36	c	37	d	38	b	39	a	40	b	41	c	42	c
43	c	44	a	45	b	46	b	47	c	48	a	49	b
50	a	51	b	52	b	53	c	54	b	55	a	56	d
57	b	58	a	59	d	60	c	61	b	62	d	63	b
64	d	65	b	66	b	67	b	68	c	69	c	70	b

9

Protozoan Diseases

Ganesh K. Sawale

Department of Veterinary Pathology, Mumbai Veterinary College, Parel, Mumbai

Introduction

The protozoa (meaning proto- first and zoa mean animals) are considered to primitive and are unicellular organism. The protozoa are **Eukaryotic** organism having nucleus in which the genetic information is stored in chromosomes of nucleus. In poultry, the protozoan disease categorized into two main group

1. Intestinal protozoan parasites include *Eimeria spp.* (Coccidiosis), Cryptosporidia (Cryptosporidiosis) Histomoniasis (*Histomonas meleagridis*), Trichomoniasis (Trichomonas spp.) and *Spironucleus* (Hexamitiasis).

Coccidiosis is important disease of poultry caused by protozoa of the genus Eimeria. The disease occurs by ingestion of sporulated oocyst ehcih upon action of trypsin rupture in gizzard and proventriculus relealeses sporozoites. The sprozoites penetrate mucosa of intestine and two generation of asexual reproduction occurs (Schizogony) and releases merozoites which mature and produces gamonts. Sexyual reproduction occurs (Gametogony) and produses zygot which mature to form oocysts. The oocysts are passed in faeces. The high moisture (exceeding 30%), immunosuppressive diseses and environmental and managemental stress lead to occurrence of disease. The birds affected with coccidiosis show depression, ruffled feathers, blood tinged diarrhoea and pale comb and wattle. Specific part of intestine is affected by each species of Eimeria. Diagnosis of coccidiosis is done by finding oocyst in faeces under microscope.

There are nine species of eimeria that infects chicken of which now seven are important in chicken. Coccidiosis in chicken is categerised intio intestinal (due to *E. acervulina, E. necatrix, E. maxima, E. mitis* and caecal coccidiosis (caused *due E. tenella*). The *E. acervulina, E. necatrix* and *E. maxima* causing intestinal coccidiois and *E. tenella* causing caecal coccidiosis are common and pathogenic.

Turkey coccidisis is caused by seven species of Eimeria of which five are important. Turkey coccidiosis is mainly caused by *E. adenoeides, E. gallopavonis*, *E. meleagrimitis, E. meleagridis* and *E. dispersa* of which *E. adenoeides* is most pathogenic of the turkey coccidia.

Cryptsopridiosis in chicken is caused by *C. balleyi* and affected intestine, bursa of Fabricious and respiratory tract. Disease occurs when birds had immunosuppression.

Histomoniasis is protozoan disease of chicken and turkey caused by Histomonas meleagridis and transmitted by *Heterakis gallinarum* (caecal worm). In turkey, disease can occur by ingestion of organism also. The affected birds show decreased feed and water intake and sulphur colour faeces. Disease is characterized by necrotic typhilitis and hepatitis with saucer shaped lesions in liver.

Trichomoniasis in chicken is caused by *T. gallinae* (affect upper GI tract) and *T. gallinarum* (affect lower GI tract) and characterized by depression, unthriftiness and yellow diarrhoea.

2. Haemoparasites: These include Leucocytozoon, Plasmodium (Avian malaria), Haemoproteus and Avian Trepanosoma. These haemoprotozoan parasites are mainly transmitted by insects (vectors). Plasmodium is transmitted by mosquitoes (*Culicidae*), Haemoproteus and avian trepanosoma is transmitted by biting midges (*Ceratopogonidae*), and Leucocytozoon is transmitted by black flies (*Simulian spp.*) and biting midges (Culicoides spp.)

1. The coccidiosis in poultry is caused by
   a) Virus b) Bacteria
   c) Helminth parasite d) Protozoan parasite
2. The "salt and pepper" appearance in intestine of birds is seen due to one of the species of Eimeria
   a) *E. acervulina* b) *E. maxima*
   c) *E. tenella* d) *E. necatrix*
3. The presence of white scattered lesions oriented tranversaly or ladder-like visible on mucus membrane of duodenual loop are mainly seen due to....
   a) E. acervulina *b) E. maxima*
   c) E. tenella *d) E. necatrix*
4. The minium prepatent period for *E. tenella* is .....
   a) 120 hour b) 138 hour
   c) 115 hour d) 90 hours
5. The minium prepatent period for E. necatrix is....
   a) 120 hour b) 138 hour
   c) 115 hour d) 90 hours
6. The minium prepatent period for E. brunetti is....
   a) 120 hour b) 138 hour
   c) 115 hour d) 90 hours
7. The minium prepatent period for E. maxima is....
   a) 120 hour b) 121 hour
   c) 115 hour d) 90 hours
8. The minium prepatent period for E. acervulina is....
   a) 120 hour b) 138 hour
   c) 115 hour d) 97 hours
9. Which one of the following has largest oocyst size ...
   a) E. acervulina *b) E. maxima*
   c) E. tenella *d) E. necatrix*

10. The characteristic white, irregular linear lesions ('zebra striping') associated with gamonts and oocystsis in duodenum occurs due to....
    a) *E. acervulina* b) *E. maxima*
    c) *E. tenella* d) *E. necatrix*
11. The white and red focal lesions on the mid intestine with ballooning and an accompanying dysentery is ssen due to ....
    a) *E. acervulina* b) *E. maxima*
    c) *E. tenella* d) *E. necatrix*
12. Haemorrhagic typhlitis with blood clot in lumen of caeca is seen due to...
    a) *E. acervulina* b) *E. maxima*
    c) *E. tenella* d) *E. necatrix*
13. Caecal coccidiosis in chicken is caused by...
    a) *E. acervulina* b) *E. maxima*
    c) *E. tenella* d) *E. necatrix*
14. The coccidiosis in chicken is most commonly observed in the age group of...
    a) Below 3 b) 3- 6 week age
    c) 10-20 weeks d) Above 20 weeks
15. The older chicken over 10 weeks of age are commonly affected due to one of species of Eimeria
    a) *E. acervulina* b) *E. maxima*
    c) *E. tenella* d) *E. necatrix*
16. The lesions in caeca of Turkey occurs due to one of the species of coccidia
    a) *E. adenoeides* b) *E. gallopavonis*
    c) *E. meleagrimitis* d) *E. dispersa*
17. The lesions in caeca of Turkey occurs due to one of the species of coccidia
    a) *E. meleagridis* b) *E. gallopavonis*
    c) *E. meleagrimitis* d) *E. dispersa*
18. The lesions in caeca in Turkey coccidioisis occurs due to
    a) *E. gallopavonis* b) *E. meleagridis & E. adenoeides*
    c) *E. meleagrimitis* d) *E. dispersa*
19. In Turkey coccidiosis, lesion in anterior and mid part of intestine are seen in.....
    a) *E. gallopavonis* b) *E. meleagridis & E. adenoeides*
    c) *E. meleagrimitis & E. dispersa* d) *E. tenella*
20. The lesion in rectum in turkey coccidiosis is seen due to
    a) *E. adenoeides* b) *E. gallopavonis*
    c) *E. meleagrimitis* d) *E. dispersa*
21. The renal coccidiosis in goslings oocurs due one of the species of cocciida
    a) *E. anseris* b) *E. truncata*
    c) *E. nocens* d) *E. dispersa*

22. The most pathogenic species of coccidia in goslings causing haemorrhagic enteritis in small intestine with diarrhoea is seen due to
    a) *E. anseris* b) *E. truncata*
    c) *E. nocens* d) *E. dispersa*
23. The most pathogenic coccidial infection that causes severe disease in ducklings under 7 weeks of age, with a haemorrhagic enteritis of the anterior small intestine, dysentery and a high mortality is...
    a) *E. anseris* b) *E. truncata*
    c) *E. nocens* d) *Tyzzeria perniciosa*
24. In pheasants, the the most pathogenic species of coccidia is
    a) *E. duodenalis* b) *E. truncata*
    c) *E. colchici* d) *E. phasiani*
25. The control of coccidiosis in chicken can be achieved by
    a) Anticoccidial in feed b) Live attenuated vaccine
    c) Maintaining hygiene on farm d) All of these
26. The following are the species of Eimeria affecting Geese Except
    a) *E. anseris* b) *Tyzzeria perniciosa*
    c) *E. nocens* d) *E. truncata*
27. The following are the species of Eimeria affecting Turkey Except
    a) *E. necatrix* b) *E. gallopavonis*
    c) *E. meleagrimitis* d) *E. dispersa*
28. Cryptosporidium spp. in chicken generally attaches to epithelial cells of
    a) Respiratiry system b) Intestine
    c) Bursaof Fabricious d) All of these
29. *Cryptosporidium meleagridis* in chicken generally attaches and causes lesions in
    a) Respiratiry system b) Intestine
    c) Lymphoid system d) None of these
30. *Cryptosporidium baileyi* in chicken generally attaches and causes lesions in
    a) Respiratiry system b) Intestine
    c) Urinary systen d) None of these
31. The prepatent period for Cryptosporidiosis in chicken is
    a) 1 day's b) 2 day's
    c) 3 day's d) 5 day's
32. The special stain used for diagnosis of cryptosporidiosis in chicken is
    a) Ziehl-Neelsen stains b) GMS stain
    c) PAS stain d) All of these
33. Histomoniasis in turkey is caused by parasite ...
    a) *Histomonas meleagridis* b) *Heterakis gallinarum*
    c) *Ascardia galli* d) None of these

34. Histomoniasis in turkey is transmitted through
    a) Freshly voided faeces   b) *Heterakis gallinarum*
    c) Earthworm   d) All of these
35. Histomoniasis in chicken is transmitted through..
    a) Freshly voided faeces   b) *Heterakis gallinarum*
    c) Both a & b   d) None of these
36. The main target organ for Histomoniasis in chicken is..
    a) Caeca   b) Liver
    c) Both a & b   d) None of these
37. Histomoniasis in chicken causes
    a) Necrotic typhlitis   b) Hepatitis
    c) Both a & b   d) None of these
38. Saucer shaped necrotic lesions with raised borders in liver and necrotic typhlitis are character lesions of
    a) Fowl typhoid   b) Caecal coccidiosis
    c) Salmonellosis   d) Histomoniasis
39. *Spironucleus (Hexamita) meleagridis* in chicken is associated with
    a) Pneumonia   b) Hepatitis
    c) Watery diarrhoea   d) All of these
40. Canker in pigeon is caused by
    a) Histomonas meleagridis   b) *Heterakis gallinarum*
    c) *S. meleagridis*   d) *Trichomonas gallinae*
41. Canker in pigeon is characterized by lesions in
    a) Necrotic mass in mouth & esophagus   b) Weight loss
    c) *S. meleagridis*   d) *Trichomonas gallinae*
42. The synoname for Trichomoniasis in chicken is
    a) Black head   b) Histomoniasis
    c) Canker   d) Hexamitiasis
43. The leucocytozoonosis in chicken is mainly caused by
    a) *L simondi*   *b) L smithi*
    c) *L caulleryi*   d) All of these
44. The leucocytozoonosis in turkey is mainly caused by
    a) *L simondi*   *b) L smithi*
    c) *L caulleryi*   d) All of these
45. The leucocytozoonosis in waterfowl is mainly caused by
    a) *L simondi*   *b) L smithi*
    c) *L caulleryi*   d) All of these
46. Clinical disease and mortality in leucocytozoonosis results from
    a) Pneumonia   b) Enteritis
    c) Anaemia   d) All of these

47. Leucocytozoon in chicken is mainly transmitted by
    a) Ticks b) Black flies and biting midges
    c) Mites d) All of these
48. Leucocytozoon in chicken is mainly transmitted by
    a) Ticks b) Mites
    c) *Simulian spp. and Culicoides spp.* d) All of these
49. Leucocytozoon in chicken is commonly observed in
    a) Asian countries b) African countries
    c) Both a & b d) None of these
50. Leucocytozoon in turkey is commonly observed in
    a) Asian countries b) America
    c) African countries d) All of these
51. The gametocyte stages of Leucocytozoon in chicken are observed in
    a) Blood b) Tissue
    c) Intestine d) All of these
52. The Schizont stages of Leucocytozoon in chicken are observed in
    a) Blood b) Tissue
    c) Intestine lumen d) All of these
53. The Schizont stages of Leucocytozoon in chicken are observed in
    a) Heart muscle b) Gizzard muscle
    c) Brain d) All of these
54. Outbreaks of Leucocytozoon in chicken in Asian countries are generally observed during the month of ..
    a) January -February b) March-April
    c) September-October d) All of these
55. The leucocytozoon affected adult birds show signs of
    a) anaemia b) drop in egg production
    c) small & thinshelled egg d) All of these
56. Avain malaria in chicken is caused by
    a) Bacteria b) Virus
    c) Protozoa d) None of these
57. Avain malaria in chicken is caused by
    a) *Leucocytozoon spp.* b) *Plasmodium spp.*
    c) Histomonas spp. d) None of these
58. Avian malaria in chicken is transmitted by
    a) Ticks. b) Mites
    c) Mosquitoes d) All of these
59. Avian malaria in chicken is transmitted by
    a) Culex. b) Ades
    c) Both a and b d) None of these

60. Following a bite of mosquitoes, which stages of avian malerial parasites are inoculated in bird's body.

a) Sporozoites. b) Gamatocytes

c) Schizont d) None of these

61. The most common blood parasitic in non-domestic bird is

a) *Plasmodium spp* b) *Haemoproteus spp.*

c) *Leucocytozzon spp* d) None of these

62. Among the domestic birds, haemoproteus infection is generally seen in

a) Turkeys b) Ducks

c) Quails d) All of these

63. *Haemoproteus* infection in most avian species is considered to be

a) Nonpathogenic b) Pathogenic

c) Highly pathogenic d) All of these

64. The antimalarial drug such as chlorquine has been used with limited success for treatment of

a) Avian maleria b) Leucocytozoonosis

c) Haemoproteus infection d) All of these

65. Species of Plasmodium that cause mortalities in zoo birds, domestic fowl and in turkey flocks is…

a) *P. relictum* b) *P. elongatum*

c) *P. gallinaceum* d) All of these

66. For treatment of avian malaria in caged birds and penguins,one of the given below medicine is recommended along with chloroquine

a) Sulphadimidine b) Primaquine

c) Oxytetracycline d) All of these

67. The absence of residual pigment (haemozoin) in the blood stages of parasites is characterstic diagnostic feature of

a) Haemoproteus spp b) Plasmodium spp

c) Leucocytozoon spp d) None of these

68. The presence of residual pigment (haemozoin) in the blood stages of parasites is seen in

a) Haemoproteus spp b) Plasmodium spp

c) Leucocytozoon spp d) Both a & b

69. Avian malaria in chicken is caused by

a) *P.gallinaceum* b) *P. relictum*

c) *P. elongatum* d) All of these

70. In Avian malaria in chicken, the merogony occurs in

a) Bone marrow b) Erythrocytes

c) Endothelial cells d) All of these

Answer Key

1	d	2	d	3	a	4	c	5	b	6	a	7	b
8	d	9	b	10	a	11	d	12	c	13	c	14	b
15	d	16	a	17	a	18	b	19	c	20	b	21	b
22	a	23	d	24	c	25	d	26	b	27	a	28	d
29	b	30		31		32	d	33	a	34	d	35	b
36	c	37	c	38	d	39	c	40	d	41	d	42	c
43	c	44	b	45	a	46	c	47	b	48	c	49	c
50	b	51	a	52	b	53	d	54	c	55	d	56	c
57	b	58	c	59	c	60	a	61	b	62	d	63	a
64	d	65	d	66	b	67	c	68	c	69	d	70	d

10

Prophylaxis

J.B. Kathiriya and B.J. Trangadia

[1]*Department of Veterinary Public Health & Epidemiology, College of Veterinary Science & A.H., Kamdhenu University, Junagadh-362001, Gujarat, India*

[2]*Department of Veterinary Pathology, College of Veterinary Science & A.H., Kamdhenu University, Junagadh-362001, Gujarat, India*

Introduction

The control of infectious diseases of bacterial etiology in food animals is often by using collective and simultaneous medication of a group, i.e. the so-called preventive uses prophylaxis and metaphylaxis. These uses are vigorously debated because they involve the mass consumption of antibiotics that is suspected to favour the emergence of resistant bacteria, especially in the gut flora, which is critical for the potential transfer of resistance to humans via the food chain. Metaphylaxis corresponds to the administration of antibiotics to animals experiencing any level of bacterial disease before overt disease occurs, with the time of intervention depending on the detection of disease outbreaks in a few animals in the group. Metaphylaxis is launched after (meta) pathogen contamination, with the goal of the bacteriological cure of infected animals, which subsequently warrants the final protection (phylaxis) against infection outbreaks. In this respect, metaphylaxis should be viewed as a curative treatment occurring early in the time scale of the infection, and should be compared to classical curative treatments of sick animals. The pathophysiological status of the animals and the size of the bacterial load at the infection site are specificities of metaphylaxis that could play an important role in antibiotic pharmacodynamics, including the reduction of resistance selection within the pathogenic inoculum. Recent advances have been made in evaluating the antibiotic doses required for clinical and bacteriological cures, depending on the size of bacterial load at the infection site. The observations that total doses were much lower for early treatments when bacterial loads were small, compared to later treatments of sick animals with higher bacterial loads, reinforces the in vivo relevance of the so-called 'inoculum effect', whatever its underlying mechanisms. In addition, the clinical development of infections is known to impact on the host defenses, and the individual food or water consumption that determines antibiotic intake in collective treatments, as well as on the pharmacokinetic behaviour of the antibiotics. Consequently, higher inter-individual variability of responses to antibiotics is expected in sick compared to healthy animals, resulting from both animal exposure to antibiotics and bug-drug interactions. Overall, these features might suggest that metaphylaxis has critical advantages compared to later curative treatments, with lower total doses resulting in a lower exposure of the gut bacterial flora. It is time now to re-evaluate metaphylaxis as an early curative treatment in order to determine if such potentially favourable characteristics might balance its so-called mass consumption drawback.

1. Which of the following is not considered as an essential amino acids for growing pullets
   a) Tryptophan b) Threonine
   c) Tyrosine d) Arginine
2. Protein efficiency ratio can be calculated by following formula
   a) g wt. gain/ g protein absorb b) g N retained/ g N absorb
   c) g wt. gain/ g protein consumed d) None of the above
3. Which of the following is a good precussor of vitamin A
   a) Myxoxanthin b) Xanthine
   c) Beta carotene d) Xanthophylls
4. Which of the following does not fall in the category of NFE
   a) Starch b) Fat
   c) Protein d) Carbohydrate
5 is essential for prevention of perosis in chicken
   a) Biotin b) Vit B_{10}
   c) Choline d) Vit B_5
6. The percent of CF should not be more than in layer ration
   a) 10 % b) 12 %
   c) 6 % d) 8 %
7. The normal ration of layers the % of lysine should be
   a) a) 0.5% b) 0.65%
   c) 1 % d) 0.3 %
8. Vitamin E deficiency in poultry causes the following condition especially when diet contain high level of unsaturated fatty acids
   a) Exudative diathesis b) Nutritional roup
   c) Crazy chick disease d) All of the above
9. The calcium and phosphorus ratio in layer's ration should be (a)
   a) 1:1 b) 2:1
   c) 3:1 d) 6:1
10. The most refined measure of food energy for poultry is
   a) ME b) DE
   c) NE d) None
11. FCR of layer is influenced by
   a) Pen temperature b) Rate of egg production
   c) Quality of ration d) All

12. Excess protein in poultry ration leads to
    a) Deposition of calcium urate crystal in liver
    b) Degeneration of the kidney
    c) Raisein blood uric acid
    d) All of the above
13. Higher fat deposition in carcass occurs due to
    a) Narrow C:P rati b) Wider C:P ratio
    c) Wider C:P rati d) Both a and b
14. For production of prothrombin, the vitamin needed is
    a) C b) B_6
    c) K d) D
15. Which of the following act as an antagonist to vitamin K, leading to haemorrhagic spots or bleeding
    a) Antibiotics b) Hormones
    c) Sulfa drugs d) B_7
16. Bowing of legs with enlargement of hock joint without slipping of achilles tendon is caused by deficiency of
    a) Calcium b) Choline
    c) Nicotinic acid d) Carotene
17. Which of the following is needed for maturation of RBC in poultry
    a) Biotin b) Pantothenic acid
    c) Folic acid d) B_6
18. Deficiency of vitamin causes rough and scaly dermatitis on the bottom of chick foot
    a) Nicotinic acid b) Ascorbic acid
    c) Biotin d) Retinol
19. The vitamin not essential in the diet of poultry but needs supplementation during summer stress is
    a) Nicotinic acid b) Biotin
    c) Ascorbic acid d) Retinol
20. The chief source of calcium in poultry diet is
    a) Bone meal b) calcium phosphate
    c) Oyster shell d) None
21. Manganese is essential for the synthesis
    a) Fatty acids b) Oxidative phosphorylation
    c) Organic matrix of bone d) All of these
22. Among the poultry feed ingredients as a source of energy which one stands at the top
    a) Rice polish b) Barley
    c) Maize d) Oats

23. The best protein feed which contain all the essential amino acid required for chicken is
   a) Meat meal b) Ground nut cake
   c) Fish meal d) Lucern meal
24. Premix should not be prepared for
   a) Vitamin b) Antibiotics
   c) Fish meal d) Coccidiostate
25. Commonest limiting amino acid in poultry
   a) Tyrosine b) Arginine
   c) Methionine d) Aspartic acid
26. Molybdenum is essential for
   a) Carbonic anhydrase b) Catalase
   c) Xanthine oxidase d) All
27. Thiamine deficiency symptom is
   a) Curled toe paralysis b) Nutritional myopathy
   c) Polyneuritis d) All
28. Phosphorus utilization enhanced by supplementing ______ in diet
   a) High protein b) Goiterogens
   c) Phytase enzyme d) All
29. Which of the following is responsible for olive coloured yolks in chicken egg
   a) Xanthophyll b) GNC
   a) Cottonseed cake d) Sesame cake
30. Which of the following is used as a flavor enhancer in poultry ration
   a) Lignocellulose b) Egg powder
   c) Monosodium glutamate d) None
31. Scurfy skin, thin hair, slow growth and a characteristic goose stepping in poultry is due to deficiency of
   a) Thiamine b) Riboflavin
   c) Pantothenic acid d) Nicotinic acid
32. Necrotic dermatitis of chicken feet is occurred due to deficiency of
   a) Mn b) F
   a) Zn d) Nicotinic acid
33. Gossypol of cottonseed meal react with
   a) Zinc b) Manganese
   c) Iron d) Selenium
34. Weight gain per unit weight of protein consumed refers to
   a) GPV b) BV
   c) PER d) EAAI

35. The first limiting amino acid in chick diets based on maize sesame meal is
    a) Threonine b) Methionine
    c) Lysine d) Tryptophan
36. To classify as animal protein supplement the ingredient has to contain a protein content of more than
    a) 55 % b) 60 %
    c) 47 % d) 30%
37. The following vitamin is a constituent of coenzyme A
    a) Biotin b) Pyridoxine
    b) (c) Pantothenic acid d) Folic acid
38. The following vitamin is required in higher quantities in breeder diets than in layer diets for chicken
    a) Biotin b) Vitamin A
    c) Vitamin E d) Folic acid
39. Energy content of an egg is
    a) 80 Kcal b) 60 Kcal
    c) 90 Kcal d) 125 Kcal
40. The following amino acid is essential for growth but not for egg production
    a) Lysine b) Methionine
    b) (c) Glycine d) Arginine
41. The major end product of nitrogen metabolism in chicken is
    a) Ammonia b) Urea
    b) (c) Uric acid d) Creatinine
42. The major end product of nitrogen metabolism in mammals is
    a) Ammonia b) Uric acid
    b) (c) Urea d) Creatinine
43. The major end product of nitrogen metabolism in fish is
    a) Uric acid b) Urea
    c) Ammonia d) Creatinine
44. The concentration of vitamin A in the ration of poultry should be highest for which class of birds
    a) Laying hens b) Broiler starter
    c) Breeding hens d) Broiler finishers
45. Digestibility of a feed decreases because of an increase in its
    a) Starch content b) Vitamin Content
    c) Lignin content d) NFE content
46. Increasing the level of feeding decreases digestibility because of
    a) Increased surface area b) Higher exposure time to enzymes
    c) Lower exposure time to enzymes d) Compacting of feed

47. The most important animal factors that affect digestibility of feed are
    a) level of feeding b) species of animal
    c) Physiological status of the animal d) All the above
48. The most important feed factors that affect digestibility of feed are
    a) Preparation of the fee b) Feed composition
    c) Ration composition d) All the above
49. The heat production in an animal can be measured
    a) Only by direct calorimetric b) Only by indirect calorimetric
    c) By direct and indirect calorimetric d) by slaughter studies
50. Loss of nitrogen in urine when an animal is fed protein free diet
    a) MFN b) N equilibrium
    c) EUN d) all the above
51. Loss of nitrogen in feces when an animal is fed protein free diet
    a) EUN b) N equilibrium
    a) MFN d) all the above
52. Animal origin protein supplements contain protein level
    a) Less than 20% b) Between 30% and 40%
    c) Mostly above 45% d) Between 20% and 30%
53. The deficiency of in the diet of poultry leads to lesser intake of water
    a) K b) Ca
    c) Na d) Mn
54. The number of thin shelled and soft shelled increases subsequently egg production and hatchability show marked decline
    a) Vitamin B_2 b) Vitamin B_5
    c) Vitamin D_3 d) Vitamin C
55. Chicks show Dermatitis, severe lesions of bottom of feet in early stages and mandibular lesion at a later stage is due to deficiency of
    a) Vitamin B_2 b) Vitamin B_5
    a) Biotin d) Folic acid
56. Microcytic, hypochromic anemia in chicken is due to deficiency of
    a) Na b) Mn
    c) Fe/Cu d) K
57. Microcytic, hyperchromic anemia in chicken is due to deficiency of
    a) thiamine b) Mn
    c) Na d) folacin
58. As per BIS (1992) ME Kcal/kg feed in starter broiler mesh is
    a) 3100 b) 2700
    c) 2900 d) 2800

59. Chelation is used to enhance the absorption of
   a) Protein b) Fat
   c) Mineral d) Carbohydrate
60. The rancidity developed in good quality rice polish is due to
   a) High protein b) High minerals
   c) High fat d) High carbohydrate
61. A chick needs a dietary supply of the amino acid in addition to the ten amino acids is
   a) Serine b) Alanine
   c) Glutamic acid d) Glycine
62. Nicotinic acid can be synthesized in the chicks from
   a) Tryptophane b) Ribose
   c) Thiamin d) Lysine
63. Exogenous requirements of choline in birds is influenced by the dietary level of
   a) Lysine b) Methionine
   c) Calcium d) Phosphorus
64. Xanthine oxidase involved in purine metabolism contains
   a) Zinc b) Iron
   c) Cobalt d) Molybdenum
65. Phosphoprotein in egg yolk is
   a) Phosvitin b) Provitin
   c) Ovalbumin d) Flavin
66. DCP is rich source of calcium contains approximatly
   a) 29 % b) 20 %
   c) 35 % d) 15 %
67. Which of the following feed component imparts yellow pigmentation to egg yolk
   a) Chlorophyll b) Carotene
   c) Cryptoxanthine d) Xanthophyll
68. Protein contains of a egg is:
   a) 20 % b) 18 %
   c) 9 % d) 12 %
69. Find out the Antifungal feed additives:
   a) propionic acid b) sodium propionate
   c) nystatin d) All of the above
70. Which of the following is not a reason for animal disease?
   a) Genetic diseases b) Deficiency diseases
   c) Environmental discomforts d) Hygiene and cleanliness

71. Which of the following steps should not be done for the prevention of infectious diseases?
    a) Proper disposal of dead infected animals
    b) Disinfection of the animal house
    c) Freedom of infected animals
    d) Vaccination of animals against major diseases
72. Which of the following virus causes Foot and Mouth disease?
    a) Coxsackievirus b) Cowpox virus
    c) Retrovirus d) Reovirus
73. Which of the following is not a characteristic symptom of Foot and Mouth disease?
    a) An eruption of vesicles over the lips b) Fever
    c) Increase in appetite d) Lameness
74. Cowpox is caused by cowpox virus.
    a) True b) False
75. Which of the following diseases can spread to humans while milking?
    a) Foot and Mouth disease b) Small Pox
    c) Ranikhet d) Cowpox
76. Which of the following is the highly contagious viral disease of cattle?
    a) Foot and Mouth disease b) Rinderpest
    c) Cowpox d) Ranikhet
77. Which of the following is not a method by which Rinderpest is spread amongst cattle?
    a) Contact b) Contaminatedfeed
    c) Flies d) Clean water
78. Which of the following is not a symptom of Rinderpest?
    a) Dysentery b) Fever
    c) Congestion d) Blue urine
79. Prophylaxis was initiated in India in 1954 and has effectively controlled rinderpest.
    a) True b) False
80. Which of the following is not a viral disease?
    a) Salmonellosis b) Ranikhet disease
    c) Laryngotracheitis d) Fowl Pox
81. Which of the following is incorrect about Bird Flu?
    a) Caused by H5N1 b) Bacterial disease
    c) Also known as Avian influenza d) Attacks poultry birds
82. Diseases that spread from one person to another are called _______.
    a) Communicable diseases b) Degenerative diseases
    c) Non-communicable diseases d) None of the above
83. Night blindness is caused due to the deficiencies of_______.
    a) Vitamin A b) vitamin B
    c) Vitamin C d) vitamin E

84. Which of the following diseases is an example of non-communicable diseases?
    a) Cancer
    b) Diabetes,
    c) Hypertension
    d) All of the above

85. Alzheimer's and osteoporosis are examples of _______.
    a) Communicable diseases
    b) Degenerative diseases
    c) Non-communicable diseases.
    d) None of the above

86. Excessive bleeding during an injury is a deficiency of_________.
    a) Vitamin A
    b) vitamin B
    c) Vitamin K
    d) vitamin E

87. Goiter and the enlarged thyroid gland are mainly diagnosed in patients with deficiencies of which of the following minerals?
    a) Iron
    b) Iodine
    c) Calcium
    d) Phosphorus

88. Cystic Fibrosis and Haemophilia are examples of _______.
    a) Hereditary diseases
    b) Degenerative diseases
    c) Deficiency diseases
    d) None of the above

89. Which of the following diseases is caused by various pathogenic microorganisms?
    a) Deficiency diseases
    b) Hereditary diseases
    c) Infectious diseases
    d) Degenerative diseases

90. Which of the following diseases is caused by protein deficiency?
    a) Anaemia
    b) Kwashiorkor

91. Which of the following vitamins is also known as ascorbic acid?
    a) Vitamin A
    b) Vitamin B
    c) Vtamin C
    d) Vitamin E

92. The deficiency diseases can be prevented by _____________.
    a) Prolonged cooking
    b) Eating only fruits
    c) Eating only vegetables
    d) Eating food with good nutritional value

93. AIDS, common cold, dengue fever and influenza are examples of __________.
    a) Deficiency Disease
    b) Infectious diseases
    c) Physiological Diseases
    d) Non-infectious diseases

94. Which of the following vitamins helps in blood clotting?
    a) vitamin A
    b) vitamin C
    c) vitamin D
    d) vitamin K

95. Which of the following vitamins functions as both hormone and visual pigment?
    a) Thiamine
    b) Retinal
    c) Riboflavin
    d) Folic acid

96. Which of the following vitamin is also known as niacin and plays a vital role in many digestive tract functions?
    a) vitamin B1
    b) vitamin B2
    c) vitamin B3
    d) vitamin B12
97. The Deficiency of vitamin E leads to _______
    a) Soft Bones
    b) Bleeding in gums
    c) Weakness in muscles
    d) Neurological disorders
98. Xerophthalmia caused due to the deficiency of __________.
    a) vitamin A
    b) vitamin B
    c) vitamin C
    d) vitamin E
99. Which of the following is not an infectious disease?
    a) Dengue
    b) Scurvy
    c) Typhoid Fever
    d) Whooping cough
100. Which of the following is the main cause of blindness in children worldwide?
    a) Glaucoma
    b) Cataracts
    c) Protein deficiency
    d) vitamin A deficiency
101. Amoxicillin, Doxycycline Azithromycin, & Penicillin are some examples of _____.
    a) Bacteria
    b) Pathogens
    c) Antibiotics
    d) Vaccinations
102. Which of the following is true for rabies?
    a) Rabies is prevented by pre-exposre prophylaxis
    b) The death rate is highest in the elderly
    c) All the vaccines can be used intradermally
    d) Deaths have occurred post transplant
103. The risk of rabies is in?
    a) Dogs more than bats, worldwide.
    b) Greater in children than adults
    c) Dogs in Asia more than Europe
    d) all the above
104. Rabies Immunoglobulin?
    a) Is only manufactured as a human immunoglobulin
    b) At least half the dose should be infiltrated around the wound
    c) Can only be given within 1 week of a bite
    d) If you are really concerned can be given IV in very high risk cases
105. Which of the following is true regarding intradermal rabies vaccine versus intramuscular routes?
    a) ID gives lower antibody titres using the same time schedule (days 0, 7, and 28) as IM administered vaccines
    b) An ID schedule is less effective in the long term than an IM one
    c) ID vaccine is less effective in post-exposure prophylaxis than IM vaccine
    d) Five injections of ID vaccine are required (days 0, 3, 7, 14 and 28) compared to two IM injections (days 0 and 3) in post-exposure cases where the traveller has had a full pre-exposure prophylaxis by either the ID or the IM routes.

106. The rabies vaccine?
   a) Is a live vaccine
   b) Is cell cultured, freeze dried and reconstituted prior to administration
   c) Is a polysaccharide vaccine derived from culture on human diploid cells
   d) Can not be given to breast feeding mothers
107. Which of the following is false regarding the rabies vaccine?
   a) The rabies vaccine should never be given intravenously
   b) The dosage is the same for children as it is for adults
   c) Human diploid cell vaccine can lead to ulceration if given intradermally
   d) The vaccine is safe to give with live vaccines
108. A traveller comes to your clinic after getting two doses of a vaccine 6 months ago and next week is travelling to an endemic area for rabies. What should you do?
   a) Start the scheduling again and get him to cancel his trip
   b) Give one dose of vaccine and assume he has good cover
   c) Order the same vaccine he used and give him one extra dose
   d) Assume he already has enough cover
109. The clinical disease?
   a) The incubation period is proportional to the time the virus takes to travel from the inoculation site to the brain and/or spinal cord
   b) The incubation period is normally 3-6 months
   c) The autonomic nervous system is usually spared
   d) The clinical disease mostly begins as a flu-like illness
110. Rabies virus?
   a) Is a flavivirus
   b) Is transmitted by aerosolised secretions
   c) Is a reverse-zoonosis
   d) Is more likely to cause paralytic rabies in dogs than in other non-human animals
111. The best public health measure is?
   a) Kill all stray dogs
   b) Vaccinate all dogs
   c) Add the rabies vaccine to the countries immunisation schedule
   d) Capture all animals that bite to observe them for 15 days to guide medical management
112. The purpose is to limit the incidence of disease by controlling causes & risk factors
   a) Primordial prevention
   b) Primary prevention
   c) Secondary prevention
   d) Tertiary prevention
113. The property of a test to identify the proportion of truly ill persons in a population who are identified as ill by a screening test
   a) Sensitivity
   b) Specificity
   c) Positive predictive value
   d) Negative predictive value

114. The probability of a persons having the disease when the test is positive
a) Sensitivity b) Specificity
c) Positive predictive value d) Negative predictive value

115. The extent to which a test is measuring what it is intended to measure
a) Reliability b) Validity
c) Sensitivity d) Specificity

116. A study that measures the number of persons with influenza in a calendar year
a) Cohort study b) Case control
c) Cross sectional d) Case report

117. Stage by which the presence of factors favors the occurrence of disease
a) Stage of susceptibility b) Stage of presymptomatic disease
c) Stage of clinical disease d) Stage of disability

118. Modes of horizontal transmission of disease, except
a) Contact b) Vector
c) Common Vehicle d) Genetic

119. An infected person is less likely to encounter a susceptible person when a large proportion of the members of the group are immune
a) Active immunity b) Passive immunity
c) Herd immunity d) Specific immunity

120. Occurrence in the community of a number of cases of disease that is unusually large or unexpected
a) Endemic b) Epidemic
c) Pandemic d) Infection

121. Measures of central tendency, except
a) Mean b) Median
c) Mode d) Variance

122. Range of values surrounding the estimate which has a specified probability of including the true population values
a) Standard deviation b) Standard error
c) Confidence interval d) Correlation coefficient

123. The probability of rejecting the null hypothesis when it is true
a) Type 1 error b) Type 2 error
c) Power of a statistical test d) Level of significance

124. The following are measures of disease frequency, except
a) Incidence rate b) Prevalence
c) Cumulative incidence d) Relative risk

125. The proportion of cases of a specified disease or condition which are fatal within a specified time
a) Morbidity rate b) Case fatality rate
c) Proportionate mortality d) Death rate

126. The relation between exposure and disease is considered to be causal or etiological in the following, except
a) Dose response relation b) Cessation of exposure
c) Temporal relation d) No confounding

127. A study that measures the incidence of a disease
a) Case report b) Cross sectional
c) Case control d) Cohort

128. A study wherein bias is less likely to occur
a) Case report b) Cross sectional
c) Case control d) Cohort

129. The proportion of disease incidence that can be attributed to a specific exposure
a) Relative risk b) Odds ratio
c) Attributable risk d) Potential risk

130. All of the following are potential benefits of a randomized clinical trial, except
a) The likelihood that the study groups will be comparable is increased
b) Self-selection for a particular treatment is eliminated
c) External validity of the study is increased
d) Assignment of the next subject cannot be predicted

131. Recall is an example of what type of bias
a) Selection bias b) Information bias
c) Confounding d) Systematic

132. Type of design where both exposure and disease are determined simultaneously for each subject
a) Case study b) Cross sectional study
c) Case control study d) Cohort study

133. A study is conducted to determine the proportion of persons in the population with PTB using AFB sputum for diagnosis
a) Case study b) Cross sectional study
c) Case control study d) Cohort study

134. Randomization is the best approach in designing a clinical trial in order to
a) Achieve predictability b) Achieve unpredictability
c) Achieve blinding d) Limit confounding

135. Type of sampling whereby subjects are assigned according to a factor that would influence the outcome of a study
a) Simple random sampling b) Systematic sampling
c) Stratified random sampling d) Cluster sampling

136. The extent to which a specific health care treatment, service, procedure, program, or other intervention produces a beneficial result under ideal controlled conditions is its
a) Effectiveness b) Efficacy
c) Efficiency d) Effect modification

137. Leading cause of Diarrheal disease
   a) Enterotoxigenic Escherichia coli
   b) Salmonella (non-typhoid)
   c) Rotavirus
   d) Campylobacter jejuni
138. Mammography should be done annually in women of what age?
   a) 50 years old and above
   b) 60 years old and above
   c) 45 years old and above
   d) 30 years old and above
139. APGAR family assessment is interpreted by means of
   a) Scoring
   b) Comparing with a standard table
   c) Using a scale of wellness
   d) Consultation with a family psychologist
140. How are infectious diseases, such as colds and influenza, most commonly spread?
   a) Breathing viruses in air
   b) Hand-to-face contact
   c) Drinking infected water
   d) Eating contaminated food
141. Public health surveillance includes which of the following activities:
   a) Soliciting case reports of persons with symptoms compatible with SARs from local hospitals
   b) Creating graphs of the number of dog bites by week and neighborhood
   c) Writing a report on trends in seat belt use to share with the state legislature
   d) All of the above
142. The hallmark feature of an analytic epidemiologic study is: (Choose one best answer)
   a) Use of an appropriate comparison group
   b) Laboratory confirmation of the diagnosis
   c) Publication in a peer-reviewed journal
   d) Statistical analysis using logistic regression
143. Comparing numbers and rates of illness in a community, rates are preferred for: (Choose one best answer)
   a) Conducting surveillance for communicable diseases
   b) Deciding how many doses of immune globulin are needed
   c) Estimating subgroups at highest risk
   d) Telling physicians which strain of influenza is most prevalent
144. For the cruise ship scenario described in Question 7, how would you display the time course of the outbreak? (Choose one best answer)
   a) Endemic curve
   b) Epidemic curve
   c) Seasonal trend
   d) Secular trend
145. For the cruise ship scetnario described in Question 7, if you suspected that the norovirus may have been transmitted by ice made or served aboard ship, how might you display "place"?
   a) Spot map by assigned dinner seating location
   b) Spot map by cabin
   c) Shaded map of United States by state of residence
   d) All of the above

146. Which variables might you include in characterizing the outbreak described in Question 7 by person?
   a) Age of passenger
   b) Detailed food history (what person ate) while aboard ship
   c) Status as passenger or crew
   d) A and C both
147. When analyzing surveillance data by age, which of the following age groups is preferred? (Choose one best answer)
   a) 1-year age groups
   b) 5-year age groups
   c) 10-year age groups
   d) Depends on the disease
148. A key feature of a cross-sectional study is that:
   a) It usually provides information on prevalence rather than incidence
   b) It is more useful for descriptive epidemiology than it is for analytic epidemiology
   c) It is synonymous with survey
   d) All of the above
149. The epidemiologic triad of disease causation refers to: (Choose one best answer)
   a) Agent, host, environment
   b) Time, place, person
   c) Source, mode of transmission, susceptible host
   d) John Snow, Robert Koch, Kenneth Rothman
150. Indirect transmission includes which of the following?
   a) Mosquito-borne
   b) Foodborne
   c) Doorknobs or toilet seats
   d) All of the above
151. Disease control measures are generally directed at which of the following?
   a) Eliminating the reservoir
   b) Eliminating the vector
   c) Interrupting mode of transmission
   d) All of the above
152. A propagated epidemic is usually the result of what type of exposure?
   a) Point source
   b) Continuous common source
   c) Intermittent common source
   d) Person-to-person

Answer Key

1	c	2	c	3	c	4	c	5	c	6	d	7	b
8	c	9	d	10	a	11	d	12	d	13		14	
15		16		17		18		19		20		21	
22		23		24		25		26	c	27	c	28	c
29	c	30	c	31	c	32	c	33	c	34	c	35	c
36	c	37	c	38	c	39	c	40	d	41	c	42	c
43	c	44	c	45		46		47	d	48		49	c
50	c	51	c	52	c	53	c	54	c	55	c	56	c
57	d	58	d	59	c	60	c	61	d	62		63	b
64		65		66		67	d	68	d	69	d	70	d
71	c	72	a	73	c	74	a	75	d	76	b	77	d
78	a	79	a	80	a	81	b	82	a	83	a	84	d
85	b	86	c	87	b	88	a	89	c	90	b	91	c
92	d	93	b	94	d	95	b	96	c	97	c	98	a
99	b	100	d	101	c	102	d	103	d	104	b	105	a
106	b	107	c	108	b	109	a	110	b	111	b	112	b
113	a	114	c	115	b	116	c	117	a	118	d	119	c
120	b	121	b	122	d	123	c	124	a	125	d	126	b
127	d	128	d	129	d	130	c	131	c	132	b	133	b
134	b	135	b	136	c	137	b	138	c	139	a	140	a
141	b	142	d	143	a	144	c	145	b	146	d	147	d
148	d	149	d	150	a	151	d	152	d	153	d		

11

Collection, Preservation, Processing and Dispatch of Clinical Materials

J.B. Kathiriya[1], B.B. Javia[2], S.N. Ghodasara[2] and D.B. Barad[2]

[1]*Department of Veterinary Public Health & Epidemiology, College of Veterinary Science & A. H., Kamdhenu University, Junagadh-362001, Gujarat, India*

[2]*Department of Veterinary Microbiology, College of Veterinary Science & A. H. Kamdhenu University, Junagadh-362001, Gujarat, India*

Introduction

The quality of interaction between clinicians and microbiologists has an enormous influence on the effectiveness of the laboratory service. An accurate diagnosis is based on the interpretation of both clinical and laboratory data. Investigation of disease is solely dependent on the quality and appropriateness of the specimens collected. The diagnosis depends on the skill and care with which the clinicians select, collect and transport the specimen to the laboratory. Clinical history, including the tentative diagnosis, should always accompany the specimen. If available, a detailed post-mortem report must also be sent. These set of information will help the microbiologist to select the most appropriate procedure and to furnish a meaningful interpretation of the results.

Specimens need to be collected for establishing a disease diagnosis or monitoring of vaccine response or surveillance. The knowledge of the pathogenesis of the infectious disease is the most important factor for determining the most suitable specimen. The samples need to be appropriate, and adequate in number and amount to provide a statistically valid result. Samples must be taken with care, to avoid undue stress or damage to the bird or danger to the operator. Careful consideration must be given to the collection, containment, and storage of the specimens, including biosafety measures to prevent spillage to the environment or exposure of other birds and humans.

Strict sterile precautions must be observed while collecting and handling materials for isolation. The chance of isolating a microbe depends critically on the knowledge, care, and attention of the veterinarian collecting the specimen. Specimens taken as a last resort after failed antibiotic therapy are invariably a waste of effort in case of bacterial disease. Having obtained suitable material, it must be carefully packaged, labeled, and transmitted to the laboratory by the fastest practicable method. Relevant shipping regulations must be followed. If material is sent to a laboratory of another country, the laboratory must be consulted in advance about its willingness to receive the material. All samples must be accompanied by a written note indicating the origin of the material, the relevant history, and the tests required.

General guidelines for the collection of specimens

Laboratory results are directly dependent on the mode of collection, preservation, and shipment of the specimen. Therefore, the samples are to be collected and handled in a manner that permits a high rate of recovery of the microorganisms present.

- Collect specimens from live sick or recently dead birds. Just prior to death and shortly thereafter, a number of intestinal bacteria may invade the host tissues. Some of the potential pathogens are difficult to assess when tissues have been invaded. Hence, for best results, fresh tissues must be collected as soon as feasible.
- Collect samples as aseptically as possible to avoid cross-contamination.
- Collect samples from affected sites as soon as the appearance of clinical signs. This is very important in the case of viral infections as the shedding of the virus is more pronounced during the early phase of infection. This holds true for enteric bacterial infection also.
- It is better to collect samples from clinical cases and in-contact birds. The later may shed large numbers of microorganisms.
- While investigating diseases of unknown cause, collect multiple different specimens that represent the different stages of the disease progression (e.g. the pre-clinical, early clinical, active clinical, chronically affected and convalescent phases).
- Collect samples from edge of the lesions and include some normal tissue. Microbial replication is more active at lesion's edge.
- Collect specimens before treatment. Samples taken from treated birds are of little value.
- If the specimens are not collected in time and/or before the start of treatment, the same should be intimated to the laboratory so that the laboratory can opt for other molecular tests than isolation work.
- Specimen should be relevant to the suspected disease. If not, a wide range of tissues should be sent in order to avoid failure of isolation of significant organisms.
- Obtain a tentative diagnosis. If not, collect specimens for several disciplines such as bacteriological, mycological, virological, and pathological examination.
- Specimen on the dry swabs is liable to desiccation and hence more amounts of samples should be taken and sent to the laboratory as soon as possible. If needed, they can be sent in commercial swabs containing transport medium.
- Discuss the unexpected result with the laboratory.
- If a sample shows negative, it may not be considered due to intermittent shedding. Thus repeated sampling may yield actual results.
- The presence of commesal might not be considered unless pathogenic factors of such isolate are revealed
- Submit a detailed history of the case along with samples.
- The samples in water-tight, screw-capped jars clearly indicating the tissue enclosed, animal identification and the date of collection are preferable.
- Send the samples at 4°C and not frozen, if delay in transportation is expected.

Transportation of clinical materials

Specimens should always be placed in the plastic biohazard transport bag attached to the request form and the bag should be sealed. Multiple specimens should be transported in impervious transport containers (green transport bags) and should not be carried by hand or in plastic or paper bags. Specimens must not be sent in standard envelopes via the internal post.

Specimen packaging

It is the responsibility of all persons sending samples to the laboratory to adhere to national and international regulations ensuring that specimens sent to the laboratory do not present a risk to anyone coming in contact with them during transportation or on receipt in the laboratory.

Packaging Clinical materials

- The packaging must be of good quality, and strong enough to withstand the shocks and loadings normally encountered during carriage.
- The packaging must consist of at least three components:
- A leakproof primary receptacle e.g. blood collection tube, MSU container;
- A secondary sealable package to enclose and protect the primary container(s), e.g. plastic specimen bag.
- Outer package: the secondary package is placed in an outer transport container with suitable cushioning that protects it and its contents from external influences such as physical damage and water while in transit.

Few points about antibacterial sensitivity test (ABST)

1. First of all, it has to be clear that the outbreak must be due to bacteria alone. Or else it will lead to obfuscating result, as commensal bacteria/opportunistic pathogen might intercept.
2. The specimen such as heart blood swab shall have to be obtained from birds that have died not before three hours in order to prevent contaminating microbes.
3. It is not guaranteed that the bacterial growth obtained for performing ABST is always pure and the growth may even comprise the causative bactera. In such cases, the outcome of the treatment based on ABST may not result in fruitful end.
4. It is pertinent to isolate the causative bacteria and then perform ABST, although this process may be time-consuming.
5. Bacteria such as streptococci or *Avibacterium paragallinarum* does not grow in the media used in regular ABST.
6. Despite taking all the care mentioned in the above points, there is a possibility of *in vitro* and *in vivo* differences which may lead to ineffective therapy.
7. Based upon the experience, a clinician must decide the correct choice of antibiotics when more than one antibiotic are found to be sensitive or intermediate sensitive in ABST.

Conclusion

It can be concluded that the collection and despatch of specimens with correct labeling determine the efficiency of the laboratory data. The rapidity in collection and despatch of the specimens to the willing laboratory with good expertise is another factor that decides fruitful laboratory output. Moreover, it is mandatory to follow the Nation's guidelines in the despatch of the specimens.

MCQ

1. Select all the important procedures that are required when performing the routine collection method of microbial specimens
   a) A specimen should be collected in a sterile container
   b) A specimen should be properly labeled with the patient's name, date, and time of collection
   c) A specimen should be collected by using a sterile cotton swab or collection needles
   d) All of above
2. Which of the following is the correct volume size of blood specimen taken from the adult patient for the routine laboratory diagnosis of the infection and the identification of the possible pathogen?
   a) 1 ml b) 10 ml
   c) 20 ml d) 0.5 ml
3. Which of the following specimens are appropriate clinical specimens and are commonly used for the proper diagnosis of Salmonellosis?
   Select all the correct options
   a) Blood specimen b) Throat swab
   c) Urine specimen d) Stool specimen
4. Which of the following specimen collection procedure can give accurate results for the laboratory diagnosis of Tuberculosis?
   a) Throat swab specimen each morning for 3 consecutive days
   b) Sputum specimen each morning for 3 consecutive days
   c) Blood specimens once a week for 2 weeks
   d) Skin biopsy test before the start of antibiotics therapy
5. Name the routine method used for the direct microscopic examination of a urine sample taken from a person suspected of urinary tract infection?
   a) Wet mount method b) Hanging drop method
   c) Thin and thick smear method d) Widal test method
6. Herpes simplex virus is one of the contagious viral diseases, HSV 1 is can spread from person to person.
   Which of the following cells appear as multinucleated cells taken from the lesion specimen and can be observed by the direct microscopy method?
   a) b) Buruli ulcer cells
   c) Schizont cells d) Tzanck cells

7. Which of the following temperature can be optimal for the storage of swab specimens taken from the Coronavirus infected patient while performing the Covid-19 test method?
   a) 2 to 4 degrees Celsius for up to 24 hours after the specimen collection
   b) 25 degrees celsius for up to 3 days after the specimen collection
   c) 2 to 4 degrees Celsius for up to 72 hours after the specimen collection
   d) 5 to 10 degrees Celsius for up to a week after the specimen collection
8. Which of the following microorganism can be detected by their ability to produce a toxin and can be identified by Elek's test method?
   a) *Cryptococcus neoformans* b) *Corynebacterium diphtheria*
   c) *Mycobacterium tuberculosis* d) *Bacillus anthracis*
9. Which of the following chemical compound is commonly used to clean and decontaminate the infected skin area or nail before the collection of the specimens and laboratory diagnosis?
   a) Iodine solution b) KOH solution
   c) Warm water d) 70% alcohol
10. Which of the following is the most widely used test for the detection of genetic material in the Covid-19 swab sample?
   a) PCR test (Polymerase chain reaction)
   b) Western blot test
   c) ELISA (Enzyme-linked immunosorbent assay)
   d) Animal inoculation test
11. Which of the following specimen is appropriate for the laboratory diagnosis of meningitis?
   a) Throat swab b) Hair and skin samples
   c) Cerebrospinal fluid d) Urine specimen
12. Direct microscopy is a common laboratory diagnosis procedure performed for the detection of spores or mycelia present in fungi.

   Select all the correct methods or steps for the procedure
   a) 1- 2 drops of potassium hydroxide are added to the slide that contains the specimen (skin, hair, or sputum)
   b) The slide is covered with the coverslip
   c) a, b, and d) are the correct answers.
   d) The slide is observed under the microscope
13. Name all the common types of cell culture methods most frequently used in the isolation of a virus
   a) Animal inoculation b) Tissue culture
   c) Embryonated eggs d) All of above

14. A blood smear is considered the gold standard diagnosis for identification of malarial parasite.

    Name the commonly used stain for the identification of the material parasite and detection of the life stages of the parasite?

    a) Lactophenol cotton blue
    b) Giemsa stain
    c) Gram stain
    d) Malachite green

15. Select all the important laboratory techniques and methods used for the identification of different microorganisms

    a) Microscopic methods
    b) Culture methods
    c) Serological methods
    d) Animal inoculation
    e) Antigen detection test
    f) Molecular methods
    g) All of above

16. What is the ideal time period limit for the transportation of the specimen to the laboratory after the collection method?

    a) 2 minutes
    b) 30 minutes
    c) 1 hour
    d) 2 hours

17. Which of the following preservatives is commonly used to preserve urine specimen?

    a) Boric acid
    b) Ethyl alcohol
    c) Formalin
    d) Hydrogen peroxide

18. Which of the following anticoagulant is used for the preservation of blood and bone marrow specimens?

    a) Boric acid
    b) Ethyl alcohol
    c) Polyvinyl alcohol
    d) Sodium polyanethol sulfonate (SPS)

19. What is the correct standard method used by a microbiologist for the storage of specimens such as urine, stool and swabs?

    a) Storage at frozen -80 degree Celsius
    b) Storage at refrigerator at 4 degree Celsius
    c) Storage at room temperature at 25 degree Celsius
    d) None of the above

20. Which of the following is the appropriate oxygen and carbon dioxide levels for the incubation and culture of capnophilic bacteria such as Haemophilus influenzae and Neisseria gonorrhoeae?

    a) 0.03% CO2 and 21% O2
    b) 5% to 10% CO2 and 0% O2
    c) 5% to 10% CO2 and15% O2
    d) 0.03% CO2 and 0% O2

21. Gram stain also known as differential stain is the principle stain mainly used in the microscopic identification and differentiation of which of the following group of pathogens?
    a) Gram positive and gram negative bacteria
    b) Mold, yeast and Fungi
    c) DNA and RNA Viruses
    d) Helminths and protozoa
22. All of the following are macroscopic morphology in culture/agar media that should be observed by a microbiologist in the identification process of the bacteria, Except
    a) Colony shape and size
    b) Pigmentation of the colony
    c) Surface appearance of the colony
    d) Microscopic observation of the colony
23 When a surgeon wants to send the autopsy specimen for virological examination, it should be preserved in:
    a) 50% glycerine
    b) 10% formalin
    c) Rectified spirit
    d) Saturated solution of common salt
24. Which of the following blood cells play an important role in blood clotting?
    a) Thrombocytes
    b) Neutrophils
    c) Leucocytes
    d) Erythrocytes
25. Serum differs from blood as it lacks
    a) antibodies
    b) clotting factors
    c) albumins
    d) globulins
26. Which of the following is correct?
    a) Serum contains blood and fibrinogen
    b) Plasma is blood without lymphocytes
    c) Blood comprises plasma, RBC, WBC and platelets
    d) Lymph is plasma with RBC and WBC
27. This plasma protein is responsible for blood coagulation
    a) Fibrinogen
    b) Globulin
    c) Serum amylase
    d) Albumin
28. DNA is not present in
    a) an enucleated ovum
    b) hair root
    c) a mature spermatozoa
    d) mature RBCs
29. Globulins of the blood plasma are responsible for
    a) defence mechanisms
    b) blood clotting
    c) oxygen transport
    d) osmotic balance
30. Lymph differs from blood in having
    a) no plasma
    b) more RBCs and less WBCs
    c) more WBCs and no RBCs
    d) plasma without proteins

31. WBCs which release heparin and histamine
    a) Basophils
    b) Neutrophils
    c) Monocytes
    d) Eosinophils
32. WBCs which are the most active phagocytic cells
    a) lymphocytes and macrophages
    b) neutrophils and eosinophils
    c) neutrophils and monocytes
    d) eosinophils and lymphocytes
33. Find the correct statement for WBCs
    a) can squeeze through blood capillaries
    b) produced only in the thymus
    c) deficiency leads to cancer
    d) do not contain a nucleus
34. Name all the common physical methods used for the sterilization process in healthcare facilities such as microbiology laboratories, hospitals, and biotechnology industries
    a) Dry heat
    b) Ionizing gamma Radiation
    c) Filtration
    d) All of above
35. Autoclave is the example of moist heat method which is common and reliable sterilization method used in the microbiology laboratory.
    Which of the following is the recommended heat temperature and time period for the moist heat sterilization method used in an autoclave?
    a) 180 degree C for 5 minutes
    b) 121 degree C for 15 minutes
    c) 126 degree C for 3 minutes
    d) 160 degree C for 45 minutes
36. What is the correct statement for the term 'Bioburden'?
    a) The number of microorganisms present on the surface
    b) The bacterial spores present on the surface after the sterilization of the surface
    c) The process of elimination of microorganisms by using physical agents
    d) The aseptic process for the maintenance of the sterility of the surface
37. Which of the following best describes the process of 'Disinfection'?
    a) The elimination of all forms of microorganisms and bacterial spores
    b) The elimination of all forms of bacterial spores
    c) The reduction or elimination of microorganisms and bacterial spores
    d) The reduction or elimination of many microorganisms and some bacterial spores
38. Name the sterilization method that is most frequently used in hospitals and clinical laboratories for the heat-labile liquid substances or antibiotics.
    a) Dry heat
    b) Radiation
    c) Filtration
    d) Formaldehyde
39. Which of the following methods has been found safe and effective in the elimination of COVID-19 virus?
    Select all that apply:
    a) Use of 60-70 % isopropyl alcohol
    b) Use of antibacterial ointments
    c) Hand wash with Soap and water
    d) Intake of antibiotics when symptoms appear

40. Which of the following "water purification" methods is most common in the rural parts of the countries like India, Nepal, and Africa that is also a simple, reliable, and economical method?
   a) Solar disinfection
   b) Chlorination
   c) Advanced purifiers
   d) Salt

41. All of the following chemical disinfectants used in laboratories and healthcare industries have been found to be effective against many bacteria, fungi, and viruses, Except?
   a) Alcohols
   b) Ethylene oxide
   c) Formaldehyde
   d) Chlorine
   e) Steam heat

42. Which of the following sterilizing agent is found to have less or no sporicidal activity?
   Select all the correct options:
   a) Hot air oven
   b) Ethyl alcohol
   c) Pasteurization
   d) Autoclave

43. Name the spore containing the pathogen which shows resistance to heat and is usually not destroyed by using heat at 100 degrees Celcius.
   a) E. coli
   b) Candida albicans
   c) Vibrio cholera
   d) Clostridium perfringens

44. Joseph Lister first introduced the use of antiseptics in hospitals, what is the name of the chemical he used for the antisepsis process?
   a) Ethyl alcohol
   b) Carbolic acid
   c) Hydrogen peroxide
   d) Chlorohexidine

45. The Quality and Safety of products in pharmaceutical industries, food, and other biotechnology companies are mainly controlled by which of the following regulation departments in the USA?
   a) Food and drug administration
   b) International Standard Organization 9001
   c) Good manufacturing practices
   d) Center for Disease Control and prevention

46. Which of the following is the correct definition for the 'pasteurization' process of milk and fermented products?
   a) The sterilization method that uses heat at a boiling temperature of 100 degrees Celcius
   b) The sterilization method that uses heat at 100 to 120 degrees Celcius
   c) The sterilization method that uses moist heat below 100 degrees Celcius
   d) The sterilization method that uses moist heat above 100 degrees Celcius

47. Nonionizing radiation and ionizing radiation are sterilization methods mainly used in hospitals. Ultraviolet radiation is one example of nonionizing radiation, name the ionizing radiation?
   a) Infrared
   b) X-rays and gamma rays
   c) Halogens
   d) Ethylene oxide

48. Identify the temperature and time period commonly used for the hot air oven while sterilizing glassware in the laboratory
    a) 180 degrees Celcius for 30 mins
    b) 63 degrees Celcius for 30 mins
    c) 121 degrees Celcius for 15 mins
    d) 160 degrees Celcius for 45 mins
49. An outbreak of enteric infection occurred in 1996 in the USA . Numerous children got sick after the consumption of a specific juice company, investigation was done and the reports showed lack of good sanitation practices and elimination of the pasteurization process by that company, this led to foodborne infection.
    Name the bacteria identified as the cause of the outbreak?
    a) *E. coli* O157:H7
    b) *Vibrio cholerae*
    c) *Bacillus subtilis*
    d) *E. coli* O121
50. Select all the common and effective methods that can help in reducing the highly transmissible waterborne infections like typhoid and cholera
    a) Boiling of the water
    b) Using chlorine for purification
    c) Pasteurization process
    d) Use of water filters
51. Which one of the following level is maintained in body by Parathyroid gland :-
    a) Sodium
    b) Potassium
    c) Magnessium
    d) Calcium
52. Direct bilirubin is also called as :
    a) Unconjugated bilirubin
    b) Conjugated Bilirubin
    c) Water soluble bilirubin
    d) Both "2" and "3"
53. Increase Cortisol level is seen in which syndrome ?
    a) Addison's disease
    b) Cushing Syndrome
54. Different between N. Meningitis and N. Gonorrhea is that N. Meningitis ferment only :
    a) Glucose
    b) Maltose
    c) Sucrose
    d) Lactose
55. Chinese letter arrangement, Metachromatic granules, tellurite hydrolysis and elek test is characteristic of which bacteria ?
    a) Listeria monocytogenes
    b) Bacillus anthracis
    c) Corynebacterium diphtheriae
    d) Moraxella catarrhalis
56. Which of the following bacteria is urase positive, Indole Positive, and H2S Positive?
    a) Proteus
    b) Escherchia
    c) Salmonella
    d) Shigella
57. Seagull appears is characteristic of which bacteria ?
    a) Campylobacter Jejuni
    b) Vibrio cholerae
    c) *E. coli*
    d) Salmonella
58. Which of the following bacteria Stain which silver impregnation and can be seen by Dark field microscopy ?
    a) Treponema pallidum
    b) Homeopathic influenza
    c) Streptococcus pyogenes
    d) Spirillum minus

59. Lowenstein-Jensen (LJ) is used for the growth of which of the following :
    a) Staphylococcus b) Streptocossus
    c) Neisseria d) Mycobacteria
60. A cause of acute factitious infantile diarrhea is :
    a) hantavirus b) HIV
    c) Rhabdovirus d) Rotavirus
61. Specimen for viral culture should be transported in :
    a) Anaerobic Container b) Bovine Albumin
    c) Nutrient medium with antibiotic d) Sheep blood (5 – 10 %)
62. In order to prove a yeast is dimorphic, which of the following test is performed ?
    a) Carbohydrate assimilation b) Growth on Corn Meal Agar,
    c) Incubate yeast subculture at 37°C d) Urease
63. The infrective stage for strongyloides stercoralis is :
    a) Ovaf b) Filariform larvae
    c) Rhabditiform Larvah d) Free living adult
64. If human ingest the egg of taenia Solium , they may devolp :
    a) Hydatid Disease b) Sparganosis
    c) Trichinosis d) Cysticercosis
65. Good sanitation practices have played a vital role in reducing the spread of Covid-19 infection and other respiratory diseases.

    All of the following are important sanitation practices that can help in killing or reducing viable pathogens, Except?
    a) Handwashing and use of an oral mask for personal hygiene
    b) Use of chemical disinfectants to clean the surface area
    c) Fumigation of area for the decontamination of air
    d) Getting the recommended vaccine shot against the disease
    e) Cleaning of objects with chemical agents
66. What is the correct meaning of the term known as the 'terminal sterilization process?
    a) The initial sterilization of the raw materials for the product
    b) The final sterilization of the healthcare products and medical devices
    c) The decontamination of the environmental bioburden
    d) The aseptic technique used during the manufacturing process of the product
67. Name the chemical in a 'bleach' (a disinfectant) used to eliminate bacteria, fungi, and viruses?
    a) Sodium chloride b) Ethylene oxide
    c) Sodium hypochlorite d) Ethyl alcohol
68. Which of the following is a recommended method for sterilizing surgical instruments?
    a) Wiping with alcohol b) Cleaning with soap and water
    c) Autoclaving d) Soaking in disinfectant solution

69. What is the minimum recommended concentration of bleach for disinfection purposes in healthcare facilities, home spaces and public places?
    a) 5% b) 10%
    c) 50% d) 100%
70. Select all the common and effective 'physical disinfection method' used for the elimination pathogens?
    a) Boiling (100 oC for 15 minutes)\
    b) Pasteurization (70 oC for 30 minutes)
    c) Ultraviolet rays (nonionizing radiation)
    d) Alcohols
71. Which of the following is the standard safety precautions that is required and essential while working in the laboratory?
    a) Avoid mouth pipetting
    b) Avoid eating or chewing in the lab
    c) Thoroughly wash hands and other skin surfaces after removing gloves and immediately after any contamination
    d) Always wear proper Protective Personal equipment (PPE)
    e) All of the above
72. All of the following statements are correct regarding the Biological Safety Cabinet in a microbiology laboratory, Except?
    a) Used while handling hazardous microorganisms
    b) Categorized into three classes (I, II and III)
    c) Consists of UV light, HEPA filters for sterilization
    d) Standard Personal protective equipment (PPE) may not be required while using the cabinet
73. On collecting blood, what solution is added to it?
    a) sodium citrate b) potassium citrate
    c) sodium phosphate d) potassium phosphate
74. Which of the following tests can be performed on the extracted blood?
    i) HIV ii) Diabetes
    iii) Hepatitis B surface antigen iv) Malaria
    v) Antibody to Hepatitis C vi) Serological test for Syphilis
    vii) Dengue viii) Creatinine
    a) i, iii, v, vi b) i, ii, iii, iv, v, vi, viii, viii
    c) ii, iv, vii, viii d) i, v, viii
75. How much blood does the body have in reserve and where is it stored?
    a) 150 ml stored in liver b) 10 ml stored in gall bladder
    c) 100 ml stored in the spleen d) 15 ml stored in the heart
76. How is dengue detected in blood?
    a) Low level of RBCs b) Low level of WBCs
    c) Low level of Platelets d) Low level of fibrin

77. What machine is used to test the blood?
   a) Auto analyzer b) Hemodialyzer
   c) Diathermy machine d) Ventilator
78. Anaemia is caused due to deficiency of
   a) Haemoglobin b) Fibrin
   c) Thrombin d) Neutrophils
79. Hemophilia is more dominant in
   a) Males b) Females
   c) Young children d) Transvestite
80. Soft fats in milk fat are ________________
   a) Lauric & Stearic b) Capric & Lauric
   c) Oleic & Butyric d) Oleic & Lauric
81. Principal protein in milk is _____________
   a) Albumin b) Lactalbumin
   c) Casein d) Lactoglobulin
82. Percentage of mineral matter in milk is about ___
   a) 1 % b) 0.7 %
   c) 1.5 % d) 0.05 %
83. Whey is the by-product in the manufacture of?
   a) Skimmed milk b) Butter
   c) Cheese d) Yogurt
84. Which of the following is an example of soft cheese is?
   a) Cheddar b) Swiss
   c) Brick d) Cottage
85. How many indigenous enzymes have been reported in bovine milk?
   a) 30 b) 60
   c) 50 d) 40
86. Destruction of which enzyme is used as an index of super-HTST pasteurization?
   a) Catalase b) Lipase
   c) Lactoperoxidase d) Pepsin
87. Rennet belongs to ___________
   a) Lipases b) Catalase
   c) Proteinases d) Phosphatases
88. Temperature used in UHT treatment is _____
   a) 90-100 °C b) 100-120 °C
   c) 120-125 °C d) 130-140 °C
89. Lactose is a disaccharide which contains?
   a) Glucose & Fructose b) Glucose & Glactose
   c) Glucose & Glucose d) Glucose & Maltose

90. $CaCl_2$ is added at the rate of ______________
   a) 0.5 %   b) 0.8 %
   c) 0.02 %   d) 0.08 %
91. Which one is used as an emulsifying agent in process cheese blend?
   a) Paprika   b) Pectin
   c) Glycerides   d) Whey Powder
92. People with high blood pressure or edema are advised to take___________
   a) Multivitamin Mineral Milk   b) Low Sodium Milk
   c) Sterile Milk   d) Low Lactose Milk
93. Normal bovine milk contains what amount of protein?
   a) 7.5%   b) 5.5%
   c) 3.5%   d) 9.5%
94. The aim of pasteurization milk is to _______
   a) Improve flavor   b) Kill disease producing organisms
   c) Improve color   d) Oxidation

Answer Key

1	d	2	b	3	a	4	b	5	a	6	d	7	c
8	b	9	d	10	a	11	c	12	c	13	d	14	b
15	g	16	d	17	a	18	d	19	b	20	c	21	a
22	a	23	a	24	a	25	b	26	c	27	a	28	d
29	a	30	c	31	a	32	c	33	a	34	d	35	b
36	a	37	d	38	c	39	a	40	a	41	e	42	c
43	d	44	b	45	a	46	c	47	b	48	d	49	a
50	a	51	d	52	d	53	e	54	b	55	c	56	a
57	a	58	a	59	b	60	d	61	b	62	c	63	b
64	d	65	d	66	b	67	c	68	c	69	b	70	a
71	e	72	d	73	a	74	a	75	c	76	c	77	a
78	a	79	a	80	c	81	c	82	b	83	c	84	d
85	c	86	c	87		88	d	89	b	90	c	91	c
92	b	93	c	94	b								

12

Emerging, Re-emerging and Exotic Diseases

***Sabarinathan Akambaram*[1], *Chhavi Gupta*[2] *and Balagangadharathilagar M.*[1]**

[1]*Department of Veterinary Clinical Complex, Veterinary College and Research Institute, TANUVAS, Tirunelveli - 627358, India*

[2]*Department of Veterinary Gynaecology and Obstetrics, Veterinary College and Research Institute, TANUVAS, Tirunelveli - 627358, India*

Introduction

The current health situation in poultry farming is dotted with cases where these emerging or re-emerging diseases attack birds. A large majority of them are of viral origin and a powerful immunosuppressive effect is observed, sometimes accompanied by bacterial infections. Most of the important infectious diseases of poultry have been known for many years and are controlled by medication, vaccination, eradication and bio-security. Examples of such diseases that were known before the intensive commercial poultry industry development are infectious bronchitis (IB), newcastle disease (ND), infectious bursal disease (IBD), lymphoid leucosis and so on. From time to time, new diseases emerge to provide fresh challenges for diagnosis, control and understanding of their epidemiology.

World Health Organization (WHO) definition of an emerging disease is defined as a disease that has appeared in a population for the first time, or that may have existed previously but is rapidly increasing in incidence or geographic range. Diseases that reappear after a period of absence can be considered as re-emerging. Some of these include runting/stunting syndrome and inclusion body hepatitis. In addition, other well-established diseases evolve in different ways and can also present problems for diagnosis and control. In the wider sphere, it is recognized that emerging viral infections in both humans and animals have been reported with increased frequency in recent years. Examples are SARS, avian influenza, West Nile virus and the Nipah virus. The more recent diseases of viral origin, others that have re-emerged and some experiences from previous emerging diseases are living examples for threat to the poultry industries. In addition, infectious bronchitis is an example of a disease which the causal virus is showing constant evolution. The impact of infections caused by the avian metapneumovirus (aMPV) is an example of recently emerged viral agent.

The two most prominent viral emerging diseases to affect poultry in recent years are PEMS and hepatitis E virus infection, associated with hepatospelenomegaly or big liver and spleen disease (BLS). PEMS is a highly infectious disease of young turkeys defined by spiking mortality, diarrhea, growth depression, stunting and immune suppression. It was first described in young turkeys in the southwestern U.S. It appears to be multifactorial in nature and can be transmitted using gut extracts and also with bacteria-free extracts of thymus. Because of the uncertainty of the aetiology, and particularly the role of viruses, control is best achieved by basic disease prevention principles such as all-in all-out and thorough cleansing and disinfection.

Emerging EDS was caused by a virus that could easily be grown in the laboratory and, it hemagglutinated erythrocytes, immediately providing a convenient serological test. Further work on the virus showed that it was of duck origin. A disease in which evolution can be followed by constant surveillance is IB. The coronavirus constantly generates variants because of the instability of a hypervariable region in the S1 spike gene. The S1 spike is biologically very important, with roles in cell attachment, virus immunity and induction of immunity. Variants occurring due to mutations or recombinants can arise against which existing vaccines are poorly protective.

It can be expected that new viral diseases will continue to emerge from time to time in the poultry industry, in the various ways listed above. Indeed it may be that some of these are already present in domestic poultry. Perhaps new diseases will emerge caused by viruses in genera not yet recognized as pathogens in domestic poultry such as pestiviruses, toroviruses or lentiviruses. It will be necessary to use all available diagnostic methods to determine the viral causes. Although frequently overlooked in the rush to use modern methodologies, full characterization of the gross and microscopic pathology of a new disease is imperative to obviate confusion when similar outbreaks and to have clear strategies to overcome the disease outbreak and their impact on the economy.

Multiple Choice Questions

1. Pathogenic strains of new castle disease cause high mortality with depression and death within 3 to 5 days is

    a) Velogenic b) Mesogenic

    c) Lentogeneic d) All of the above

2. Causative viral agent for Lymphoid Leucosis is

    a) Alphaherpesvirus b) Retrovirus

    c) Paramyxovirus d) None of the above

3. Etiological factor of avian influenza

    a) Adenovirus b) Avian paramyxovirus type 1.

    c) Paramyxovirus d) All of the above

4. Etiological factor of infectious laryngotracheitis Gallid herpesvirus 1.

    a) Paramyxovirus b) Circovirus

    c) Reovirus d) Gallid herpes virus 1.

5. Caseous cast in the proximal trachea adjacent to the glottis is characteristic of

    a) Laryngotracheitis b) Infectious bronchitis

    c) IBD d) Fowl pox

6. Confirmatory diagnostic method for the Avian Influenza is

    a) AGID b) ELIZA

    c) RT-PCR assay d) Cell culture

7. Subcutaneous hemorrhage is characteristic of strain with highly pathogenic avian influenza

a) H5N2	b) H3N5
c) H5N7	d) H5N1

8. Etiological factor of Infectious Bronchitis is

a) Avian coronavirus	b) Circo virus
c) IBD	d) Paramyxovirus

9. The two significant Mycoplasma species affecting commercial chickens

a) M. gallisepticum	b) M. synoviae
c) Both a and b	d) None of the above

10. Chronic respiratory disease in poultry caused by

a) M. synoviae	b) M. gallisepticum
c) Both a and b	d) None of the above

11. Synovitis and airsacculitis caused by

a) M. synoviae	b) Salmonella pullorum
c) E.coli	d) Salmonella gallinarum

12. Mycoplasmosis is transmitted by ----------- route from infected parent flocks to progeny

a) Horizontal	b) Direct contact
c) Vertical	d) All of the above

13. Lateral transmission occurs by ------------ between clinically affected or recovered carriers and susceptible flocks.

a) Parent flocks to progeny	b) Fomites
c) Feed	d) Direct contact

14. Acute foamy airsacculitis and caseous airsacculitis due to

a) Mycoplasma gallisepticum	b) M. synoviae
c) E.coli	d) Salmonella gallinarum

15. Etiological factor of fowl typhoid is

a) Salmonella pullorum	b) Mycoplasma gallisepticum
c) *E. coli*	d) Salmonella gallinarum

16. Etiological factor of Fowl Cholera is

a) Salmonella gallinarum	b) Mycoplasma gallisepticum
c) *E. coli*	d) Pasteurella multocida

17. Etiological factor of avian encephalomyelitis

a) Picornavirus	b) Reo virus
c) Circo virus	d) Poxvirus

18. Infectious Stunting Syndrome caused by

a) Circo virus	b) Reovirus strains
c) Picornavirus	d) Poxvirus

19. Which of the following bacteria is most commonly isolated from exudates of egg peritonitis
    a) *E. coli*
    b) Salmonella pullorum
    c) Mycoplasma gallisepticum
    d) Pasteurella multocida
20. Which of the following Newcastle disease virus strains can be used for vaccinating one-day-old chicks by the coarse-spray method
    a) Lasota
    b) Lentogenic
    c) Velogenic
    d) Hitchener B1
21. What is recommended amount of powdered skim milk that needs to be added to the water used for vaccinationvia drinking water
    a) 5 grams per liter
    b) 1 grams per liter
    c) 2.5 grams per liter
    d) 25 grams per liter
22. Compared to the lentogenic, the mesogenic strains of Newcastle disease virus are strains
    a) More pathogenic and less immunogenic
    b) More pathogenic and more immunogenic
    c) Less pathogenic and more immunogenic
    d) None of the above
23. Mature chickens infected laterally with avian encephalomyelitis virus shed the virus in the
    a) Faeces
    b) Egg and faeces
    c) Egg and respiratory secretions
    d) Eggs, faeces, and respiratory secretions
24. Infectious coryza is characterized by all of the following clinical signs / gross lesions except
    a) Diffuse hemorrhage in the tracheal mucosa
    b) facial subcutaneous edema
    c) serous or mucoid nasal discharge
    d) conjunctivitis
25. With coarse-spray vaccination, the size of the droplet would be
    a) 150 -300 microns
    b) 300 - 400 microns
    c) 200 - microns
    d) 100-50 microns
26. What is the major type of antibody found in the yolk
    a) IgE
    b) IgA
    c) IgG
    d) IgM
27. In chickens affected with chicken infectious anemia, lesions are consistently and characteristically found in the bone marrow and
    a) Spleen
    b) Liver
    c) Thymus
    d) Bursa of Fabricius

28. Which of the following neoplasm-induce viruses is egg-transmitted
    a) Lymphoid leukosis virus and reticuloendotheliosis virus
    b) lymphoid leukosis virus
    c) Marek's disease virus
    d) Marek's disease virus and lymphoid leukosis virus
29. Which of the following live vaccines can be administered by the wing- web stab method
    a) Mareks vaccine
    b) fowl cholera and viral arthritis vaccines
    c) Avian encephalomyelitis and fowl cholera vaccines
    d) avian encephalomyelitis vaccine
30. Which type of influenza virus does cause avian influenza
    a) Types A and B
    b) Type A
    c) Type B
    d) Type C
31. If a bird is infected with S. pullorum-typhoid diseases, the antigen should agglutinate (clump) when mixed with the bird's blood within
    a) 90 – 105 sec
    b) 30 – 45 sec
    c) 50 – 60 sec.
    d) 65 – 75 sec
32 IBD is characterized by destruction of the lymphoid cells of the bursa of fabricius which leads to
    a) B cell suppression
    b) B cell stimulation
    c) B and T cell suppression
    d) None of the above
33 Number of distinct serotypes of IBD identified
    a) Four
    b) Two
    c) Five
    d) Six
34 Mycoplasma meleagridis is associated with airsacculitis in
    a) Turkeys
    b) Guinea fowl
    c) Pea fowl
    d) All of the above
35 Mycoplasma synoviae is the cause of infectious synovitis in
    a) Guinea fowl
    b) Pea fowl
    c) Chickens and Turkeys
    d) Turkeys
36 Mycoplasma gallisepticum causes
    a) Chronic respiratory disease
    b) Fowl typhoid
    c) Pullorum disease
    d) None of the above
37 Avian chlamydiosis is caused by
    a) C. psittaci
    b) C. avium
    c) C. allinacean
    d) None of the above
38. Chlamydia psittaci is known to infect more than avian species
    a) 100
    b) 150
    c) 200
    d) 400

39. Chlamydia psittaci can affect mammals, including
    a) Humans b) cattle
    c) Buffal d) All of the above
40. The recently recognized species Chlamydia are
    a) C. avium and C. gallinacean,
    b) Chlamydia psittaci and C. gallinacean
    c) C. avium and Chlamydia psittaci
    d) None of the above
41. Avian chlamydiosis in humans called as
    a) Psittacosis b) Ornithosis
    c) a and b d) Parrot fever
42. The genus Chlamydia are coccoid, obligate intracellular organism belongs to
    a) Gram negative bacteria b) Gram positive bacteria
    c) Fungi d) Rickettsia
43. Chlamydiae have a unique life cycle namely
    a) Elementary body b) Reticulate body
    c) a and b d) None of the above
44. c) psittaci" associated with mammals were later renamed as
    a) C. pecorum b) C. abortus
    c) C. felis d) All of the above
45 c) psittaci has been found in various mammals including
    a) Dogs b) Cats
    c) Cattle d) All of the above
46. C. gallinacea has been described in poultry including
    a) Chickens b) Turkeys
    c) Guinea fowl d) All of the above
47. c) psittaci can be acquired by birds through
    a) Inhalation infectious dust particles b) Ingestion infectious material
    c) a and b d) Direct contact
48. C. psittaci organism transmitted through biting flies, mites and lice by means
    a) Mechanical transmission b) Vertical transmission
    c) Horizontal transmission d) All of the above
49. The elementary body of Chlamydiae organism may remain viable in the environment for
    a) Five days b) One week
    c) Fifteen days d) One month
50. Humans are usually infected by direct contact with infected birds, or from the environment when
    a) Inhale contaminated dust b) Aerosolized excretion
    c) Aerosolized secretions d) All of the above

51. The disinfectants effective against c) psittaci
    a) Quaternary ammonium compounds b) Aldehydes
    c) a and b d) Detergents
52. C. psittaci is susceptible to moist heat of
    a) 121°C for 15 minutes b) 121°C for 5 minutes
    c) 110°C for 5 minutes d) 105°C for 15 minutes
53. C. psittaci is susceptible to dry heat of
    a) 150°C for 1 hr b) 160-170°C for 30 minutes
    c) 125°C for 2 hrs d) 160-170°C for 1 hr
54. Neurological signs with chlamydiae organisms are
    a) Torticollis b) Opisthotono
    c) a and b d) Status epilepticus
55. Chlamydial infections diagnostic methodologies include
    a) Detection of nucleic acids b) Detection of antigens
    c) Culture d) All of the above
56. Method to distinguish different species of Chlamydia
    a) DNA microarray hybridization tests b) Serological tests
    c) ELIZA d) All of the above
57. Chlamydial antigens identification methods are
    a) Immuno-staining methods b) Antigen capture ELISAs
    c) a and b d) None of the above
58. One of the most important agents of mycoplasmosis in terrestrial poultry
    a) Mycoplasma gallisepticum b) Mycoplasma bovis
    c) Mycoplasma cynos d) Mycoplasma pneumonia
59. Pathogenic mycoplasma in poultry include
    a) M. synoviae b) M. meleagridis
    c) M. iowae d) All of the above
60. Pathogenic mycoplasma affecting ring necked pheasants
    a) M. synoviae b) Mycoplasma gallisepticum
    c) M. meleagridis d) M. iowae
61. The M. gallisepticum lineage maintained in finches was first reported in the
    a) Eastern US b) New zealand
    c) Austraila d) Africa
62. M. gallisepticum occurs in
    a) Respiratory and ocular secretions b) Semen
    c) Eggs d) All of the above
63. Vertical transmission is more frequent in birds infected during
    a) Laying b) Direct contact
    c) Aerosol d) Fomites

64. M. gallisepticum can form biofilms, which are thought to enhance the
    a) Survival of mycoplasmas
    b) Enhance the growth of mycoplasmas
    c) Inhibit growth of mycoplasmas
    d) No any changes
65. Mycoplasmas can be inactivated by
    a) 1% sodium hypochlorite b) Cresylic acid
    c) Iodophors d) All of the above
66. Mycoplasma incubation period in finches
    a) 4 to 14 days b) 30 days
    c) 5 days d) 10 days
67. Turkeys and game birds affected with mycoplasma may develop
    a) Epilepsy b) Paranasal sinusitis
    c) Paralysis d) Hepatitis
68. The postmortem lesions in poultry and game birds affected M. gallisepticum
    a) Airsacculitis b) Salpingitis
    c) a and b d) None of the above
69. Common sampling sites for identification of mycoplasmosis through culture and PCR
    a) Oropharynx b) Cloaca
    c) Feathers d) Skin
70. Isolation medium for M. gallisepticum
    a) Nutrient agar b) Tryptic soy agar
    c) Brain heart infusion agar d) Frey's medium
71. Mycoplasma species can be distinguished with tests
    a) PCR-RFLP b) Culture test
    c) Serological tests d) Grams staining
72. The microscopic lesions in M. gallisepticum meningoencephalitis in turkeys
    a) Multifocal parenchymal necrosis b) Meningitis
    c) Perivascular cuffing and vasculitis d) All of the above
73. Commonly used assays for the screening of Mycoplasma in poultry is
    a) Rapid serum agglutination b) Hemagglutination test
    c) Gram staining d) All of the above
74. More specific test for the identification of Mycoplasma
    a) Rapid serum agglutination b) Hemagglutination inhibition test
    c) Hemagglutination test d) Gram staining
75. Percentage of drop in egg production is common during outbreak of mycoplasmosis
    a) 10-20% b) 30-40%
    c) 5-10% d) 30-35%

76. Meningoencephalitis in turkeys associated with
    a) *E. coli* b) M. gallisepticum
    c) S. pullorum d) S. gallinarum
77. The causative agent of egg drop syndrome which leads to significant economic loss in poultry industry
    a) Duck atadenovirus A b) Orthomyxovirus
    c) Avipoxvirus d) Paramixovirus
78. Egg drop syndrome 76 was first described in in the year 1970.
    a) Ducks b) Finches
    c) Chickens d) Grey parrot
79. Highly host specific viral disease of poultry
    a) Orthomyxovirus b) Paramixovirus
    c) Picornavirus d) Avipoxvirus
80. The main target organ of IBDV is the
    a) Lymph nodes b) Bursa of Fabricius
    c) Spleen d) Liver
81. Duck atadeno virus A can be transmitted by
    a) Vertically b) Horizontally
    c) a and b d) None of the above
82. The most obvious postmortem lesions in the duck adenovirus
    a) Plug of gelatinous material in the trachea
    b) Lungs edematous
    c) Atrophy of oviducts
    d) All of the above
83 Duck atadenovirus A can be isolated in
    a) Embryonated duck egg b) Embryonated goose eggs
    c) Cell culture d) All of the above
84 Fowl typhoid and pullorum disease are common in
    a) Central and South America b) Africa and Asia
    c) a and b d) All of the above
85 The incubation period in fowl typhoid
    a) 10 days b) 4 - 6 days
    c) 30 days d) 14 days
86 Clinical signs of recently hatched birds affected with salmonella
    a) Drooping wings b) Labored breathing
    c) a and b d) Paralysis
87. Postmortem lesions in birds affected with fowl typhoid
    a) Unabsorbed yolk sacs b) Congested lungs
    c) Peritonitis d) All of the above

88. Most consistent gross lesion in adult carriers of Salmonella Pullorum
   a) Misshapen /discolored ovaries   b) Air sacculitis
   c) Hydronephrosis   d) Parasinusitis
89. A flock test or to identify chronically infected birds in control program
   a) Serological test   b) Histopathology
   c) Gram staining   d) Postmortem lesion
90. Pullorum disease causes outbreaks
   a) Young birds   b) Growing birds
   c) Adult birds   d) None of the above
91. Fowl typhoid disease causes outbreaks
   a) Young birds   b) Growing birds
   c) Adult birds   d) b and c
92. Highly pathogenic avian influenza contained
   a) H5 hemagglutinin   b) H7 hemagglutinin
   c) a and b   d) None of the above
93. The vast majority of low pathogenic viruses are maintained in
   a) Wild birds   b) Wetland birds
   c) Aquatic birds   d) All of the above
94. Influenza A viruses are susceptible to
   a) Aldehydes   b) Povidone-iodine
   c) Phenols   d) All of the above
95. Avian influenza viruses, their nucleic acids and antigens can be found in
   a) Oropharyngeal swabs   b) Cloacal swabs
   c) Tracheal swabs   d) All of the above
96. The World Organization for Animal Health (OIE) has defined Newcastle disease as an infection caused by
   a) Pigeon paramyxovirus type 1   b) Highly virulent APMV-1 viruses
   c) a and b   d) None of the above
97. Necropsy lesions caused by velogenic APMV-1 viruses are
   a) Swollen periorbital region   b) Hemorrhages of tracheal mucosa
   c) Petechiae in proventriculus   d) All of the above
98. Avian encephalomyelitis pathognomonic microscopic changes are
   a) Diffuse gliosis   b) Marbling of lungs
   c) Cystic kidney   d) Cystic changes in the ovary
99. Reovirus causes in domestic fowls
   a) Arthritis   b) Tenosynovitis
   c) a and b   d) Pneumonia
100. Circovirus in domestic fowl causes
   a) Aplasia of the bone marrow   b) Atrophy of the thymus
   c) Atrophy of spleen   d) All of the above

Answer Key

1	a	2	b	3	b	4	d	5	a	6	c	7	a
8	a	9	c	10	b	11	a	12	c	13	d	14	a
15	d	16	d	17	a	18	b	19	a	20	d	21	c
22	b	23	d	24	a	25	d	26	c	27	c	28	a
29	c	30	b	31	a	32	a	33	b	34	a	35	c
36	a	37	a	38	d	39	d	40	a	41	c	42	a
43	c	44	d	45	d	46	d	47	c	48	a	49	d
50	d	51	c	52	a	53	d	54	c	55	d	56	d
57	c	58	a	59	d	60	b	61	a	62	d	63	a
64	a	65	d	66	a	67	b	68	c	69	a	70	d
71	a	72	d	73	a	74	b	75	a	76	b	77	a
78	c	79	d	80	b	81	c	82	d	83	d	84	d
85	b	86	c	87	d	88	a	89	a	90	a	91	d
92	c	93	d	94	d	95	d	96	c	97	d	98	a
99	c	100	d										

13

Diagnostic Techniques in Disease Diagnosis

J.B. Kathiriya[1] and Dr. B.J. Trangadia[2]

[1]Department of Veterinary Public Health & Epidemiology, College of Veterinary Science & A.H., Kamdhenu University, Junagadh-362001, Gujarat

[2]Department of Veterinary Pathology, College of Veterinary Science & A.H., Kamdhenu University, Junagadh-362001, Gujarat

Any abnormal condition, which affects the normal functioning of cells, tissues, organs and any other system in an individual, is called a disease. In all living organisms, including plants, animals, birds and humans, diseases can be caused due to infectious or non-infectious agents and various other factors. Laboratory tests may identify organisms directly (eg, visually, using a microscope, growing the organism in culture) or indirectly (eg, identifying antibodies to the organism). Some tests (eg, Gram stain, routine aerobic culture) can detect a large variety of pathogens and are commonly done for many suspected infectious illnesses. However, because some pathogens are missed on these tests, clinicians must be aware of the limitations of each test for each suspected pathogen. In such cases, clinicians should request tests specific for the suspected pathogen (eg, special stains or culture media or advise the laboratory of the suspected organism(s) so that it may select more specific tests. The main causative factors of diseases in humans include internal factors, genetic irregularities, allergies, poor immune system, external factors and a lot more.

Based on the causes, these diseases can be further classified into:

- Allergies
- Epidemic Diseases
- Infectious Diseases
- Deficiency Diseases
- Neoplastic diseases
- Degenerative Diseases
- Non-infectious Diseases

1. Widal test is commonly used for detection of

   a) AIDS b) Tuberculosis

   c) Sexually transmitted diseases d) Typhoid

2. Balloon pump is used in disease concerned with
   a) Brain b) lungs
   c) liver d) heart
3. Blood dialyser is also called
   a) Artificial heart b) Artificial kidney
   c) Artificial lung d) Artificial liver
4. Artificial arteries are made of
   a) rubber b) silver
   c) glass d) daclon or teflon
5. the technique involving the as of positron emitting radio isotopes is
   a) CT scanning b) PET scanning
   c) NMR imaging d) SQUID
6. Grafting between two members of the same species is
   a) autograft b) allograft
   c) xenograft d) none of these
7. Scientist pipointed the location of colour processing centres in human visual cortex by means of
   a) PET scanning b) NMR imaging
   c) CT scanning d) Ultra sound imaging
8. Relative biological effectiveness is related to
   a) soil b) water
   c) radiation d) pollution
9. The pacemaker of heart is
   a) Bundle of His b) SA node
   c) AV node d) Purkinje fibres
10. Intra aortic balloon is filled with
   a) hydrogen b) Helium
   c) nitrogen d) oxygen
11. Blood dialysis is also called
   a) artificial heart b) artificial lungs
   c) artificial liver d) artificial kidney
12. Southern blot technique is related to
   a) DNA profiling b) Widal test
   c) Blood test d) Sonography
13. Father of electrocardiography
   a) Einthoven b) Hook
   c) Odum d) Roseline
14. A fully pacemaker was introduced in 1960 by
   a) Bloch and Purcell b) Chardack
   c) Sir Godfrey Hounsfield d) Hans Berger

15. Blood dialyser works on the physical laws of ?
    a) Imbibition and osmosis b) plasmolysis
    c) Imbibition and diffusion d) Diffusion and Osmosis
16. Diagnostic test of the body fluids help the physician to
    a) screen for a disease yet to show its symptoms.
    b) Confirm an earlier diagnosis
    c) Monitor the course of the disease
    d) all the above
17. Which of the following is not the common morphological characteristics of spirochetes?
    a) They are gram-negative helical bacteria
    b) They are motile and have periplasmic flagella (endo flagella)
    c) They reproduce by transverse binary fusion
    d) They are obligate aerobes
18. Which of the following subspecies of Treponema pallidum causes endemic syphilis?
    a) Treponema carateum b) Treponema endemicum
    c) Treponema pertenue d) None of the above
19. The RPR test (Rapid Plasma Reagin test) is a nontreponemal test method that is a common screening test for syphilis, which of the following statement correctly describes the test?
    a) A screening test used for the detection of syphilis antibodies in the urine
    b) A screening test used for the detection of syphilis antibodies in the blood
    c) The test results for RPR are identified by using the microscope
    d) All of the above
20. A 30 year old man infected with syphilis developed a skin lesion on his prepuce, the lesion was oval in shape and painless.
    What is the specific name for this type of lesion?
    a) Nodules b) Papule
    c) Eczema d) Hard chancre
21. Epidemic Relapsing fever in humans is caused by the infected body louse that acts as a vector and transfers the pathogen to humans.
    Which of the following is the most likely spirochete?
    a) Borrelia recurrentis b) Leptospira interrogans
    c) Borrelia burgdorferi d) Borrelia hermsii
22. The following pathogen is transmitted to humans through the bite of infected ticks, flu like symptoms and ringlike skin rashes occur which is also known as Lyme disease.
    Name the most likely pathogen
    a) Leptospira interrogans b) Bordetella pertusis
    c) Borrelia burgdorferi d) Enterococcus faecali

23. Which of the following statements is most correct about the dark field microscopy for the diagnosis of spirochetes?
   a) Performed for the identification and detection of spirochetes from the specimen collected from the oral cavity
   b) The specimen is stained and detected under the compound microscope
   c) The color of the spirochetes appears grey when observed under the dark background
   d) Performed for the observation and detection of thin spirochetes suspended in a liquid

24. Which of the following organisms is NOT commonly found as a part of normal flora in the oral cavity?
   a) Streptococcus mutans
   b) Borrelia buccalis
   c) Spirillum minor
   d) Candida albicans

25. What stain is mostly used for the detection of Borrelia spp that causes Relapsing fever?
   a) Gram stain
   b) Ziehl-Neelsen stain
   c) Giemsa stain
   d) Methylene blue

26. The bacteria causing Leptospirosis are difficult to isolate from urine, blood, or CSF specimens by culture method, therefore a confirmation test should be performed. Which of the following statement is most correct in the diagnosis of the disease?
   a) RPR tests for the detection of serogroup antigens from the acute or convalescent phase
   b) Antibodies are tested against the serogroup antigens from the acute or convalescent phase
   c) Darkfield microscopy method is done to detect the pathogen from serum samples
   d) All of the above

27. The diagnosis of Lyme disease is done by performing two serological tests after the screening test, one is a positive confirmatory ELISA test, what is the other test?
   a) Western blotting assay
   b) PCR
   c) Immunofluorescent assay
   d) Southern blotting assay

28. The following spirochetes causes skin disease known as Pinta prevalent in Latin America and primarily seen in individuals who have dark skin color, the human transmission is by direct contact or vectors such as flies.

   Name the possible pathogen?
   a) Borrelia hermsii
   b) Spirillum minor
   c) Treponema pallidum subspecies pertenue
   d) Treponema carateum

29. Which of the following pathogen causes sexually transmitted diseases?
    a) Treponema pallidum subspecies endemicum
    b) Treponema pallidum subspecies pallidum
    c) Borrelia recurrentis
    d) Borrelia hermsii
30. Which of the following statements is not correct about 'congenital syphilis'?
    a) The spirochetes are transferred from mother to fetus across the placenta
    b) The early manifestations occur in children during the birth
    c) Five to ten percent of infected children can develop cutaneous lesions
    d) The infection can lead to stillbirth
31. What is the most likely pathogen related to rat-bite fever?
    a) Leptospira interrogans
    b) Borrelia hermsii
    c) Treponema pallidum subspecies endemicum
    d) Spirillum minor
32. Which of the following infections are transmitted through the non-sexual route caused by the Treponema spp?
    a) Yaws, Bejel and Pinta   b) Visceral leishmaniasis
    c) Shingles   d) Donovanosis
33. 'Syphilis' is caused by Treponema spp.
    What is the other major disease that is caused by the bacteria?
    a) Lyme disease   b) Tularemia
    c) Periodontal disease   d) Infectious mononucleosis
34. Which of the following test is a simple, low-cost, and commonly used test for screening syphilis infection around the world?
    a) Western blot   b) VDRL test
    c) Agglutination test   d) None of the above
35. Penicillin is the drug of choice for the treatment of syphilis, but in recent years it has been found to be highly resistant.
    Which of the following types of antibiotic is recommended for early as well as late-stage syphilis that show resistance to Penicillin?
    a) Macrolides   b) Ceftriaxone
    c) Tetracyclines   d) Fluoroquinolones
36. Endemic syphilis is mainly transmitted through nonsexual contact and has been found to be prevalent in which of the following country?
    a) USA   b) Europe
    c) Spain   d) South Africa
37. Which one of the given diseases is caused by protozoa?
    a) Malaria   b) Diphtheria
    c) Cholera   d) Pneumonia

38. Which of the given organs are affected by malaria?
    a) Heart b) Kidney
    c) Spleen d) Stomach
39. Which of the given human organs is responsible for alcohol detoxification?
    a) Lung b) Liver
    c) Kidney d) Intestines
40. Which of the substances are responsible for Arthritis in the joints of the body?
    a) Albumin b) Cholesterol
    c) Urea d) Uric acid
41. Dropsy disease is caused by which of the given substances?
    a) Mustard oil b) kerosene oil
    c) Sugar d) Salt
42. Diarrhoea is caused by which of the given vectors?
    a) Amoeba b) Bacteria
    c) Fungus d) Rotavirus
43. Hysteria is the disease commonly found in which among the given options?
    a) Young men b) Young women
    c) Old women d) None of these
44. Name the disease caused by swelling of the membrane over the spinal cord and brain.
    a) Paralysis b) Leukaemia
    c) Meningitis d) Sclerosis
45. Anthophobia is the fear of which of the given options?
    a) Cats b) Water
    c) Fruits d) Flowers
46. Hydrophobia is caused by which of the following options?
    a) Virus b) Bacteria
    c) Protozoan d) Fungus
47. Which of the given is responsible for yellow fever?
    a) Housefly b) Mosquito
    c) Water d) Bacteria
48. What happens in the body of a person who is suffering from dengue fever?
    a) His platelets decrease b) His sugar level increases
    c) His sugar level decreases d) His platelets increase
49. Which of the given diseases caused due to the deficiency of iodine?
    a) Cancer b) Night Blindness
    c) Goitre d) Rickets
50. What is the full form of MRI, a tool for diagnosis?
    a) Magnetic Resonance Index b) Magnetic Resonance Imaging
    c) Magnetic Resonance Information d) None of these

51. Which of the given is responsible for Ergotism disease?
    a) Polluted water b) Uncooked food
    c) Rotting vegetables d) Contaminated grains
52. Which of the given is responsible for Itai-Itai disease?
    a) Cadmium b) Lead
    c) Nickel d) Mercury
53. For which of the given, BMD tests are performed?
    a) Arthritis b) Osteomalacia
    c) Osteoporosis d) None of these
54. In medical terms, "Golden Hour" is related to which of the given options.
    a) Heart attack b) Cancer
    c) AIDS d) Childbirth
55. Which of the following diseases are not treated under DPT vaccines?
    a) Poli b) Diphtheria
    c) Tetanus d) Typhoid
56. When any disease spread across the world then what it is called?
    a) Endemic b) Pandemic
    c) Epizootic d) None of these
57. Deficiency of which vitamin causes Scurvy disease?
    a) Vitamin D b) Vitamin C
    c) Vitamin K d) Vitamin A
58. Which one of the following is used in the treatment of blood cancer?
    a) Iodine 131 b) Sodium 24
    c) Phosphorus 32 d) Cobalt 60
59. Where is the Indian Veterinary Research institute located?
    a) Bareilly b) Mathura
    c) Karnal d) Patna
60. Which of the following is an important source of vitamin E?
    a) Palm oil b) Coconut oil
    c) Mustard oil d) Wheat germ oil
61. Who discovered vitamins?
    a) Gerardus Johannes Mulder b) Miller and Urey
    c) funk d) Anselme Payen
62. Where is vitamin stored in the body?
    a) Skin b) Liver
    c) Lungs d) Kidney
63. Which type of cells increases leukaemia?
    a) Bone cells b) Platelets
    c) Red blood cells d) White blood cells

64. What do you call someone who can't stop eating?
    a) Bulimia b) Diabetes
    c) Anorexia Nervosa d) Hyperacidity
65. Which vitamin is obtained from sun rays?
    a) Vitamin A b) Vitamin C
    c) Vitamin K d) Vitamin D
66. Which mirror is used by the dentist to see the image of the teeth of a patient?
    a) Concave mirror b) Convex lens
    c) Convex mirror d) Plane mirror
67. Which mosquito causes the Zika virus?
    a) H1N1
    b) Tick-transmitted virus
    c) The varicella zoster virus
    d) It transmitted by Aedes Mosquitoes
68. What species causes typhoid fever?
    a) Virus b) Bacteria
    c) Fungus d) Allergy
69. What is the reason behind the defect of presbyopia?
    a) Gradual weakening of ciliary muscles only
    b) Diminishing flexibility of the eye lens only
    c) Both gradual weakening of ciliary muscles and Diminishing flexibility of the eye lens
    d) Sudden dysfunction of ciliary muscles and eye lens
70. Which is not caused by viruses?
    a) Cholera b) Chickenpox
    c) Hepatitis d) Measles
71. Which among the following is the richest source of protein?
    a) Beetroot b) potato
    c) Soybean d) wheat
72. What is break fever most commonly known as?
    a) Typhoid b) Rhinitis
    c) Yellow fever d) Dengue
73. The immunization technique was developed by whom?
    a) Louis Pasteur b) Robert Koch
    c) Joseph lister d) Edward Jenner
74. Malfunctioning of which one of the following causes diabetes?
    a) Liver b) pancreas
    c) Kidney d) Heart

75. A medicine bottle containing tablets or capsules, and a small pouch of silica gel are kept to?
    a) Absorb moisture b) Absorb gases
    c) Keep the bottle warm d) kill bacteria
76. Dropsy is a disease caused due to adulteration in?
    a) Ghee b) Turmeric powder
    c) Mustard oil d) Argon oil
77. Widal test is commonly used for detection of
    a) AIDS b) Tuberculosis
    c) Sexually transmitted diseases d) Typhoid
78. Balloon pump is used in disease concerned with
    a) Brain b) lungs
    c) liver d) heart
79. Blood dialyser is also called
    a) artificial heart b) artificial kidney
    c) artificial lung d) artificial liver
79. Artificial arteries are made of
    a) rubber b) silver
    c) glass d) daclon or teflon
80. The technique involving the as of positron emitting radio isotopes is
    a) CT scanning b) PET scanning
    c) NMR imaging d) SQUID .
81. Grafting between two members of the same species is
    a) autograft b) allograft
    c) xenograft d) none of these
82. Scientist pipointed the location of colour processing centres in human visual cortex by means of
    a) PET scanning b) NMR imaging
    c) CT scanning d) Ultra sound imaging
83. Relative biological effectiveness is related to
    a) soil b) water
    c) radiation d) pollution
84. The pacemaker of heart is
    a) Bundle of His b) SA node
    c) AV node d) Purkinje fibres
85. Intra aortic balloon is filled with
    a) hydrogen b) Helium
    c) nitrogen d) oxygen

86. Blood dialysis is also called
a) artificial heart b) artificial lungs
c) artificial liver d) artificial kidney
87. Southern blot technique is related to
a) DNA profiling b) Widal test
c) Blood test d) Sonography
88. Father of electrocardiography
a) Einthoven b) Hook
c) Odum d) Roseline
89. A fully pacemaker was introduced in 1960 by
a) Bloch and Purcell b) Chardack
c) Sir Godfrey Hounsfield d) Hans Berger
90. Blood dialyser works on the physical laws of ?
a) Imbibition and osmosis b) plasmolysis
c) Imbibition and diffusion d) Diffusion and Osmosis
91. Widal test is commonly used for detection of
a) AIDS b) Tuberculosis
c) Sexually transmitted diseases d) Typhoid
92. Balloon pump is used in disease concerned with
a) Brain b) lungs
c) liver d) heart
93. Blood dialyser is also called
a) artificial heart b) artificial kidney
c) artificial lung d) artificial liver
94. Artificial arteries are made of
a) rubber b) silver
c) glass d) daclon or teflon
95. The technique involving the as of positron emitting radio isotopes is
a) CT scanning b) PET scanning
c) NMR imaging d) SQUID
96. Grafting between two members of the same species is
a) autograft b) allograft
c) xenograft d) none of these
97. Scientist pipointed the location of colour processing centres in human visual cortex by means of
a) PET scanning b) NMR imaging
c) CT scanning d) Ultra sound imaging
98. Relative biological effectiveness is related to
a) soil b) water
c) radiatio d) pollution

99. The pacemaker of heart is
   a) Bundle of His b) SA node
   c) AV node d) Purkinje fibres
100. Intra aortic ba lloon is filled with
   a) hydrogen b) Helium
   c) nitrogen d) oxygen
101. Blood dialysis is also called
   a) artificial heart b) artificial lungs
   c) artificial liver d) artificial kidney
102. Southern blot technique is related to
   a) DNA profiling b) Widal test
   c) Blood test d) Sonography
103. Father of electrocardiography
   a) Einthoven b) Hook
   c) Odum d) Roseline
104. A fully pacemaker was introduced in 1960 by
   a) Bloch and Purcell b) Chardack
   c) Sir Godfrey Hounsfield d) Hans Berger
105. Blood dialyser works on the physical laws of ?
   a) Imbibition and osmosis b) plasmolysis
   c) Imbibition and diffusion d) Diffusion and Osmosis

Answer Key

1	d	2	d	3	b	4	d	5	b	6	b	7	a
8	c	9	b	10	b	11	d	12	a	13	a	14	b
15	d	16	d	17	d	18	b	19	b	20	d	21	a
22	c	23	d	24	c	25	c	26	b	27	a	28	d
29	b	30	c	31	d	32	a	33	c	34	b	35	a
36	d	37	a	38	c	39	b	40	d	41	a	42	d
43	b	44	c	45	d	46	a	47	b	48	a	49	c
50	b	51	d	52	a	53	c	54	a	55	d	56	b
57	b	58	d	59	a	60	d	61	c	62	b	63	d
64	a	65	d	66	a	67	d	68	b	69	c	70	a
71	c	72	d	73	d	74	b	75	a	76	c	77	d
78	b	79	d	80	b	81	b	82	a	83	c	84	b
85	b	86	d	87	a	88	b	89	b	90	d	91	d
92	d	93	b	94	d	95	b	96	b	97	a	98	c
99	b	100	b	101	d	102	a	103	a	104	b	105	d

14

Prevention and Control of Diseases

Felix Uchenna Samuel[1], Ibrahim Mohammed Abdul[2] and Ama Adadzewa Eshun[3]

[1]*Animal Science Program, Alabama Cooperative Extension*
Alabama A&M University, Normal
[2]*National Animal Production Research Institute, Ahmadu Bello University, Nigeria*
[3]*Department of Food and Animal Sciences, Alabama A&M University, Normal*

Introductioin

Poultry diseases can be caused by bacteria, viruses, fungi, parasites, or a combination of these pathogens. Common poultry diseases include Newcastle disease, avian influenza, infectious bronchitis, infectious bursal disease, coccidiosis, and salmonellosis, among others (Grace *et al.*, 2024). These diseases can affect various organs and systems in poultry, including the respiratory, gastrointestinal, and immune systems, leading to a wide range of clinical signs and symptoms (Dunislawska *et al.*, 2024). Prevention and control of diseases in poultry is paramount for maintaining the health and welfare of poultry flocks and ensuring the sustainability of the poultry industry. Poultry diseases can have devastating effects on production, leading to decreased productivity, increased mortality rates, and significant economic losses. Therefore, implementing effective prevention and control measures is essential for poultry producers to mitigate the risks associated with diseases (George & George, 2023).

Prevention and Control of poultry Diseases

This explores various aspects of disease prevention and control in poultry, including biosecurity measures, vaccination programs, management practices, and disease surveillance.

1. Biosecurity Measures

Biosecurity is a set of practices designed to prevent the introduction and spread of diseases within poultry flocks. Implementing robust biosecurity measures is the first line of defense against disease outbreaks (Subasinghe *et al.*, 2023). Key biosecurity practices include:

Restricted Access: Limiting access to poultry facilities to essential personnel only helps prevent the introduction of pathogens from outside sources.

Cleaning and Disinfection: Regular cleaning and disinfection of poultry houses, equipment, and vehicles help eliminate disease-causing organisms and reduce the risk of contamination.

Quarantine: Quarantining new birds before introducing them to the existing flock allows for observation and testing to detect any potential diseases before they spread.

Rodent and Pest Control: Implementing measures to control rodents, insects, and other pests helps reduce the risk of disease transmission.

Biosecurity Education: Educating farm workers about the importance of biosecurity and proper hygiene practices helps ensure compliance with biosecurity protocols.

2. Vaccination Programs

Vaccination is an effective strategy for preventing infectious diseases in poultry. Vaccines stimulate the bird's immune system to produce antibodies against specific pathogens, providing immunity against infection. Vaccination programs should be tailored to the specific disease risks in each region and poultry operation (Abdallah *et al.*, 2023). Key considerations for vaccination programs include:

Vaccine Selection: Choosing the right vaccines based on the prevalent diseases in the area and the age and type of poultry being vaccinated.

Vaccine Administration: Ensuring vaccines are administered correctly according to the manufacturer's instructions, including dosage, route of administration, and timing.

Vaccination Schedule: Developing a vaccination schedule that takes into account the age of the birds, the risk of disease exposure, and the duration of immunity provided by each vaccine.

Vaccine Storage and Handling: Proper storage and handling of vaccines are essential to maintain their efficacy. Vaccines should be stored at the correct temperature and protected from light and contamination.

Monitoring and Evaluation: Regular monitoring of vaccine efficacy and disease incidence helps ensure that vaccination programs are effective in controlling disease outbreaks.

3. Management Practices

Good management practices play a crucial role in disease prevention and control in poultry. Proper nutrition, housing, and husbandry practices help maintain optimal health and immunity in poultry flocks (Serbessa *et al.*, 2023). Key management practices include:

Nutrition: Providing a balanced diet with adequate levels of essential nutrients, vitamins, and minerals helps support the bird's immune system and overall health.

Housing: Maintaining clean and well-ventilated housing facilities with adequate space and bedding reduces stress and minimizes the risk of disease transmission.

Sanitation: Implementing strict sanitation protocols, including regular cleaning and disinfection of feeders, waterers, and housing facilities, helps prevent the buildup of pathogens.

Water Quality: Providing clean and uncontaminated water is essential for maintaining hydration and preventing the spread of waterborne diseases.

Stocking Density: Avoiding overcrowding and maintaining appropriate stocking densities help reduce stress and minimize the risk of disease transmission within the flock.

4. Disease Surveillance

Regular monitoring and surveillance of poultry flocks are essential for early detection and control of disease outbreaks (Grace *et al.*, 2024). Disease surveillance involves:

Clinical Observation: Monitoring birds for signs of illness, including changes in behavior, appetite, and productivity, helps identify potential disease outbreaks early.

Diagnostic Testing: Conducting diagnostic tests, such as blood tests, fecal examinations, and necropsies, helps confirm the presence of diseases and identify the causative agents.

Epidemiological Investigations: Investigating disease outbreaks to determine the source of infection and the mode of transmission helps implement targeted control measures and prevent further spread.

Reporting: Reporting suspected or confirmed cases of reportable diseases to the appropriate authorities helps facilitate rapid response and control efforts.

Conclusion

Prevention and control of diseases in poultry are essential for maintaining the health and productivity of poultry flocks and ensuring the sustainability of the poultry industry. By implementing robust biosecurity measures, vaccination programs, management practices, and disease surveillance, poultry producers can minimize the risks associated with diseases and safeguard the welfare and profitability of their operations. It is essential for poultry producers to work closely with veterinarians, extension agents, and other industry stakeholders to develop and implement comprehensive disease prevention and control strategies tailored to their specific needs and circumstances. With proactive management and diligent adherence to best practices, poultry producers can effectively mitigate the impact of diseases and maintain healthy and productive flocks for years to come.

References

Grace, D , Knight-Jones, T. J., Melaku, A , Alders, R., & Jemberu, W. T. (2024). The Public Health Importance and Management of Infectious Poultry Diseases in Smallholder Systems in Africa. Foods, 13(3), 411.

Dunislawska, A., Pietrzak, E., Bełdowska, A., & Siwek, M. (2024). Health in poultry-immunity and microbiome with regard to a concept of one health. Physical Sciences Reviews, 9(1), 477-495.

George, A. S., & George, A. H. (2023). Optimizing poultry production through advanced monitoring and control systems. Partners Universal International Innovation Journal, 1(5), 77-97.

Subasinghe, R., Alday-Sanz, V., Bondad-Reantaso, M. G., Jie, H., Shinn, A. P., & Sorgeloos, P. (2023). Biosecurity: Reducing the burden of disease. Journal of the World Aquaculture Society, 54(2), 397-426.

Abdallah, N., Tekelioğlu, B. K., Kurşun, K., Baylan, M., & Ümit, E. L. Ç. İ. (2023). Vaccination and Poultry (chicken) Production. Journal of Agriculture, Food, Environment and Animal Sciences, 4(1), 119-136.

Serbessa, T. A., Geleta, Y. G., & Terfa, I. O. (2023). Review on diseases and health management of poultry and swine. International Journal of Avian & Wildlife Biology, 7(1), 27-38.

Multiple Choice Questions and Answers

1. What is the primary purpose of implementing biosecurity measures in poultry farms?

   a) Increase egg production b) Enhance poultry welfare

   c) Prevent disease outbreaks d) Reduce feed costs

2. Which of the following is NOT a key biosecurity practice?
   a) Restricted Access
   b) Rodent and Pest Control
   c) Free-range farming
   d) Cleaning and Disinfection
3. What does quarantine involve in the context of poultry farming?
   a) Isolating sick birds from healthy ones
   b) Limiting access to poultry facilities
   c) Observing and testing new birds before introducing them to the flock
   d) Regular cleaning and disinfection
4. Why is biosecurity education important on poultry farms?
   a) To increase egg production
   b) To reduce labor costs
   c) To ensure compliance with biosecurity protocols
   d) To improve meat quality
5. What is the purpose of rodent and pest control in biosecurity?
   a) Improve poultry welfare
   b) Enhance farm aesthetics
   c) Reduce the risk of disease transmission
   d) Increase egg production
6. Which of the following is NOT a key component of biosecurity measures?
   a) Vaccination programs
   b) Restricted Access
   c) Cleaning and Disinfection
   d) Quarantine
7 What is the role of cleaning and disinfection in biosecurity?
   a) Increase disease transmission
   b) Reduce the risk of contamination
   c) Enhance egg production
   d) Improve poultry welfare
8. Why is restricted access important in biosecurity?
   a) To increase disease spread
   b) To improve meat quality
   c) To prevent the introduction of pathogens
   d) To decrease feed costs
9. What is the purpose of implementing biosecurity measures?
   a) To maximize mortality rates
   b) To minimize egg production
   c) To prevent disease outbreaks
   d) To reduce farm profitability
10. What is the significance of educating farm workers about biosecurity?
   a) To increase feed costs
   b) To ensure compliance with biosecurity protocols
   c) To reduce vaccination costs
   d) To improve meat quality
11. How do vaccines work in preventing diseases in poultry?
   a) By directly killing pathogens
   b) By stimulating the immune system to produce antibodies
   c) By providing vitamins and minerals
   d) By increasing stocking density

12. What is a key consideration for vaccine selection in poultry?
    a) Brand popularity b) Price
    c) Disease prevalence in the region d) Vaccine color
13. Why is correct vaccine administration important?
    a) To improve egg quality b) To reduce labor costs
    c) To avoid adverse effects on poultry d) To increase farm profitability
14. What should be considered when developing a vaccination schedule?
    a) Employee schedules b) Weather conditions
    c) Bird age and disease risk d) Market demand
15. What is essential for proper vaccine storage and handling?
    a) Exposure to sunlight b) Incorrect labeling
    c) Maintaining correct temperature d) Mixing vaccines
16. How does monitoring and evaluation contribute to vaccination programs?
    a) By increasing feed costs
    b) By reducing vaccination frequency
    c) By ensuring program effectiveness
    d) By improving meat quality
17. What is the purpose of vaccine storage and handling procedures?
    a) To maximize disease spread b) To increase egg production
    c) To maintain vaccine efficacy d) To minimize poultry welfare
18. Why is it important to tailor vaccination programs to specific poultry operations?
    a) To reduce labor costs b) To increase feed costs
    c) To maximize mortality rates d) To address specific disease risks
19. What is the significance of vaccine administration according to manufacturer's instructions?
    a) To reduce vaccination costs b) To improve meat quality
    c) To ensure vaccine efficacy d) To decrease farm profitability
20. How does vaccination contribute to disease prevention and control?
    a) By increasing disease transmission b) By reducing the risk of infection
    c) By minimizing egg production d) By maximizing mortality rates
21. Why is proper nutrition important for disease prevention in poultry?
    a) To increase feed costs b) To reduce egg production
    c) To support the immune system d) To decrease farm profitability
22. What role does housing play in disease prevention?
    a) Increase stress levels
    b) Enhance disease transmission
    c) Provide protection from weather conditions
    d) Reduce water consumption

23. What is the purpose of sanitation protocols in poultry farming?
    a) To attract pests
    b) To reduce cleaning frequency
    c) To prevent pathogen buildup
    d) To increase disease spread
24. Why is providing clean water important for poultry health?
    a) To increase mortality rates
    b) To reduce egg production
    c) To maintain hydration and prevent disease spread
    d) To decrease feed costs
25. How does stocking density affect disease transmission?
    a) Higher stocking density reduces stress
    b) Lower stocking density increases the risk of disease spread
    c) Higher stocking density decreases disease transmission
    d) Stocking density does not affect disease transmission
26. What is the purpose of nutrition management in poultry farming?
    a) To maximize mortality rates
    b) To improve meat quality
    c) To support growth and immunity
    d) To reduce labor costs
27. Why is maintaining proper ventilation important in poultry housing?
    a) To increase disease transmission
    b) To reduce egg production
    c) To prevent respiratory diseases
    d) To decrease farm profitability
28. How does sanitation contribute to disease prevention in poultry farming?
    a) By increasing pathogen buildup
    b) By decreasing water quality
    c) By reducing disease transmission
    d) By minimizing egg production
29. What is the role of water quality in disease prevention?
    a) To increase mortality rates
    b) To reduce egg production
    c) To maintain hydration and prevent disease spread
    d) To decrease feed costs
30. How does stocking density impact poultry welfare?
    a) Higher stocking density improves welfare
    b) Lower stocking density increases stress
    c) Stocking density has no effect on welfare
    d) Stocking density reduces feed costs
31. What is the primary goal of disease surveillance in poultry farms?
    a) Increase egg production
    b) Identify sick birds for culling
    c) Early detection and control of disease outbreaks
    d) Reduce vaccination costs
32. Which method is used for monitoring birds for signs of illness?
    a) Blood tests
    b) Fecal examinations
    c) Clinical observation
    d) Vaccination

33. What is the purpose of diagnostic testing in disease surveillance?
    a) To improve egg quality
    b) To confirm the presence of diseases
    c) To increase feed costs
    d) To reduce labor costs
34. Why are epidemiological investigations conducted during disease outbreaks?
    a) To increase egg production
    b) To identify the source of infection and mode of transmission
    c) To reduce vaccination costs
    d) To improve meat quality
35. Why is reporting suspected cases of diseases important?
    a) To increase feed costs
    b) To improve egg quality
    c) To facilitate rapid response and control efforts
    d) To decrease farm profitability
36. What is the significance of clinical observation in disease surveillance?
    a) To improve meat quality
    b) To detect signs of illness in birds
    c) To increase egg production
    d) To minimize mortality rates
37. How does diagnostic testing contribute to disease control?
    a) By increasing disease transmission
    b) By confirming the presence of diseases
    c) By minimizing egg production
    d) By maximizing mortality rates
38. Why are epidemiological investigations important during disease outbreaks?
    a) To reduce labor costs
    b) To identify the causative agent
    c) To decrease feed costs
    d) To maximize mortality rates
39. What is the role of reporting suspected cases of diseases?
    a) To increase egg production
    b) To improve meat quality
    c) To facilitate rapid response and control efforts
    d) To decrease farm profitability
40. How does disease surveillance contribute to poultry health management?
    a) By increasing disease spread
    b) By reducing the impact of outbreaks
    c) By minimizing egg production
    d) By maximizing mortality rates
41. Why is prevention and control of diseases essential in poultry farming?
    a) To increase mortality rates
    b) To reduce egg production
    c) To maintain the health and productivity of poultry flocks
    d) To decrease farm profitability

42. What are the potential consequences of disease outbreaks in poultry farms?
    a) Increased profitability
    b) Enhanced poultry welfare
    c) Decreased productivity and economic losses
    d) Improved meat quality

43 How can effective prevention and control measures mitigate the risks associated with diseases?
    a) By increasing disease transmission
    b) By maximizing mortality rates
    c) By minimizing the impact of outbreaks
    d) By decreasing vaccination costs

44. Why is collaboration with veterinarians and industry stakeholders important in disease prevention?
    a) To maximize mortality rates
    b) To improve meat quality
    c) To develop comprehensive prevention strategies
    d) To increase egg production

45. What is the role of proactive management in disease prevention and control?
    a) To minimize mortality rates
    b) To increase disease spread
    c) To ensure rapid response to outbreaks
    d) To decrease farm profitability

46. How can poultry producers safeguard the welfare of their flocks?
    a) By increasing disease transmission
    b) By implementing biosecurity measures
    c) By reducing stocking density
    d) By decreasing feed costs

47. What measures can be taken to ensure the sustainability of the poultry industry?
    a) Maximizing mortality rates
    b) Minimizing disease outbreaks
    c) Reducing egg production
    d) Increasing feed costs

48. Why is it important to tailor disease prevention and control strategies to specific poultry operations?
    a) To increase feed costs
    b) To improve meat quality
    c) To address specific disease risks
    d) To maximize mortality rates

49. How can disease prevention and control measures contribute to the sustainability of the poultry industry?
    a) By increasing disease spread
    b) By minimizing economic losses
    c) By maximizing mortality rates
    d) By decreasing feed costs

50. What is the long-term benefit of implementing effective disease prevention and control measures?
    a) Increased profitability
    b) Enhanced poultry welfare
    c) Sustainable poultry production
    d) Decreased productivity.

Answer Key

1	c	2	c	3	c	4	c	5	c	6	a	7	b
8	c	9	c	10	b	11	b	12	c	13	c	14	c
15	c	16	c	17	c	18	d	19	c	20	b	21	c
22	c	23	c	24	c	25	b	26	c	27	c	28	c
29	c	30	b	31	c	32	c	33	b	34	b	35	c
36	b	37	b	38	b	39	c	40	b	41	c	42	c
43	c	44	c	45	c	46	b	47	b	48	c	49	b
50	c												

15

General Clinical Examination

Abbas Rabiu Ishaq

Paws and Claws Specialist Veterinary Clinic, Al-Sahafa District Riyadh Kingdom of Saudi Arabia

Introduction

A thoroughly performed physical examination in poultry and avian clinical practice is of great importance. Most avian species happen to be prey animals, with the exception of a few raptors that tend to be predatory. This makes them try to appear healthy, in preparation to escape from potential predators, and as such, makes it difficult for their owners, keepers and veterinarians to detect early diseases. Physical examination when carefully performed in detail, increases the chances of obtaining fewer differential diagnosis that are likely to be harboring the confirmatory diagnosis after laboratory works are being performed. In essence, a thorough physical examination brings about cost efficiency in poultry/avian clinical practice. Take for instance, a farm with over 50,000 layers, having lowered productivity. It will be cumbersome to go ahead and start blood sampling, faecal sampling or oral cavity swabs for laboratory analysis as the starting point. The disadvantages will be high labour demands, high capital demands, more stress on the animals and of course, long time till feasible outcome is to be obtained.

On the other hand, a clinician with an approach that is more oriented towards clinical observation, leading to possible further diagnostics will consider overall avian presentation, faecal appearance (Colour, consistency, smell, presence of adult worms or ova, blood droplets, etc., posture, gait, wing positioning, and feather (contour, colour, presence of nits, etc. Thorough examination of the aforementioned will offer some vital information, which may serve as a tentative diagnosis in many cases.

A thorough physical examination (Hands on observation) is in the order of head, nares, beak, mouth/buccal cavity, eyes, ears, neck, crop, chest, abdomen, vent, legs and ends with the wings.

Head examination begins by evaluating the feathers on the head, looking for normal feather development and good quality feathers. The presence of bare patches or poor feather development may be indicating nutritional, metabolic, systemic diseases or due to trauma. Excessive head region feather flakiness can be due to nutritional condition such as a vitamin A deficiency.

Nares should be checked for presence of any exudates/discharges, discolouration, flakiness, dryness or excessive moisture. Though subject to some variations even within same species, the nares colour can be used for aging and sexing, especially in budgies. Hypertrophied nares in female birds can be an indication for breeding, while in males can be due to estrogen-producing testicular tumours. Another important thing that should not be ignored during nares examination is the symmetry, any size or shape difference can be suggesting a defect. For instance, remarkable enlargement can be due to chronic rhinitis of trauma.

Multiple Choice Questions

1. Routine avian examination may comprise all except one of below
   a) 'hands on' physical examination
   b) weight check
   c) laboratory tests of the droppings and the blood
   d) FNA for histopathology
2. One of the following is not true about what to be examined in all avian species by a veterinarian.
   a) Ability to fly in all avian species b) Gait
   c) Body condition score d) None
3. When examining the head, one of below is not applicable in avian
   a) Feather condition b) Beak appearance
   c) External nares d) Muzzle color
4. An abnormal crest feather in cockatoos and parrots may be suggestive of
   a) Aspergillosis
   b) Psittacine beak and feather disease
   c) Chlamydiasis
   d) All above
5. Missing fe athers from the head of traumatic cause such as fights can be ascertained by
   a) Presence of green stumps b) Presence of black stumps
   c) Presence of light-red stumps d) No possible clues at all
6. Skin flakiness on head region can be due to all except
   a) Vitamin A deficiency b) Vitamin E deficiency
   c) Photosensitization d) hyperventilation
7. Another term used to describe the external nares in avian is
   a) core b) dorso
   c) cere d) dorsum
8. Normal appearance of external nares in avian is
   a) Always moist b) Dry and slightly flaky
   c) Moist and pinkish d) Moist and yellowish
9. When examining the external nares in budgies, which of below is false decision
   a) Blue suggests a male
   b) Brown hypertrophy suggests a female with breeding hypertrophy
   c) Color should be white in all cases
   d) Light blue, brown or dark brown may indicate a female

10. A confirmed male budgerigar is brought for examination, which of below is true decision
    a) enlarged brown nare may indicate testicular tumor secreting estrogen
    b) color variation has no sexing significance
    c) a and b
    d) none
11. Which of below can be untrue about the beak
    a) little flakiness is normal
    b) excessive flakiness is suggestive of nutritional deficiencies
    c) flakiness is species related, not find in some
    d) all above
12. black/brown hemorrhages on beaks and toes may be due to
    a) excitation
    b) prolonged thirst
    c) fatty liver disease
    d) none above
13. Beak malocclusions can be from all except
    a) Trauma
    b) Genetic
    c) Malnutrition
    d) Thrush
14. Which of the below can be used to hold the beaks open during mouth examination?
    a) Mouth speculum
    b) Gauze strips
    c) Scissors
    d) All above
15. One of the following is not true about the epithelial lining of avian oral cavity
    a) It should be smooth
    b) There should be papillary spikes evenly distributed
    c) Off-white lesions may suggest hypovitaminosis A
    d) Greyish flakes may be due to bacterial infection
16. Oral cavity lesions can be caused by all except one of the following
    a) Bacterial infections
    b) Avian pox
    c) Trichomoniasis
    d) Schistosomiasis
17. One of the statements is false about avian candidiasis
    a) Is more encountered in young birds
    b) Incidence is more on captive birds
    c) Abscesses may be seen on sides of tongue
    d) Incidence is more in adult birds, owing to lifecycle of fungus
18. Blunt, round-edged choanal slit, devoid of papillae is indicative of
    a) Aspergillosis
    b) Hypovitaminosis C
    c) Hypovitaminosis A
    d) Hypovitaminosis k
19. Which one of the following is true about the third eyelids in avian
    a) Is deleted permanently during embryonic stage in all species
    b) Is well developed to extent that it functionally closes the eye when needed
    c) Present but not offering any physiological functions
    d) Is the only eyelid present in avian

20. Periophthalmitis, ocular discharges, and conjunctivitis may be due to
    a) Mycoplasmosis b) Erysipellosis
    c) Hemoproteos infection d) None
21. One of below is not true about ear infections in avian
    a) Is one of commonest conditions
    b) Otitis external is most frequent type
    c) Is a rare condition
    d) Discharges may be encountered
22. When examining the neck/trachea, one of the following is the least to be expected in an active avian
    a) Cervical vertebra fractures b) Presence of air sac mites
    c) Presence of unusual swellings d) Skin lacerations
23. Crop palpation is aimed at checking for all except
    a) Fistula b) Fluid/gas
    c) Foreign bodies d) Microbes
24. A thickened crop wall can be
    a) A normal finding b) Suggestive of moniliasis
    c) Due to crop parasites d) Compensatory hypertrophy to aid a weak gizzard
25. Crop fistulas can be detected by all except
    a) Food outflow b) Fistula visualization
    c) Presence of scab d) Injecting air using a syringe
26. Chest muscles condition can be helpful in
    a) Detecting early disease conditions b) Obesity detection
    c) Hydration status of avian d) All above
27. Which of below is true about the abdomen in avian
    a) Is relatively small
    b) Cranial boarder at base of sternum runs caudally to the ribs
    c) Cranial boarder at apex of sternum runs caudally to the ribs
    d) a and b
28. Which one of the following is an abnormal finding during abdominal palpation in avian
    a) gizzard palpation on the left side of the abdomen
    b) palpation of the right lobe of the liver
    c) egg palpation
    d) palpation of the sternum
29. Massively enlarged abdomen could be due to all except one of the following
    a) excessive water uptake b) ascites
    c) egg-binding d) obesity

30. One of below is false about massive enlargement of abdomen as described above
    a) mishandling can cause abdominal air sac rupture
    b) compromised respiration
    c) needle and syringe aspiration relieving in all cases
    d) death may occur
31. Fecal staining of vent may suggest
    a) Abdominal mass irritation
    b) Due to gastrointestinal viral infections
    c) Gastrointestinal bacterial infection
    d) All above
32. Hemorrhagic staining of cloaca can be due to all except one of below
    a) Cloacal papilloma b) Cloacal prolapse
    c) Egg binding d) Estrus
33. An enlarged and dilated vent is indicative of
    a) Hormonal stimulation b) Reproductive readiness
    c) a and b d) Excessive environmental temperature
34. Normal feet/legs appearance should be any of below except one
    a) Presence of some scales b) Scales to be similar to reptilian
    c) Devoid of scales in some avian d) a and b
35. Presence of crustiness may be suggestive of mites infection, commonly
    a) *Cheylitiella species* b) *Cnemidocoptes species*
    c) *Pneumonyssoides species* d) All above
36. Presence of pressure sores/ulcerations on bottom of feet may be due to
    a) Poor perches b) Vitamin A deficiencies
    c) Hypervitaminosis A d) A and b
37. An 8 months old turkey presented small blister like lesions on the comb, wattles, and corners of the beak and around the eyelids. Which of the following is the least likely cause
    a) Turkey pox b) Chicken pox
    c) Mosquito bite d) a and b
38. Psittacine integumentary lesions on non-infectious origin can be due to all except one of below
    a) Nutritional deficiencies b) Hormonal imbalances
    c) Slime d) Neoplasia
39. Which of below is true about avian skin biopsy
    a) Is difficult due to thinness of skin
    b) Thinness makes it easy to process
    c) Skin biopsies have limited significance
    d) B and c

40. one of the following is not normal finding in avian skin
    a) pale/bluish pink coloration b) opacity
    c) translucency d) elasticity
41. one of below is abnormal findink
    a) firm attachment of skin over skull
    b) loose attachment of skin around the feet
    c) firm skin attachment near wint tips
    d) loose skin around the thigh
42. heart disease can be a differential by seeing all except one of below, during clinical examination
    a) skin cyanosis b) jugular distension
    c) jaundice d) ascites
43. lungs auscultation can be best achieved via
    a) ventral chest b) dorsal thorax
    c) on the carinal apex d) ventral thoraco-abdominal junction
44. one of the following can be helpful in assessing peripheral blood circulation
    a) skin color b) skin temperature
    c) vessel turgidity d) all above
45. Whole body radiographs can be helpful in detecting all except one of the following
    a) opacified vessels b) pulmonary effusion
    c) liver enlargement d) none
46. which of the following is false about avian plain radiograph
    a) heart size changes with the cardiac cycle
    b) increased basilar to apical dimension suggests cardiomegaly
    c) heart size is independent of its cycle
    d) prominence of the left atrium suggests cardiomegaly
47. Which of below can be true about wattles in avian
    a) It is expected to be rigid
    b) Can be flexible or rigid depending on species
    c) Normal wattles should be flexible
    d) Texture depends on breeding cycle
48. One of below is not true with respect to the combs
    a) Should be thick
    b) Mostly upright
    c) Paired combs above eyes of adult grouse (Moorbird)
    d) Should be thin and elastic
49. One of below may be an abnormal coloration of the comb
    a) Red b) Yellow
    c) Orange d) Blue

50. The skin covering all except one of below should be heavily keratinized, as such appears tough
    a) Carinal apex
    b) Feet
    c) Beak
    d) Spurs
51. Irrespective of the avian species presented, one of below is termed abnormal during examination of the feather
    a) Color
    b) Arrangement
    c) Growth
    d) None
52. Which of the following is true about the visible glandular nature of the avian skin
    a) It has abundant sweat glands that moisten the feathers
    b) Has numerous sebaceous glands to lubricate the contour feathers
    c) It is devoid of both sebaceous and sweat glands
    d) a and b
53. Which of below is an abnormal epidermal modification with respect to species
    a) Smooth surfaced bare skin covering head of rockfowl
    b) Tubercles widespread on thick skin covering head of guineafowl
    c) Smooth surfaced thin skin covering head of vulture
    d) Thick, tubercle-covered skin around head of stork
54. One of the combinations is an abnormality during physical examination of avian eye
    a) Abundant skin around eyes of a falcon
    b) Abundant skin around eyes of a parrot
    c) Eyes devoid of skin, except the nictitating membrane on a broadbill
    d) All above
55. Two birds were brought to you, expected to be a couple for sexing. Which of below can be a close to accurate decision, based on integumentary modifications
    a) Significant outgrowths are mostly on head and neck
    b) Bird with larger and brighter ones is likely a male
    c) a and b
    d) Bird with larger and brighter ones is likely a female
56. A flock of storks are to be examined and sorted for breeding maturity, which of the following can be a misguiding judgement
    a) Those that have rudimentary or no integumentary outgrowths are matured enough for breeding
    b) The outgrowths are permanent once formed and can guide for maturity assessment
    c) There is size and color variation during breeding
    d) The outgrowths replaced an initially feather-covered areas upon maturity

57. One of below is a wrong decision during examination of throat/neck in avian
    a) A distensible, bare and loose neck skin on a duck shows airsacculitis
    b) Massive throat pouch on a pelican is a normal modification for feeding
    c) An inflatable oral sac in male great bustards could be from a leaking crop
    d) a and c

58. which of below findings is unusual during avian examination, with respect to the caruncles
    a) is always present in adult turkeys
    b) It is expected to be rounded
    c) Only present in males, irrespective of the species
    d) a and b

59. One of the following is true about the rictus
    a) It is soft border of the mouth from its angle
    b) It is expected to have an exclusively smooth surface, any other is termed abnormal
    c) Is expected to have very thick epidermis, any thin area is due to atrophy
    d) Molting does not occur in all species

60. When examining an avian for a suspected ear problem, which of the following can be applicable
    a) Look for the earlobes, which are always soft
    b) Look for rigid cartilaginous earlobes
    c) External ear canal is directly dorsal to the earlobes
    d) a and c

61. when examining birds, special considerations should be taken with regards to the fact that;
    a) birds, irrespective of species, share same vitals with other mammals
    b) birds may mask early illnesses owing to survival extinct from predation
    c) birds have higher metabolic rates compared to other animals
    d) b and c

62. The beak in all avians can also be called
    a) Beal
    b) Bill
    c) Rhamphotheca
    d) b and c

63. Which of below decisions is wrong, with respect to avian practice
    a) prior to diagnosis, trial medications can be administered
    b) whenever first diagnosis is termed to be wrong, new diagnosis should offer all desired results
    c) avian patients brought overnight can be kept till the next morning for a thorough diagnosis before medication
    d) all above

64. Which of the following is the MOST APPROPRIATE when bringing avian patient to the clinic
    a) look for a cleaner cage to bring your bird
    b) a box with minimal openings to avoid scaring the bird
    c) bring in the original cage of the bird as it is to the clinic
    d) a and b
65. Which of the recommendations is significant with respect to wildlife birds presented to the clinic
    a) bring in first to examine and release so as to minimize stressing the bird
    b) should be given no priority, as birds have similar mentality
    c) owners should wait with the birds at the clinic car park till their turn, to avoid mixing with home pets
    d) they can be kept till end of the dsy, so they get maximal attention
66. There is a need for sticking to safety tip(s) in clinics meant to be handling avian to avoid casualties, one of the options below can be applicable
    a) avoid using stainless steel tools to avoid heavy metal poisoning
    b) avoid using tools made from polytetrafluoroethylene (PTFE) to avoid poisoning
    c) air freshners can be helpful to calm birds from smells coming from others
    d) a and c
67. During examination, a female budgie nares appeared to be dark brown, which of below is true
    a) Is due to aflatoxins
    b) Is a sign of malnutrition
    c) Is normal
    d) A and b
68. A hypertrophied nares in female bird can be commonly due to
    a) Breeding season
    b) Fatty liver
    c) Renal failure
    d) None
69. Blue colouration of nares in a confirmed male budgie can be
    a) Sex variation
    b) Cyanosis
    c) Poisoning
    d) None
70. Presence of grooves on upper beak can be due to all except
    a) Chronic nasal discharges
    b) Poor beak polishing
    c) Sex variation
    d) None
71. Beak malocclusion can be from all except one of the following
    a) Malnutrition
    b) Hereditary
    c) Trauma
    d) Ornamental
72. Which of the following can be applicable to malocclusion in beaks
    a) Regular trimming is indicated
    b) Surgical correction can be done
    c) Beak replacement
    d) A and b
73. Presence of black/brown areas of hemorrhage on the beak and toenails may indicate
    a) Fatty liver disease
    b) Heat stress
    c) Brooding stress
    d) Avitaminosis B

74. All except one of the following birds are expected to have thin margins of the beak
   a) Macaw   b) Cockatoos
   c) Grey African parrots   d) All above
75. Presence of grayish cast, with a pungent odor in oral cavity of bird indicates
   a) Blocked crop   b) Bacterial infection
   c) Viral infection   d) Hypocalcaemia
76. The most common nutritional deficiency sign noticed in oral cavity of birds is
   a) Vitamin A deficiency   b) Vitamin E deficiency
   c) Iron deficiency   d) Riboflavine deficiency
77. Abscesses evident on the sides of the tongue of a young bird can be due to
   a) Warts virus   b) Candidiasis
   c) Crop worms   d) None of above
78. All except one of the following can cause mouth lesions in avian
   a) Aphtho's fever   b) Candidiasis
   c) Trichomoniasis   d) avian pox
79. Oral vesicles on young birds being hand raised are likely due to
   a) Aphtho's fever   b) Candidiasis
   c) Trichomoniasis   d) avian pox
80. A normal choanal slit margin should be
   a) Sharp   b) Blunt
   c) Rectangular   d) None
81. A non-defective choanal slit margin appears to be
   a) bordered by numerous sharp papillae   b) Slimy and smooth
   c) Rough and slimy   d) B and c
82. A blunted choanae indicates
   a) Normal finding   b) Vitamin A deficiency
   c) Choline deficiency   d) High carbohydrate diet
83. Absence of papillae on choanae is suggestive of
   a) Normal finding   b) Vitamin A deficiency
   c) Choline deficiency   d) High carbohydrate diet
84. Severely thickened edges of choanae with white plaques indicate
   a) Normal finding   b) Vitamin A deficiency
   c) Choline deficiency   d) High carbohydrate diet
85. Which of the following is true about the third eyelids in avians
   a) Is absent   b) Is present but vestigial
   c) Is highly functional   d) None
86. Corneal ulceration and eyelid lesions are commonly associated with
   a) Avian pox   b) Chicken pox
   c) Salmonellosis   d) Egg drop syndrome

87. Ocular discharges, conjunctivitis, matting of feathers around the eyes, and periophthalmic swellings are all indications of ___________ infections
a) Toxoplasma b) Anaplasma
c) Mycoplasma d) Mycobacteria

88. Ear infections are ________ in birds
a) Most common b) Uncommon
c) Seen only in sea avians d) Untreatable

89. Trachea transillumination in smaller birds such as finches can help in detecting ________
a) air sac mites b) Trachea lice
c) Cutaneous polyp d) None

90. Which of the following can be a complication during crop examination
a) Regurgitation b) Aspiration
c) A and b d) Anorexia

91. Which of the followingis true about the texture of a normal crop
a) Wall should be thin
b) Wall should be thick
c) Thickeness depends on species, some have rigid
d) None

92. Which of the following is suggestive of candidiasis during crop examination
a) A thin wall b) Thickened wall
c) Gritty feeling d) Presence of gas

93. Presence of food on the lower aspect of the crop may indicate
a) Brooding b) Aspiration
c) Crop fistula d) None

94. Presence of crop fistula can be demonstrated by all except one of the following
a) during feeding b) visualizing the actual fistula
c) routing d) scabbing

95. pectoral muscles and keelbone examination can be vital for;
a) knowing the type of avian b) knowing age
c) sexing of avian d) early disease diagnosis

96. Pectoral skin fold elasticitycan be used in
a) Detecting foreign body b) Hydration status
c) Seasonal variation d) Sexing

97. A dark trunk skin with no or little elasticity is an indication for
a) Ageing b) Dehydration
c) Seasonal variation d) Sexing

98. Reproductive tract disorders palpable during abdominal examination can be due to
a) egg-binding b) cystic ovaries
c) a and b d) not palpable

99. Rough palpation of the abdomen can cause
   a) Air sac rupture   b) Death
   c) Egg rupture   d) All above
100. A normal abdominal enlargement can be due to
   a) Presence of abdominal pebbles   b) Presence of eggs
   c) Presence of fluids   d) Presence of gases
101. A firm mass on the left side of the abdomen can be
   a) A tumour   b) Air sac
   c) Gizzard   d) None
102. One of the following is true about the liver during examination
   a) Is always palpable
   b) palpation of the right lobe indicates enlargement
   c) has no clinical significance
   d) a and c
   e. none
103. Ascites can be due to all except one of the following
   a) Heart disease   b) Reproductive tract disorder
   c) Liver enlargement   d) Neoplasms
104. Staining of the vent with droppings can be an indication of
   a) Diarrhea   b) Abdominal mass irritation
   c) Cloacal prolapse   d) Anorexia
105. The presence of an enlarged dilated vent can be due to;
   a) Reproductive hormonal stimulation   b) Anorexia
   c) Tachypnea   d) All above
106. Which of the following is true about a normal avian foot
   a) foot has scales similar to reptilian skin   b) smooth
   c) shining   d) all above
107. An observed pressure sores/ulcerations are commonly caused by
   a) Malnutrition   b) Bad perches
   c) A and b   d) Excessive light
108. Hyperkeratosis of the feet is commonly associated with
   a) Hypovitaminosis A   b) Hypervitaminosis A
   c) Hypovitaminosis D   d) Hypervitaminosis D
109. Crustiness of the feet/legs is an indication of
   a) Flea infestation   b) Cheylitiella infestation
   c) Cnemidocoptic infestation   d) None
110. Another name for condition above is
   a) Scaly leg/ face   b) Walking dandruff
   c) Xeroderma   d) Pyoderma

111. Tattoo for surgically sexed birds are placed mostly on
   a) Neck b) Foot
   c) Beak d) Wing web
112. Sexed males are marked at the_______
   a) Left side b) Right side
   c) Both sides d) Not marked
113. Sexed females are marked at the_______
   a) Left side b) Right side
   c) Both sides d) Not marked
114. Feather follicles filled with brownish debris suggests
   a) Acanthosis b) Xeroderma
   c) Mites d) None
115. Confirmation of condition above can be achieved by
   a) Allergy tests b) Bacterial culture
   c) Microscopically d) None
116. Which of the following is true about avian heart examination
   a) Difficult to examine due to high heart rates
   b) Heartbeats are inaudible
   c) Only 'lubb' sounds heard
   d) Only 'dubb' sounds heard
117. One of below options is true about respiratory auscultation in avian
   a) Stethoscopes are not helpful b) Can be readily checked
   c) Airsacs make it difficult d) A and c
118. One of the following is true about pectoral muscles in non-flying birds
   a) They are well-developed b) They are less developed
   c) They are absent d) None
119. One of the following is/are true about flying birds' pectoral muscles
   a) They are well-developed b) They are least developed
   c) They are absent d) None
120. One of the following is true about the pectoral muscles in layer chicken
   a) They are more developed compared to broiler
   b) They are less developed compared to broiler
   c) They are absent
   d) Seen only during laying
121. One of the following is true about the pectoral muscles in broiler chicken
   a) They are more developed compared to layers
   b) They are less developed compared to layers
   c) They are absent
   d) Seen only during laying

122. For a flying avian with normal body condition score__________ is true
   a) Muscles should protrude beyond keel bone
   b) Muscles should not protrude beyond keel
   c) Keel-muscle position not useful
   d) None
123. Presence of layer of fat between keel skin and the keel is_____________
   a) obesity
   b) Good body condition
   c) Nutritional deficiencies
   d) Cachexia
124. Massive and chronic alteration in vocalization is most likely due to
   a) Toxocariasis
   b) Colibacillosis
   c) Crop worms
   d) Aspergillosis
125. Dyspnea is seen as
   a) Heavy breathing
   b) Shortness of breathing
   c) Abnormal breathing sounds
   d) All above
126. Dyspnea is associated with
   a) Lung diseases
   b) Air sac diseases
   c) Both
   d) None
127. One of the following is/are true about vomiting in avian
   a) more violent action in which the contents of the stomach/crop are expelled out the mouth
   b) a less violent action in which food from the throat or crop appears to spill over
   c) it results in less mess
   d) all above
128. One of the following is/are true about regurgitation in avian
   a) more violent action in which the contents of the stomach/crop are expelled out the mouth
   b) less violent action, making food contents from throat or crop to spill over
   c) less threatening
   d) b and c
129. Which of the following is/true about intoxications in avian
   a) become hyperactive
   b) becoming irritated
   c) become weak
   d) all above
130. A significant reduction in the amount of feces may indicate
   a) inadequate food intake
   b) indigestion
   c) excessive digestion
   d) none
131. Red or black discoloration of the feces may indicate
   a) Gastrointestinal bleeding
   b) Gastrointestinal Eimeria
   c) Dietary causes
   d) All above
132. Bright red blood seen in the stools likely comes from
   a) Rectum
   b) Cloaca
   c) Both a and b
   d) None

133. One of the following is not a normal component of bird droppings
   a) Watery urine   b) Urates
   c) Faeces   d) Ova

134. Presence of uric acid crystals in bird droppings can
   a) Sign of kidney failure   b) Normal finding
   c) Gout   d) None

135. One of the following is/are untrue about polyuria in avian
   a) Can be due to increased water uptake   b) May result from diabetes
   c) May be from renal issues   d) None

136. Endoscopy with a rigid endoscope can be used in visualizing all except one of the following
   a) Trachea   b) syrinx
   c) air sacs   d) periosteum

137. The blood to be collected from a healthy bird for diagnostics can be up to ________ percent of total body weight
   a) 5   b) 10
   c) 1   d) 0.5

138. One of the following is not true about blood urea nitrogen increase in birds
   a) It suggests over-dehydration
   b) It is confirmatory for kidney failure
   c) It comes from massive water uptake
   d) All above

139. One of the following is/are true about radiology in avian
   a) Superimposition is a limitation   b) Cannot detect ova in-utero
   c) Good positioning not possible   d) All above

140. One of the following is/true about computed tomography in avian
   a) No superimposition
   b) Tissues tend to overlap
   c) Cannot visualize the less-density avian bones
   d) B and c

141. One of the following is true about the normal avian
   a) High metabolic rates   b) High body temperature
   c) Big surface area to body weight ratios   d) All above

142. Pink discoloration of droppings can occur with___________
   a) Poisoning   b) Severe renal problems
   c) A and b   d) Heart disease

143. Very pale feces may indicate____________
   a) Severe pancreatitis   b) Anorexia
   c) Hypoventilation   d) Excessive digestion

144. A waterfowl presented with acute paralysis can be due to___________
a) Clostridium septicum
b) Clostridium botulinum
c) Clostridium novyi
d) None

145. All except one of the following, can affect the body condition scoring
a) Heavy bones
b) Cysts
c) Tumour
d) Ascites

146. Rough handling during examination can affect one of the analytes
a) Glutamate dehydrogenase (GLDH)
b) Aspartate aminotransferase (AST)
c) Creatine kinase (CK)
d) Bile acid

147. A hanging hemorrhagic mass at the vent following laying may likely be
a) Cloacal prolapse
b) Dystocia
c) Haemorrhoid
d) Ova

148. Panting in avian may be associated with
a) Hyperthermia
b) Fear
c) Excitation
d) All above

149. A massive swe/lling seen under the feet of avians under deep-litter system is likely____________
a) Colobroma
b) Multiple myeloma
c) Bumble-feet
d) None

150. A huge reddish wattles and comb noticed on female avian that laid the day before is likely
a) Haemorrhagic syndrome
b) Early avian influenza
c) Normal reproductive changes
d) Fowl cholera

References

Burgmann, P. M. (1995). Common psittacine dermatologic diseases. Seminars in Avian and Exotic Pet Medicine, 4(4), 169-183. https://doi.org/10.1016/S1055-937X(05)80015-5

Chaitanya, Y., Deepti, B., & Ramesh, P. Management of Avian Pox in Turkeys.

Harvey, P. (2010). Avian casualties: Wildlife triage. Veterinary Times. September, 20-26.

Hunt, C. (2018). History taking and examination. In BSAVA Manual of Avian Practice (pp. 125-155). BSAVA Library.

Menon, G. K. (1984). Glandular functions of avian integument: an overview. Journal of the Yamashina Institute for Ornithology, 16, 1-12.

Murphy, B. (2023). Conducting avian fecal assessments.

Nett, C. S., Hodgin, E. C., Foil, C. S., Merchant, S. R., & Tully, T. N. (2003). A modified biopsy technique to improve histopathological evaluation of avian skin. Veterinary Dermatology, 14(3), 147-151. https://doi.org/10.1046/j.1365-3164.2003.00333.x

Perry, S. M., Sander, S. K., & Mitchell, M. A (2015). Integumentary system. Current Therapy in exotic pet practice. St. Louis: Elsevier, 17-75.

Sakas, P. S. (2002). Basic Avian Anatomy. Sakas PS. Essentials of avian medicine: a guide for practitioners Amer Animal Hospital Assn.

Sakas, P. S. (2002). Basic pet bird care. Essentials of Avian Medicine: A Guide for Practitioners, Second Edition. American Animal Hospital Association Press Publ. Niles, IL.

Speer, B. L. (2011). The Business of Wellness Management of the Avian Patient and the Physical Examination. Advancing and Promoting Avian Medicine and Stewardship, 59.

Stettenheim, P. R. (2000). The Integumentary Morphology of Modern Birds—An Overview. Integrative and Comparative Biology, 40(4), 461-477. https://doi.org/10.1093/icb/40.4.461

16

Electrolyte Balance and Fluid Therapy

E. Madhesh

Department of Veterinary Medicine, TANUVAS, Veterinary college and Research Institute, Ramayanpatti, Tirunelveli-627 358

ELECTROLYTE BALANCE

Electrolytes like sodium, potassium, and chloride are substances that dissolve into positively and negatively charged particles when mixed with a liquid. The interaction between these substances, referred to as the 'dietary electrolyte balance (DEB), can be influenced by either the electrolyte itself or the additional salt source used.

Dietary inclusion of potassium and chloride has shown positive effects on heat-stressed broilers. Among various salt options for broiler diets, sodium bicarbonate and potassium chloride have been identified as the optimal choices, especially during hot summer conditions.

Electrolyte balance is often quantified by the uncomplicated equation Na + K – Cl expressed in terms of mEq/kg of diet. An ideal overall dietary equilibrium ranging from 240 to 260 mEq/kg is generally deemed optimal for normal physiological functioning. The body's buffering systems play a pivotal role in maintaining a close-to-normal physiological pH, thus preventing deviations in electrolyte levels. The principal function of electrolytes pertains to the regulation of body water and ionic equilibrium. Consequently, the requisites for elements like sodium, potassium, and chloride can't be viewed in isolation; it's the collective equilibrium that holds significance. The term "electrolyte balance," synonymous with acid-base balance, is influenced by three factors:

1. The equilibrium and proportion of these electrolytes in the diet.
2. Endogenous production of acids.
3. The pace of renal clearance.

In most instances, the body sustains a healthy equilibrium between positively and negatively charged ions to uphold physiological pH. If a shift towards acidic or alkaline conditions occurs, metabolic mechanisms restore the body to a normative pH. Genuine electrolyte imbalances are rare, as regulatory mechanisms inherently maintain optimal cellular pH and osmolarity. Thus, electrolyte balance is better defined as the adjustments that inevitably arise in bodily processes to restore regular pH levels. In extreme cases, these adaptations in regulatory mechanisms can negatively impact other physiological systems, potentially giving rise to incapacitating conditions.

Electrolyte disparity leads to various metabolic disorders in avian species, most notably tibial dyschondroplasia and respiratory alkalosis in layers. The anomalous formation of a cartilaginous plug at the tibial growth plate can be triggered by several factors, with its incidence heightened by metabolic acidosis stemming from substances like NH4Cl. Tibial dyschondroplasia appears to occur more frequently when sodium excessively outweighs potassium in the diet, accompanied by elevated chloride levels. Addressing the latter concern is facilitated by substituting sodium chloride with sodium bicarbonate in the diet.

Total electrolyte balance holds constant importance but becomes paramount when chloride or sulfur levels are elevated. When dietary chloride levels are low, adjustments in electrolyte balance often elicit minimal response. However, during high dietary chloride circumstances, it becomes essential to modulate dietary cations to preserve overall equilibrium. Alternatively, chloride levels can be reduced, although chickens require ~0.12%–0.15% of the diet to prevent deficiency symptoms from manifesting at levels < 0.12%.

The sodium content in drinking water can significantly influence a bird's total sodium intake. Water with sodium content exceeding 300 ppm may necessitate a reduction in dietary sodium levels. The addition of external phytase has implications on electrolyte balance. Although this frequently used enzyme aims to decrease reliance on inorganic phosphorus supplements, it concurrently curtails renal sodium excretion. As a result, diets containing phytase require reduced supplemental sodium levels.

FLUID THERAPY

The primary goal of fluid therapy is to rectify fluid deficits and meet daily maintenance requirements. Fluids are necessary for dehydrated birds and for stabilizing hypovolemic shock and electrolyte imbalances. Before administration, fluids should be warmed to body temperature. Birds in the initial stages of shock often exhibit signs like hypothermia, hypotension, prolonged capillary refill time (>1 second), and tachycardia. The fluid deficit can be calculated using this formula:

Fluid deficit (ml) = Estimated dehydration (%) x Bodyweight (g)

Routes for Administration

Fluids can be delivered through enteral, intravenous, or intraosseous routes, Subcutaneous fluid administration is not recommended due to the minimal subcuticular space. The intracelomic route is not suitable for birds due to air sac presence. Continuous infusion of fluids is possible, but bolus delivery is more common due to the challenge of safeguarding the infusion line.

Enteral Administration

Enteral rehydration suffices for stabilized birds with mild dehydration and for maintaining requirements. However, this method carries a risk of aspiration. A curved stainless steel feeding tube is preferred for ease of use. The tube should be attached to a preloaded syringe and passed to the right of the glottis into the crop, while the bird is held upright.

Intravenous Administration

Birds with significant blood loss (loss >25–30% of total blood volume) benefit from intravenous fluid administration. This route rapidly replaces substantial fluid volumes. Intravenous jugular catheter placement is recommended for collapsed birds, and plucking feathers is usually unnecessary due to the apterium covering the puncture site.

Intraosseous Administration

Intraosseous administration may be favored for small birds or those extremely debilitated with collapsed veins that hinder venipuncture. Any bone with a bone marrow cavity is suitable. Preferred sites include the distal ulna and proximal tibiotarsus.

FLUID TYPES

Crystalloids

Crystalloids like isotonic glucose saline, Hartmann's solution, and lactated Ringer's solution are ideal for reversing dehydration and providing maintenance fluids during recovery. Lactated Ringer's and Hartmann's solutions help correct acidosis through bicarbonate production in the liver. Crystalloids are administered intravenously or intraosseously at a rate of 3 ml/kg.

Colloids:

Colloids are vital for treating hypovolemic shock as they replace deficient plasma proteins. Combining colloids and crystalloids reduces the crystalloid fluid requirement by 40–60%. Synthetic colloids expand intravascular volume by around 1.4 times the infused volume. Oxygen-carrying colloids are effective resuscitation fluids for hypovolemic shock. Blood transfusion (natural colloids) may stabilize chronic anemia cases.

It's important to consult a veterinarian for the proper application of fluid therapy to ensure the bird's well-being.

RESTORATION OF NORMOTHERMIA

Hypothermia is frequently noted in moderately to severely ill birds. Measuring body temperature accurately in birds poses challenges, but it's feasible in unconscious birds using a flexible temperature probe inserted into the crop and proximal proventriculus. Established temperature ranges may not be available for all bird species.

Methods for externally delivering warmth encompass heated incubators, warming pads, radiant heat lamps, circulating warm water or air blankets, and administering warmed subcutaneous fluids. Administering warmed IV or IO fluids contributes to raising core body temperature.

VASCULAR ACCESS

In avian medicine, vascular access can be achieved through two primary routes: intravenous (IV) and intraosseous (IO). The decision of which route to use depends on the patient's size, condition, and the veterinarian's preference. In some cases, catheters can be successfully placed using only manual restraint and local anesthesia, particularly in calm or minimally responsive patients. However, patients prone to struggling during the procedure benefit from low-dose sedation, as previously discussed, along with the infusion of local lidocaine at the catheter insertion site. Injecting sodium bicarbonate-buffered lidocaine (with a ratio of 1 part sodium bicarbonate to 10 parts lidocaine) beneath the skin, rolling it back over the venipuncture site, and allowing a few minutes for the drug to dissipate are essential steps. The use of general anesthesia for intravenous catheterization is rare and can pose increased risks, especially for critical patients.

For routine placement, IV catheters are commonly inserted into cockatiels and larger birds using 24- to 26-gauge catheters. Suitable sites include the right jugular, basilic (or ulnar), and medial metatarsal veins. However, sites other than the jugular vein are mainly useful for larger birds. The smallest IV catheters routinely employed are 25- to 26-gauge catheters placed into the jugular vein of a cockatiel or small conure. A notable complication associated with jugular catheterization in birds is the inadvertent infusion of fluid or blood leakage into adjacent air sacs, which, if occurring in significant volumes, could result in fatality.

Medial metatarsal catheters can be secured using tape alone. In contrast, basilic and jugular catheters are typically sutured in place. To mitigate the risk of fatal hemorrhage due to catheter disruption, no bird should be left unattended with an IV catheter in place.

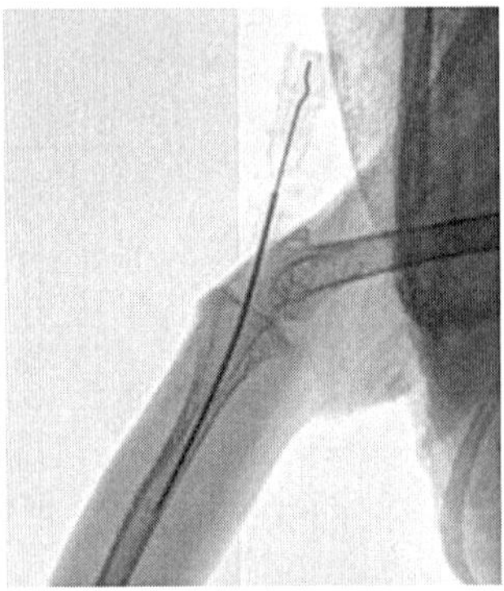

Gray-scale reverse radiographic image of a 22-gauge spinal needle placed in the ulna of a military macaw (Ara militaris). The needle is inserted into the medullary space distal to the condyle of the dorsal ulna, avoiding the joint

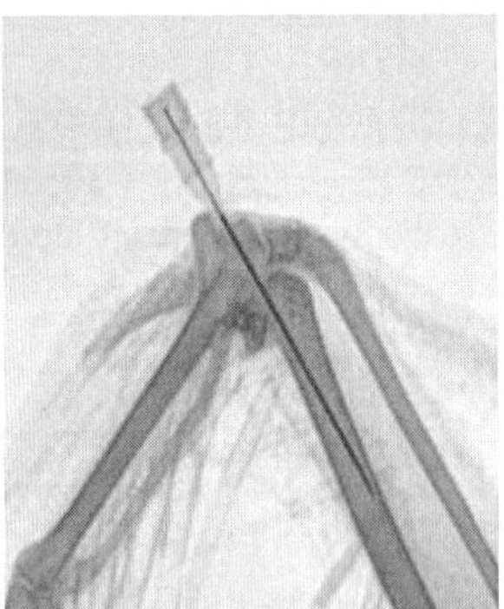

Gray-scale reverse radiographic image of a 22-gauge spinal needle placed into the proximal tibiotarsus of a military macaw (Ara militaris). The needle is inserted to the side of, or through, the patellar tendon into the medullary space

IO catheterization is well-documented in birds and can even be performed in patients as small as a finch. Sites for IO catheterization includes the proximal tibiotarsus at the cnemial crest and the distal ulna. Thanks to the relatively soft bone cortex in most birds, standard injection needles can be used as IO catheters, with needle sizes ranging from 22 to 27 gauge.

Ensuring proper IO catheter placement requires confirmation through two orthogonal radiographic views, as single views are prone to misleading results. Firm seating of the needle isn't always indicative of success, given that the needle can pass through both bone cortices. Injected fluids that accumulate in the wrong places can be detected. However, it's important to avoid excessive movement during placement, which could lead to a large entry point in the bone causing fluid leakage during infusion. Correct ulnar catheter placement may result in the blanching of the basilic vein during fluid administration. The IO catheter can be capped with a standard IV injection cap and secured by taping it to the limb.

The use of IO catheters in pet birds is largely anecdotal. While studies in human patients and some animal models suggest that IO vascular access is equivalent to IV access in terms of the onset and peak levels of therapeutic agents, it's recommended to maintain the catheter for no more than 72 hours. Complications in humans are uncommon and include catheter displacement and fluid extravasation into soft tissue. Serious complications like compartment syndrome and osteomyelitis are rare. Over a span of more than 10 years, the authors have encountered no complications using this technique in clinical practice. However, there's awareness of a single case of infection at the catheter placement site and fatal hemorrhage following self-removal of the catheter. Notably, successfully placing a functional IO catheter in female birds with hyperostotic endostosis of long bones is challenging or nearly impossible.

For conscious patients, all catheters should be securely wrapped using elastic-style tape. Wing catheters are protected by wrapping the wing with a typical figure-8 style bandage, either with or without securing the wing to the body.

Effective fluids used for resuscitation in birds encompass crystalloids (lactated Ringer's solution, normal saline, hypertonic saline), synthetic colloids like hydroxyethyl starch (HES), and natural colloids (whole blood, plasma, albumin). Hypertonic saline quickly draws fluid from other body compartments into the intravascular space, aiding in raising blood pressure. All fluids must be warmed to body temperature before administration, typically around 102° to 103° F (39° C). Although hypoglycemia is rare in birds, dextrose solutions can be added to crystalloid solutions if needed. Confirming hypoglycemia through blood glucose measurement is crucial. To address hypoglycemia, a starting bolus of 50% dextrose diluted in a 1:4 ratio with saline can be administered, with subsequent frequent monitoring of blood glucose levels.

FLUID THERAPY: SAMPLE PROBLEM

Patient: Adult female red-tailed hawk with an open fracture of the humerus

Bodyweight: 1040 g

PCV: 28%

TP: 2.6

Hydration state: 10% dehydrated

Fluid deficit (ml) = Estimated dehydration (%) x Bodyweight (g)

Fluid: *Fluid deficit:* 1040 g × 0.10 = 104 ml

Requirements: *Maintenance:* 50 ml/kg/day

Plan: Replace 50% of deficit (+ maintenance) in the first 24 hours; the remainder (+ maintenance) over the next 48 hours

Therapy	Administration
Day 1: 50% of deficit = 52 ml Maintenance = 50 ml Total = 102 ml	Administer 25 ml i.v. q.i.d. = total of 100 ml
Day 2: 25% of deficit = 26 ml Maintenance = 50 ml Total = 76 ml	Administer 25 ml i.v. t.i.d. = total of 75 ml Start oral alimentation
Day 3: 50% of deficit = 26 ml Maintenance = 50 ml Total = 76 ml	Administer 25 ml i.v. t.i.d. = total of 75 ml
Day 4: Maintenance = 50 ml	Provide maintenance fluids in two doses, i.e. 25 ml i.v. b.i.d.Oral alimentation as indicated Increase solid intake to near normal levels

FLUID OVERLOAD

Symptoms of excessive fluid administration or fluid overload become apparent when fluids are administered too quickly. These symptoms encompass clear nasal discharge, rapid breathing, difficulty breathing, fluid accumulation in the abdomen, persistent coughing, excessive urination, accelerated heart rate, trembling, and edema lungs. Anticipated corresponding results from laboratory tests include a decline in packed cell volume and total solids values, along with a rise in body weight.

BLOOD TRANSFUSION

Birds exhibit impressive tolerance to blood loss. In a study involving ducks, the onset of hypovolemic shock due to acute blood loss was only evident after approximately 60% of the blood volume had been removed. Instances of chronic blood loss have been observed in birds, leading to packed cell volumes (PCV) as low as 6% to 7%. Situations warranting blood transfusion include continuous blood loss, PCV dropping below 12% to 15% accompanied by signs of weakness linked to anemia, presence of coagulopathy, or planned surgery in the presence of preexisting significant anemia.

Obtaining whole blood for bird transfusion poses challenges. Research indicates that blood transfusion between birds of the same species (homologous) results in prolonged erythrocyte lifespan. When a suitable homologous species isn't available, transfusion from a closely related species should be considered. Some veterinary clinics collaborate with bird rescues and clients willing to bring donor birds in exchange for clinic credit. While cross-matching is ideal, its application in birds lacks extensive study.

Blood collection is carried out on a healthy donor bird through cautious restraint, sedation, or anesthesia via the jugular vein. Different anticoagulants such as sodium citrate, heparin, and acid-citrate dextrose (ACD) can be utilized. Heparin is commonly used at a ratio of 0.25 mL per 10 mL of blood, or other anticoagulants as per the manufacturer's recommendation. Using a filter to eliminate aggregated debris is recommended. The amount collected should not surpass 10% of the donor's blood volume.

Donor blood is administered as a slow bolus over 10 minutes or through an IV or IO catheter using a syringe pump. In cases of significant hemorrhage, blood administration can be expedited, even within minutes. All collected whole blood must be administered within 4 hours to prevent bacterial growth, aligning with the standards set by the American Association of Blood Banks.

Multiple Choice Questions

1. Which organ in birds plays a critical role in regulating electrolyte balance and maintaining fluid homeostasis?
   a) Kidney b) Heart
   c) Spleen d) Pancreas
2. Which of the following is a common electrolyte found in avian blood?
   a) Glucose b) Urea
   c) Sodium d) Hemoglobin
3. A bird that consumes a diet high in seeds may be at risk of developing which electrolyte imbalance?
   a) Hypernatremia b) Hypokalemia
   c) Hypocalcemia d) Hyperkalemia
4. What is the primary function of the salt glands in birds?
   a) Regulation of body temperature b) Excretion of excess salt
   c) Synthesis of electrolytes d) Production of bile
5. Dehydration in pet birds can lead to:
   a) Increased appetite b) Decreased thirst
   c) Increased urination d) Enhanced feather coloration
6. The hormone that plays a key role in regulating water balance and electrolyte levels in birds is:
   a) Insulin b) Thyroid hormone
   c) Aldosterone d) Cortisol
7. What is the primary purpose of fluid therapy in avian medicine?
   a) Enhance feather growth b) Promote vocalization
   c) Correct electrolyte imbalances d) Increase metabolic rate
8. Which electrolyte is crucial for maintaining nerve impulse transmission and muscle function in birds?
   a) Sodium b) Potassium
   c) Calcium d) Magnesium
9. Overhydration in pet birds can lead to:
   a) Hypokalemia b) Hypernatremia
   c) Acidosis d) Hyperkalemia
10. Which of the following is a potential cause of hypervolemia in birds?
    a) Excessive fluid loss b) Dehydration
    c) Hypokalemia d) Hyperkalemia

11. Birds that predominantly eat insects and protein-rich diets may require additional supplementation of which electrolyte ?
    a) Sodium b) Potassium
    c) Calcium d) Chloride
12. Which electrolyte is vital for maintaining proper blood clotting in pet birds?
    a) Sodium b) Potassium
    c) Calcium d) Magnesium
13. Which of the following can cause metabolic acidosis in pet birds?
    a) Hyperventilation b) Hypoventilation
    c) Excessive fluid intake d) High dietary calcium intake
14. The primary route of fluid loss in pet birds is through:
    a) Respiration b) Urination
    c) Defecation d) Salivation
15. Which electrolyte is critical for maintaining acid-base balance in pet birds?
    a) Sodium b) Potassium
    c) Chloride d) Bicarbonate
16. Which type of fluid therapy involves the injection of fluids directly into the bloodstream?
    a) Intramuscular b) Subcutaneous
    c) Intravenous d) Oral
17. A bird that consumes excessive amounts of salty foods may be at risk of developing:
    a) Hyperkalemia b) Hypokalemia
    c) Hypernatremia d) Hypocalcemia
18. What is the term for the process of water movement across cell membranes to equalize solute concentrations?
    a) Osmosis b) Diffusion
    c) Filtration d) Active transport
19. Which of the following is a potential complication of administering fluid therapy too rapidly in pet birds?
    a) Hypernatremia b) Hypervolemia or fluid overload
    c) Hyperkalemia d) Hypercalcemia
20. The function of the salt glands in marine birds is primarily to:
    a) Regulate fluid intake b) Regulate body temperature
    c) Excrete excess salt d) Regulate calcium levels
21. A bird that consumes excessive amounts of calcium supplements may be at risk of developing:
    a) Hypernatremia b) Hypokalemia
    c) Hypercalcemia d) Hypocalcemia

22. Which electrolyte imbalance can lead to muscle weakness, cardiac arrhythmias, and tetanic contractions in pet birds?
    a) Hypernatremia b) Hypokalemia
    c) Hyperkalemia d) Hypocalcemia
23. The condition characterized by abnormally high levels of uric acid in the bloodstream is called:
    a) Uremia b) Uricemia
    c) Hyperuricemia d) Urate poisoning
24. Which of the following is a potential consequence of prolonged diarrhea in pet birds?
    a) Hypokalemia b) Hyperkalemia
    c) Hypernatremia d) Hypocalcemia
25. Which type of fluid imbalance is characterized by a higher concentration of solutes in the extracellular fluid compared to the intracellular fluid?
    a) Hypertonic b) Hypotonic
    c) Isotonic d) Osmotic
26. Fluid therapy that involves the administration of fluids under the skin is known as:
    a) Intravenous therapy b) Subcutaneous therapy
    c) Oral therapy d) Intramuscular therapy
27. Which electrolyte imbalance can lead to muscle tremors, seizures, and cardiac arrhythmias in pet birds?
    a) Hypernatremia b) Hypokalemia
    c) Hyperkalemia d) Hypocalcemia
28. Which of the following is an example of a hypertonic solution?
    a) 7.2% NS b) NS
    c) D5 d) Blood
29. Which of the following hormones plays a role in regulating fluid and electrolyte balance by promoting sodium reabsorption and potassium excretion in the kidneys of birds?
    a) Insulin b) Thyroxine
    c) Cortisol d) Aldosterone
30. Which of the following is a potential cause of hypervolemia in pet birds?
    a) Excessive fluid intake b) Dehydration
    c) Hypokalemia d) Hyperkalemia
31. Birds primarily lose heat through which mechanism?
    a) Conduction b) Convection
    c) Respiration d) Perspiration
32. Which of the following conditions can lead to metabolic alkalosis in pet birds?
    a) Hyperventilation b) Hypoventilation
    c) Excessive sodium intake d) Excessive potassium intake

33. Which type of fluid imbalance is characterized by abnormally low blood pH due to an excess of hydrogen ions?
    a) Acidosis b) Alkalosis
    c) Hypokalemia d) Hyperkalemia
34. The renal system in pet birds helps regulate fluid balance and electrolytes through the production of:
    a) Bile b) Urine
    c) Saliva d) Lymph
35. A bird suffering from heat stress might exhibit signs of:
    a) Hypokalemia b) Hyperkalemia
    c) Hypernatremia d) Hypocalcemia
36. What is the term for the exchange of gases and solutes between the blood and body tissues in pet birds?
    a) Filtration b) Respiration
    c) Diffusion d) Osmosis
37. Which of the following factors can influence fluid requirements in pet birds?
    a) Altitude b) Feather coloration
    c) Nesting material d) Perch size
38. A bird that loses excess fluids through vomiting is at risk of developing:
    a) Hypernatremia b) Hypokalemia
    c) Hyperkalemia d) Hypocalcemia
39. The normal pH value of the chicken blood is ___________
    a) 5.0 - 6.0 b) 6.5 - 7.5
    c) 7.0 - 8.0 d) 7.4 - 7.5
40. Which of the following hormones plays a role in regulating fluid and electrolyte balance in pet birds?
    a) Insulin b) Thyroxine
    c) Cortisol d) Aldosterone
41. What is the primary function of electrolytes in pet bird bodies?
    a) Regulate body temperature b) Enhance feather coloration
    c) Provide energy d) Maintain fluid balance
42. In pet birds, which process is responsible for eliminating waste products and excess substances from the body?
    a) Absorption b) Filtration
    c) Digestion d) Secretion
43. In birds, a decrease in dietary intake of which electrolyte could lead to bone abnormalities?
    a) Sodium b) Potassium
    c) Calcium d) Magnesium

44. Which of the following is an example of a hypotonic solution?
    a) DNS
    b) 7.2% NS
    c) Ringer's Lactate
    d) Pentastarch
45. An avian patient with polydipsia may have an issue with which organ?
    a) Liver
    b) Heart
    c) Lungs
    d) Kidneys
46. What is the term for the condition in which a bird's body retains too much water?
    a) Hydration
    b) Dehydration
    c) Overhydration
    d) Hyperhydration
47. Which of the following is an example of an isotonic solution?
    a) 23% Calcium borogluconate
    b) 50% Dextrose
    c) 0.9% NaCl
    d) Lactated Ringer's
48. Which of the following organs helps regulate fluid and electrolyte balance through hormone secretion?
    a) Liver
    b) Spleen
    c) Heart
    d) Kidneys
49. Which avian organ plays a role in maintaining electrolyte balance through the production of bile?
    a) Kidneys
    b) Liver
    c) Lungs
    d) Spleen
50. Which of the following conditions can lead to metabolic alkalosis in pet birds?
    a) Hyperventilation
    b) Hypoventilation
    c) Excessive sodium intake
    d) Excessive potassium intake
51. Which electrolyte is involved in maintaining acid-base balance and acts as a buffer in pet birds?
    a) Sodium
    b) Potassium
    c) Calcium
    d) Chloride
52. Which avian species is known for having salt glands that help excrete excess salt from their bodies?
    a) Parrots
    b) Ducks
    c) Sparrows
    d) Falcons
53. What is the term for the process by which birds expel waste products from their bodies in the form of solid or liquid waste?
    a) Osmosis
    b) Excretion
    c) Absorption
    d) Secretion
54. A bird suffering from heat stress might exhibit signs of:
    a) Hypokalemia
    b) Hyperkalemia
    c) Hypernatremia
    d) Hypocalcemia
55. Maintenance fluid rate in bird is ______________
    a) 50 ml/kg/day
    b) 30 ml/kg/day
    c) 100 ml/kg/day
    d) 60 ml/kg/day

56. The function of the salt glands in marine birds is primarily to:
   a) Regulate fluid intake
   b) Regulate body temperature
   c) Excrete excess salt
   d) Regulate calcium levels
57. In birds, intravenous fluids should be warmed to ________°C
   a) 39°C
   b) 34°C
   c) 37°C
   d) 42°C
58. What are the signs and symptoms of heat stress in poultry?
   a) Panting, Open-mouth breathing
   b) Increased thirst, Lethargy
   c) Weakness, Death
   d) All of the above
59. What are the signs and symptoms of fluid overload in poultry?
   a) Serous nasal discharge, tachypnea, cough
   b) Dyspnea, ascites, pulmonary edema
   c) Polyuria, tachycardia, shivering
   d) All of the above
60. Which of the following fluid is most commonly used as replacement fluid in birds.
   a) Lactated Ringer's solution
   b) DNS
   c) NS
   d) Pentastarch
61. Fluids containing lactate may not be recommended for patients with severe ________ disease?
   a) Kidney
   b) Liver
   c) Eye
   d) Air sac
62. In critically ill raptors, suggested dosage of colloids is___________?
   a) 10-20ml/kg
   b) 30-40ml/kg
   c) 70-80ml/kg
   d) 90-100ml/kg
63. Isotonic sodium chloride solution is used inappropriately; the relatively increased chloride concentration can cause__________?
   a) Hyperchloremic metabolic alkalosis
   b) Hyperchloremic metabolic acidosis
   c) Hypokalemic metabolic alkalosis
   d) Hyperkalemic metabolic acidosis
64. A bird suffering from chronic vomiting needs ____________ administration.
   a) NS
   b) Blood
   c) D5
   d) Ringer's Lactate
65. The oral route of fluid administration should never be used in birds that have _________?
   a) CNS Depression
   b) Vomiting
   c) Gastrointestinal stasis
   d) All of the above
66. For maintenance fluid therapy in birds, ____________ route of fluid administration is convenient and practical?
   a) Oral
   b) Subcutaneous
   c) Intramuscular
   d) Intravenous

67. What are the complications of fluid therapy in poultry?
 a) Fluid overload
 b) Electrolyte imbalance
 c) Sepsis
 d) All of the above
68. What are the indications for fluid therapy in poultry?
 a) Dehydration, Diarrhea
 b) Vomiting, Heat stress
 c) Shock, Trauma
 d) All the above
69. What are the contraindications for fluid therapy in poultry?
 a) Hepatic failure
 b) Congestive heart failure
 c) Renal failure
 d) All the above
70. What are the monitoring parameters for fluid therapy in poultry?
 a) Hydration status, body weight
 b) Heart rate, respiratory rate,
 c) Blood pressure, electrolyte balance
 d) All the above
71. Electrolyte imbalance in poultry can result in:
 a) Improved egg production
 b) Enhanced feather growth
 c) Reduced growth rates
 d) Decreased eggshell quality
72. Which electrolyte is crucial for maintaining osmotic balance and nerve function in poultry?
 a) Magnesium
 b) Zinc
 c) Iron
 d) Potassium
73. Acid-base balance in poultry is primarily regulated by which electrolytes?
 a) Sodium and potassium
 b) Calcium and phosphorus
 c) Chloride and magnesium
 d) Iron and zinc
74. The primary electrolyte lost in poultry through urine and feces is:
 a) Sodium
 b) Potassium
 c) Calcium
 d) Chloride
75. Electrolyte supplements are particularly important during which period in poultry production?
 a) Brooding
 b) Laying
 c) Molting
 d) Slaughter
76. Which electrolyte helps in maintaining normal bone structure and eggshell quality in poultry?
 a) Sodium
 b) Potassium
 c) Calcium
 d) Magnesium
77. Electrolyte supplementation is especially crucial in hot weather to prevent
 a) Feather loss
 b) Eggshell thinning
 c) Heat stress
 d) Overfeeding?
78. The movement of electrolytes across cell membranes is primarily regulated by:
 a) Hormones
 b) Antioxidants
 c) Carbohydrates
 d) Vitamins

79. Electrolyte imbalance can contribute to a condition called "water belly," which is characterized by
   a) Feather discoloration b) Swollen abdomen
   c) Enlarged beak d) Leg paralysis
80. Which electrolyte helps in maintaining acid-base balance and nerve function in poultry?
   a) Magnesium b) Iron
   c) Phosphorus d) Chloride
81. Electrolyte imbalance can negatively impact:
   a) Egg production b) Feather color
   c) Beak length d) Respiratory rate
82. Electrolyte supplements are commonly administered to poultry through:
   a) Feeds b) Injections
   c) Fogging d) Beak trimming
83. Which electrolyte is essential for enzyme activity, oxygen transport, and energy metabolism in poultry?
   a) Sodium b) Iron
   c) Copper d) Zinc
84. Electrolyte balance is closely connected to the regulation of:
   a) Vitamin levels b) Hormone production
   c) Body temperature d) Feather color
85. Electrolyte balance is vital for maintaining overall:
   a) Egg production b) Growth and performance
   c) Feather coloration d) Beak strength
86. a) Enhancing feather coloration b) Improving eggshell quality
   c) Treating respiratory infections d) Replacing lost blood volume
87. What can happen if an incompatible blood transfusion is given to a chicken?
   a) Enhanced growth rate b) Feather loss
   c) Increased egg production d) Hemolytic reaction
88. What are the signs of adverse blood transfusion reactions in birds
   a) Regurgitation b) Hemoglobinuria
   c) Death d) All the above
89. What is the usual anticoagulant used when collecting blood for transfusion in chickens?
   a) Heparin b) Warfarin
   c) Aspirin d) Ibuprofen
90. Blood transfusion can be administered to chickens through the following routes except:
   a) Jugular vein b) Basilic vein
   c) Medial metatarsal vein d) Humerus

91. To prevent bacterial growth, what is the maximum allowable time, starting from the collection of donor blood, for a chicken blood transfusion to be completed?
    a) 2 hours b) 6 hours
    c) 8 hours d) 4 hours
92. When performing a blood collection from a single chicken, what is the maximum percentage of its body weight that should be collected to avoid adverse effects?
    a) 5% b) 15%
    c) 10% d) 1%
93. What is a potential complication of giving too much blood volume in a transfusion to a chicken?
    a) Improved immune response b) Decreased heart rate
    c) Fluid overload d) Enhanced digestion
94. What is the recommended site for blood collection in chickens for transfusion purposes?
    a) Wing vein b) Neck artery
    c) Beak vein d) Tail vein
95. What is the normal calcium concentration in the blood of a poultry?
    a) 8-10 mg/dL b) 10-12 mg/dL
    c) 12-14 mg/dL d) 14-16 mg/dL
96. Which electrolyte is the most important for fluid balance in poultry?
    a) Sodium b) Potassium
    c) Chlorine d) Calcium
97. What is the normal sodium concentration in the blood of a poultry?
    a) 145-155 mEq/L b) 155-165 mEq/L
    c) 135-145 mEq/L d) 175-185 mEq/L
98. What is the normal potassium concentration in the blood of a poultry?
    a) 3.5-5.5 mEq/L b) 5.5-7.5 mEq/L
    c) 7.5-9.5 mEq/L d) 9.5-11.5 mEq/L
99. What is the normal chloride concentration in the blood of a poultry?
    a) 95-105 mEq/L b) 105-115 mEq/L
    c) 115-125 mEq/L d) 125-135 mEq/L
100. What is the normal magnesium concentration in the blood of a poultry?
    a) 3.5-4.5 mg/dL b) 2.5-3.5 mg/dL
    c) 1.5-2.5 mg/dL d) 4.5-5.5 mg/dL

Answer Key

1	a	2	c	3	c	4	b	5	a	6	c	7	c
8	b	9	b	10	b	11	c	12	c	13	b	14	a
15	d	16	c	17	c	18	a	19	b	20	c	21	c
22	b	23	c	24	a	25	a	26	b	27	c	28	a

29	d	30	a	31	c	32	a	33	a	34	b	35	c
36	c	37	a	38	a	39	d	40	d	41	d	42	b
43	c	44	c	45	d	46	c	47	c	48	d	49	b
50	a	51	d	52	b	53	b	54	c	55	a	56	c
57	a	58	d	59	d	60	a	61	b	62	a	63	b
64	a	65	d	66	b	67	d	68	d	69	d	70	d
71	c	72	d	73	a	74	a	75	a	76	c	77	c
78	a	79	b	80	a	81	a	82		83	b	84	c
85	b	86	d	87	d	88	d	89	a	90	d	91	d
92	d	93	c	94	a	95	a	96	a	97	c	98	a
99	a	100	c										

17

Disorders of The Respiratory System

Vipin Maurya

Department of Livestock Production Management, Faculty of Veterinary & Animal Sciences, IAS, RGSC- Banaras Hindu University, Benaras, India

Introduction

Knowledge of the avian respiratory system is essential for developing a health monitoring plan for a poultry flock, recognizing problems that may occur, and taking action to correct them. The avian respiratory system begins with nostril includes trachea, bronchi (bronchus) and ends with lungs and air sacs. Respiratory diseases are the most common cause of death in a poultry flock.

The avian respiratory system is involved in the following functions:

- Absorption of oxygen (O2)
- Release of carbon dioxide (CO2)
- Release of heat (temperature regulation)
- Detoxification of certain chemicals
- Rapid adjustments of acid/base balance
- Vocalization

The most serious and paramount important economic diseases of poultry are respiratory diseases. A large number of pathogens such as bacteria, virus, and fungus are associated with respiratory infection. Viral diseases like Avian influenza (AI), Newcastle disease (NCD), Infectious bronchitis (IB), Infectious laryngotracheitis (ILT)and Avian metapneumovirus; bacterial diseases like Mycoplasmosis, Ornithobacterium rhinotracheale, Fowl cholera and Infectious coryza; and fungal disease like Aspergillosis are responsible for causing respiratory diseases. Every pathogen has unique trends regarding their infection pattern, transmission, clinical symptoms, control strategy and vaccination.

Chronic Respiratory Disease (CRD) Etiology: *Mycoplasma gallisepticum* and E. Coli. Stress, make the birds more susceptible. The condition is frequently triggered by respiratory viruses such as NCD and IB.

Transmission: Through the egg to their offspring. In addition, by contact or by airborne dust or droplets. The incubation period varies from 4 days to 3 weeks. Species affected- Chickens and turkeys.

Young chickens show respiratory distress. In adult birds the most common symptoms are sneezing, coughing and general signs of respiratory congestion. Decline in egg production. The effect is more of a chronic nature thus; overall economic loss can be very great in broilers but less dramatic in breeders and layers. Trachea is inflamed reddish and cheesy exudate in air sacs.

Infectious Coryza Etiology: *Hemophilus paragallinarum.*

Transmission: By contact and airborne infected dust particles and via the drinking water. Spread by equipment and personnel has also been reported.

Clinical signs: Inflammation of eyes and nose with foul-smelling discharges, conjunctivitis, sneezing and facial swellings. Mortality varies with the virulence of the infection.

Aspergillosis (Fungal Pneumonia) Etiology-Fungus, *Aspergillus fumigatus.*

Transmission: Inhalation of fungus spores from contaminated litter (e.g., wood shavings) or contaminated feed. Hatcheries may also contribute to infection of chicks. Young chicks are more susceptible.

Infected chicks are depressed and thirsty. Gasping and rapid breathing ("pump handle breathing") can be observed. Lesions can be primarily seen in the lungs and airsacs. Sometimes all body cavities are filled with small yellow-green granular fungus growth.

Newcastle Disease (NCD)/ Ranikhet Disease

Etiology: Paramyxovirus. The virus has mild strains (lentogenic), medium strength strains (mesogenic), and virulent strains (velogenic). A highly contagious disease & transmission occurs through infected droppings and respiratory discharge between birds. Spread between farms is by infected equipment, trucks, personnel, wild birds or air.

High mortality with depression and death in 3 to 5 days are important clinical manifestations. Mesogenic strains cause typical signs of respiratory distress. Labored breathing with wheezing and gurgling, accompanied by nervous signs, such as paralysis or twisted necks (torticollis) are the main signs. Egg production declines to 30 to 60 %. Eggs may have thin shells and eggs without shells may also be found. In well vaccinated flock's clinical signs may be difficult to find. Inflamed tracheas, pneumonia, and/or froth in the airsacs are the main lesions. Haemorrhagic lesions in the proventriculus and the intestines.

Infectious Bronchitis (IB)

Etiology: Corona-virus. Transmission Airborne route.

In young chicks IB virus infection causes cheesy exudates in the bifurcation of the bronchi, thereby causing asphyxia, preceded by severe respiratory distress. In older birds IB does not cause mortality. Egg production will decrease dramatically, deformed eggs with wrinkled shells will often be laid. Internal lesions Mucus and redness in trachea, froth in air sacs in older chickens. In young chicks a yellow cheesy plug at the tracheal bifurcation is indicative of IB infection.

Post-mortem findings, Isolation of the virus and arising antibody titre when the serum is tested against a known strain of bronchitis virus

Infectious Laryngotracheitis (ILT)

Etiology: ILT is caused by a virus belonging to the herpes group. Transmission by the respiratory route. Most outbreaks of ILT on farms are traced back to transmission by contaminated people or equipment (visitors, shoes, clothing, egg boxes, used feeders, waterers, cages, crates etc. The incubation period varies from 4 to 12 days. Species affected chickens and pheasants are natural hosts for ILT.

Respiratory distress is usually quite pronounced due to build up of blood, sloughed tracheal lining and even caseous exudates in larynx and trachea. When a caseous plug occludes the larynx or trachea, the affected chickens will have extreme difficulty breathing and will frequently die from suffocation. Mortality is approximately 1 % per day in a typical ILT outbreak. Milder forms of ILT outbreaks occur where less virulent strains of ILT virus are involved. Conjunctivitis and respiratory sounds (wheezing) can be observed, with little or no mortality in such cases. The disease spreads through a chicken house more slowly than either IB or ND Egg production in laying flocks usually decreases 10 to 50 %, but will return to normal after 3 to 4 weeks.

Multiple Choice Questions

1. Type of pneumonia seen in brooder pneumonia is
   a) Fibrinous b) Suppurative
   c) Granulomatous d) Aspiration
2. Mycoplasmal disease of poultry is
   a) Chronic respiratory disease b) Infectious coryza
   c) Avian encephalomyelitis d) Chicken infectious anemia
3. Infectious laryngotracheitis is caused by
   a) Gallid Herpesvirus - 1 b) Birnavirus
   c) Gallid Herpesvirus - 2 d) Circovirus
4. In peracute form of Infectious laryngotracheitis (ILT) main lesion is
   a) Obstructive plugs in larynx b) Hemorrhagic trachitis
   c) Caseous diphtheritic exudates d) All of the above
5. Presence of cheesy deposits in the air sacs is indicative of
   a) Fowl spirochetosis b) Avian chlamydiosis
   c) Chronic respiratory disease d) Infectious coryza
6. Caseous plug in the lower trachea and bronchi of dead chicks is observed in
   a) EDS-76 b) IB
   c) IBD d) ILT
7. Form of Fowl pox causing high mortality in layers is
   a) Diptheritic form b) Dry form
   c) Cutaneous form d) None of the above
8. Main sign of ILT is
   a) Breathe with wide open mouths and gasping
   b) Obstruction of the trachea with exudates
   c) Moist rales
   d) All of the above
9. Turkey coryza is caused by
   a) Pasteurella aviseptica b) Bordetella avium
   c) Haemophilus paragallinarum d) Salmonella gallinarum
10. Yellowish white nodules (small bumps) in the lungs are characteristic of
    a) Aspergillosis b) Favus
    c) Infectious coryza d) CRD

11. Multiple yellow to white pin point nodules scattered throughout the lung tissue is seen in
    a) Histoplasmosis
    b) Aspergillosis
    c) Favus
    d) Moniliasis
12. Cloudiness with presence of cheesy exudates in the air sac membranes and body cavities, fibrinous pericarditis and perihepatitis are lesions of
    a) Mycoplasmosis
    b) Avian Influenza
    c) Avian monocytosis
    d) Inclusion body hepatitis
13. Mode of transmission of IBR virus is
    a) Venereal
    b) Inhalation
    c) Semen
    d) All of the above
14. Diene's staining is used for
    a) Mycoplasma
    b) Bacteria
    c) Chlamydia
    d) Fungus
15. Chronic Respiratory Disease (CRD) of poultry by
    a) Mycoplasma mycoides subsp. mycoides
    b) Mycoplasma mycoides subsp. capri
    c) Mycoplasma gallisepticum
    d) Mycoplasma agalactiae
16. ________ is defined as insufficient oxygen to maintain normal metabolic functions
    a) Anoxia
    b) Hypoxia
    c) Anorexia
    d) Pneumonia
17. Hypoxia occurs when
    a) Brain is deficit in oxygen
    b) arterial oxygen is 96 mm Hg or less
    c) arterial oxygen is 60 mm Hg or less
    d) arterial oxygen is less than 20 mm Hg
18. Coughing may be non-productive if the irritation is caused by
    a) Bacterial infections
    b) Mucosal erosion
    c) Viral infections
    d) Exudative
19. Coughing is productive if caused by
    a) Copious exudate in the major airways
    b) Mucosal erosion
    c) Choking
    d) None of the above
20. Severe pulmonary oedema and emphysema causes?
    a) Respiratory insufficiency
    b) Anorexia
    c) Hyperthermia
    d) Rhinitis
21. Soft, productive and chronic cough usually originates from
    a) Pharynx
    b) Trachea
    c) Lungs
    d) Larynx

22. Common complication of phyrangitis is
    a) Bronchitis
    b) Aspiratory pneumonia
    c) Laryngitis
    d) Tracheitis
23. Infectious coryza is caused by
    a) Haemophilus paragallinarum
    b) Pasteurella multocida
    c) Aspergillus fumigatous
    d) Mycoplasma gallisepticum
24. Allergic inflammation is characterized by
    a) Lymphocytes
    b) Eosinophils
    c) Monocytes
    d) Neutrophils
25. Vertically transmitted bacterial disease of poultry is
    a) Pullorum disease and Fowl typhoid
    b) Chronic respiratory disease
    c) Colibacillosis
    d) All of the above
26. Infiltration of pleomorphic lymphoid cells is seen in
    a) Lymphoid leukosis
    b) Marek's disease
    c) IBH
    d) New castle disease
27. The disease caused by influenza virus type-A subtype H5N1 is known as
    a) Swine flu
    b) Bird flu
    c) Equine influenza
    d) Human flu
28. In Highly Pathogenic Avian Influenza virus multiple molecules of which amino acid is found at the cleavage site
    a) Lysine
    b) Arginine
    c) Tryptophane
    d) Serine
29. Type of necrosis seen in hypoxic cell death is
    a) Caseative
    b) Liquifactive
    c) Coagulative
    d) Fat necrosis
30. Accumulation of blood in the pleural sac is called as
    a) Haemothorax
    b) Hydrothorax
    c) Pneumothorax
    d) Pyothorax
31. Consequence of less supply of oxygen to brain leads to
    a) Syncope
    b) Coma
    c) Epilepsy
    d) Cerebral oedema
32 Decreased respiratory rate is termed as
    a) Apnoea
    b) Oligopnoea
    c) Orthopnoea
    d) Dyspnoea
33. Accumulation of fluid in the thoracic cavity is known as
    a) Pneumothorax
    b) Hydrothorax
    c) Both a and b
    d) None of the above
34. Frequent dry cough often in paroxysms is seen in
    a) Bronchopneumonia
    b) Interstitial pneumonia
    c) Pneumonia
    d) Bronchitis

35. Short jerky inspiration caused by stimulation of phrenic nerve is
    a) Hiccough
    b) Wheeze
    c) Roar
    d) None of the above
36. Snoring respiration is characteristic of
    a) Pneumonia
    b) Heaves
    c) Paralysis of larynx
    d) Obstruction of nasal passage
37. An example of anodyne expectorant is
    a) Codein
    b) Ammonium chloride
    c) Potassium iodide
    d) Camphor
38. Pneumonia caused by parasite is called
    a) Verminous pneumonia
    b) Bronchopneumonia
    c) Mycotic pneumonia
    d) All of the above
39. Dilatation of bronchial lumen is called
    a) Atelectasis
    b) Bronchistenosis
    c) Bronchiectasis
    d) Emphysema
40. Hypoxia affects
    a) Cells aerobic respiration
    b) Cells anaerobic respiration
    c) Both a and b
    d) Does not affect respiration
41. Which statement is incorrect?
    a) Ischaemia is a loss of blood supply due to obstructed blood flow
    b) In hypoxia glycolytic energy production can continue
    c) Hypoxia injures tissues faster than ischaemia
    d) Ischaemia injures tissues faster than hypoxia
42. Which statement is not true about avian inflammation?
    a) Chicken monocyte, basophils and thrombocytes are phagocytic
    b) Eosinophils in the chicken are not commonly found in allergic and parasitic inflammation
    c) Giant cells are absent
    d) Avian heterophil lacks myeloperoxidase
43. Most common cause of cloudy swelling
    a) Hypoxia
    b) Alteration in the physical state of the protein
    c) Toxins
    d) None of the above
44. The oedema fluid is
    a) Non-inflammatory
    b) Low in protein and other colloids
    c) Has specific gravity below 1.012
    d) All of the above
45. Tracheal worm of poultry is
    a) Heterakis gallinarum
    b) Syngamus trachea
    c) Ascaridia galli
    d) Prosthogonimus ovatus

46. Laboured breathing or Gape is characteristic of
    a) Avian influenza b) Histomoniasis
    c) Fowl pox d) Syngamiasis
47. Aspiration pneumonia is a common complication of?
    a) Stomatitis b) Phyaryngitis
    c) Choke d) All above
48. Histotoxic anoxia develops in
    a) Rape and Kale Poisoning b) Cyanide Poisoning
    c) Urget Poisoning d) All of above
49. Haemorrhegic mixed exudates originating from the lungs is
    a) Epistaxix b) Haemeatmeasis
    c) Hemoptysis d) All of them
50. Lungworm L1 spineless larvae having wavy outline of tip of tail
    a) Cystocaulus nigrescens b) Protostrongylus rufescens
    c) Muellerius capillaris d) All of the above
51. Subcutaneous odema of face (swollen face) and wattles together with conjunctivitis is seen in
    a) Pullorum disease b) Infectious coryza
    c) Fowl cholera d) Fowl Typhoid
52. Most common form of IB in poultry is
    a) Respiratory form b) Reproductive form
    c) Nephritic form d) None of the above
53. Failure of the alveoli to open and contain air is
    a) Atelectasis b) Bronchistenosis
    c) Bronchiectasis d) Emphysema
54. Parasite found in the trachea of birds is
    a) Syngamus trachea b) Cyathostoma bronchialis
    c) Cyathostoma variegatum d) All the above
55. Lungworm in which spicule have broad membranous cuticular expansions is
    a) Dictyocaulus b) Protostrongylus
    c) Muellerius d) Metastrongylus
56. Lungworm larvae which are disseminated by Pilobolus fungus is
    a) Filaroides osleri b) Dictyocaulus filaria
    c) Angistrongylus vasorum d) Dictyocaulus viviparus
57. Hourglass shaped pharynx is observed in
    a) Oxyspirura mansoni b) Oxyuris equi
    c) Heterakis gallinarum d) Contracaecum
58. Myeloperoxidase-dependent killing is seen in
    a) Monocytes b) Neutrophils
    c) Both a and b d) Basophils

59. Funnel shaped pharynx is observe in
    a) Habronema majus b) Habronema microstoma
    c) Draschia megastoma d) Habronema muscae
60. Example of inhalant expectorant include
    a) T.T. Oil b) Baladona
    c) Codeine d) Creoline
61. Accumulation of air in pericardium is called as
    a) Pneumothorax b) Pneumopericardium
    c) Hydropericardium d) Pyopericardium
62. Fowl typhoid is caused by
    a) Salmonella pullorum b) Salmonella gallinarum
    c) Salmonella typhimurium d) Salmonella typhosa
63. Small round cells of chronic inflammation are
    a) Lymphocyte and macrophage b) Neutrophil and plasma cells
    c) Macrophage and plasma cells d) Lymphocyte & and plasma cells
64. Lysis of dead tissue by enzymes derived from inflammatory leucocytes is called as
    a) Autolysis b) Heterolysis
    c) Chromatolysis d) None of these
65. Fowl cholera is caused by
    a) Haemophilus paragallinarum b) Pasteurella multocida
    c) Mycoplasma gallisepticum d) Aspergillus fumigatous
66. Gapes is a characteristic feature of
    a) Trachealis bronchi b) Heterakis galli
    c) Syngamus trachea d) Trachelis pulmoni
67. Caseous air sacculitis is observed in
    a) Infectious coryza b) Chronic respiratory disease
    c) Avian chlamydiosis d) Fowl spirochetosis
68. Defective oxygenation of blood in pulmonary circuit is known as
    a) Stagnant anoxia b) Anemic anoxia
    c) Anoxic anoxia d) Histotoxic anoxia
69. Vertically transmitted disease of poultry is
    a) Chronic Respiratory Disease b) Avian encephalomyelitis
    c) Chicken infectious anaemia d) All of the above
70. Which one is a zoonotic disease?
    a) Avian TB b) Fowl paratyphoid
    c) Campylobacteriosis d) All of above
71. Marek's disease is caused by
    a) Gallid Herpesvirus - 1 b) Gallid Herpesvirus - 2
    c) Birnavirus d) Circovirus

72. Infectious laryngotracheitis is caused by
    a) Gallid Herpesvirus - 1
    b) Birnavirus
    c) Gallid Herpesvirus - 2
    d) Circovirus
73. Brooder pneumonia is caused by
    a) Aspergillus fumigatus
    b) Aspergillus flavus
    c) Mycoplasma gallisepticum
    d) Both a and b
74. Presence of cheesy deposits in the air sacs is indicative of
    a) Infectious coryza
    b) Chronic respiratory disease
    c) Fowl spirochetosis
    d) Avian chlamydiosis
75. Death of birds after paralytic symptoms in very cloudy rainy season with high humidity, poor ventilation and overcrowding is indicative of
    a) Carbon monoxide poisoning
    b) Colibacillosis
    c) Heat stroke
    d) Smothering
76. Decline in egg production, sneezing, coughing and Caseous air sacculitis is observed in
    a) Chronic Respiratory Disease
    b) Infectious coryza
    c) Chicken infectious anaemia
    d) Avian chlamydiosis
77. Tropical pulmonary eosinophilia is mainly seen due to
    a) Cercarial reaction
    b) Nematode larvae
    c) Arthropods
    d) Pollen allergy
78. For diagnosis of Avian Influenza in chicken, inoculation done by
    a) Oral route
    b) I/m
    c) I/v
    d) Aerosol route
79. Pseudo tuberculosis is caused by
    a) Mycobacterium tuberculosis
    b) Yersinia pseudotuberculosis
    c) Mycobacterium leprae
    d) Corynebacterium pseudotuberculosis
80. Infectious bursal disease virus destroys
    a) T-cells
    b) B-cells
    c) macrophages
    d) heterophils
81. Swelling of infraorbital sinus with cheesy exudate is seen in
    a) Chronic respiratory disease
    b) Collibacillosis
    c) Infectious bursal disease
    d) Infectious coryza
82. Avian influenza or bird flu is caused by
    a) Orthomyxovirus
    b) Paramyxovirus
    c) Rhabdovirus
    d) Retrovirus
83. Mucopurulent exudates in the nares, fibrinopurulent exudates over pericardium, pleura, air sacs, hepatomegaly, marked enlargement of spleen and necrotic foci on its surface are observed in
    a) Avian influenza
    b) Mycoplasmosis
    c) Infectious bronchitis
    d) Ranikhet disease

84. Infectious bronchitis is caused by

a) Retrovirus b) Circovirus

c) Coronavirus d) Enterovirus

85. Intranuclear inclusion bodies in tracheal epithelium is characteristic of.

a) Ranikhet disease b) Infectious bronchitis

c) Infectious bursal disease d) Infectious Laryngotracheitis

86. Psittacosis is mainly a disease of

a) Elephant b) Birds

c) Horse d) Sheep

87. Characteristic lesion of chicken infectious anaemia is

a) Thymic atrophy b) Bone marrow atrophy

c) Bone marrow aplasia d) All of the above

88. Labored breathing with wheezing and gurgling, accompanied by nervous signs, such as paralysis or twisted necks (torticollis) with depression and death in 3 to 5 days are important clinical manifestations of which avian disease

a) ILT b) Avian influenza

c) Ranikhet Disease d) IB

89. Which avian disease is caused by a virus belonging to the herpes group.

a) Avian influenza b) Infectious bronchitis

c) ND d) Infectious Laryngotracheitis

90. The mild strain of Paramyxovirus virus (ND/ Ranikhet disease) is known as

a) velogenic b) lentogenic

c) mesogenic d) chromogenic

91. Transmission of which avian disease is through the egg to their offspring

a) CRD b) NCD

c) IB d) ILT

92. Major cases of fungal pneumonia in avians

a) Aspergillus fumigatus b) Aspergillus flavus

c) Candida albicans d) Mycoplasma gallisepticum

93. Infected chicks are depressed, thirsty, gasping and rapid breathing ("pump handle breathing") are signs of which avian disease

a) Fungal Pneumonia b) Fowl Typhoid

c) Marek`s Disease d) Fowl Cholera

94. All body cavities of chicks are filled with small yellow-green granular fungal growth; what may be the aetiology?

a) Aspergillus fumigatus b) Aspergillus flavus

c) Histoplasma spp. d) Mycoplasma gallisepticum

95. Vitamin A sparer is

a) Vitamin A b) Vitamin K

c) Vitamin D d) Vitamin E

96. Stage of pneumonia in which fibrin can clearly be seen is
    a) Stage of resolution b) Stage of red hepatization
    c) Stage of grey hepatization d) Stage of congestion
97. Which chemical mediator of inflammation is known as "endogenous pyrogen"
    a) PGF2α b) PGE2
    c) PGI2 d) PGG2
98. Vitamin which plays an important role in wound healing is
    a) Vitamin A b) Vitamin D
    c) Vitamin C d) Vitamin K
99. "First line of cellular defense" in inflammation is
    a) Monocyte b) Macrophage
    c) Lymphocyte d) Neutrophil
100. Swollen Head Syndrome by pnuemovirus mainly affects which avian species
    a) Japanese Quail b) Ducks
    c) Turkey d) Emu
101. Busse-Buschke`s Disease is also known as
    a) Cryptococcosis b) Yeast Meningitis
    c) Torulosis d) All of the above
102. Histoplasmosis is caused by
    a) Histoplasma capsulatum b) Histomonas meleagridis
    c) Haemonchus contortus d) None of the above
103. Hydropic degeneration is closely related to
    a) Hyaline degeneration b) Cloudy swelling
    c) Mucous degeneration d) Amyloid degeneration
104. Pneumovirus in poultry causes
    a) Turkey Rhinotracheitis b) Pneumococosis
    c) Laryngotracheitis d) Infectious bronchitis
105. Marked decline in egg production, swelling of the periorbital and infraorbital sinuses, torticollis, cerebral disorientation etc. in turkey are symptoms
    a) Coccidia b) Pneumoviral infection
    c) Fowl Pox d) Bird Flu
106. Common site for the metastasis for the primary tumor is
    a) Lungs b) Brain
    c) Liver d) Intestine
107. "Second line of cellular defense" is
    a) Neutrophils b) Plasma cells
    c) Macrophages d) Giant cells
108. In poultry Intradermal test for T. b) is performed in
    a) Skin b) Comb
    c) Wattle d) All of the above

109. Psittacosis is caused by
 a) Chlamydia b) Yeast
 c) Nematode d) Trematode
110. Swollen Head Syndrome is also called as
 a) New Castle`s Disease b) Pullorum Disease
 c) Turkey Rhinotracheitis d) Infectious bronchitis
111. Mild type of pneumonia caused by Chlamydia psittaci is
 a) Infectious Bronchitis b) CRD
 c) NCD d) Psittacosis
112. Lungworm larvae with a short "S" shaped tail is
 a) Aelurostrongylus abstrusus b) Filaroides hirthi
 c) Filaroides osleri d) Angistrongylus vasorum
113. Aspiration pneumonia in birds is
 a) Rare b) Doesn't occurs at all
 c) Common d) None of the above
114. Pneumonia caused by faulty drenching of medicine is
 a) Aspiration pneumonia b) Suppurative pneumonia
 c) Intestinal pneumonia d) Granulomatous pneumonia
115. Avian tuberculosis is a chronic wasting disease caused by
 a) Mycobacterium tuberculosis b) Mycobacterium avium
 c) Mycobacterium genavense d) Both B and D
116. Mycobacterium avium complex includes
 a) M. avium subsp. paratuberculosis b) M. avium subsp. silvaticum
 c) M. avium subsp. avium d) All of the above
117. Infectious Bursal Disease is also known as
 a) Newcastle disease b) Marek's disease
 c) Gumboro disease d) Leechi disease
118. Respiratory disease due to fungus in hatchery
 a) Aspergillosis b) brooder pneumonia
 c) mycotic pneumonia d) All of the above
119. Aspergillosis occurs as an acute disease of
 a) young birds and a chronic disease in mature birds
 b) mature birds and a chronic disease in young birds
 c) both young and mature birds
 d) None of the above
120. Mycoplasma gallisepticum causes
 a) chronic respiratory disease b) infectious sinusitis
 c) mycoplasmosis d) All of the above

121. Nutritional roup is due to deficiency of
   a) Retinol
   b) Thiamine
   c) Alpha-tocopherol
   d) Ergocalciferol

122. The disease was called psittacosis or parrot fever when diagnosed in psittacine (curve-beake d) birds, and called ornithosis when diagnosed in all other birds or in humans. It is caused by
   a) Mycobacterium avium
   b) Chlamydia psittaci
   c) Histoplasma spp.
   d) Aspergillus flavus

123. Lasota/F strain Vaccinated in poultry in first week for prevention of which disease
   a) Mareks Disease
   b) Infectious Laryngotracheitis
   c) Newcastle disease
   d) Infectious bronchitis

124. Coryza can be prevented by
   a) Adding Furazolidone to feed
   b) Rodent proof houses
   c) Avoiding overcrowding, wet litter and proper ventilation
   d) Antifungal treatment

125. Aspergillus fumigatus mainly induces airsacculitis and pneumonia, but it may also induce
   a) panophthalmitis
   b) encephalitis and panophthalmitis
   c) encephalitis and osteomyelitis
   d) encephalitis, panophthalmitis, and osteomyelitis

126 Identification of microorganisms by the polymerase-chain reaction is based on the
   a) detection of a sequence of nucleotide in a specific region of the DNA strand of the microorganism
   b) detection of a single, specific nucleotide in the DNA strand of the microorganism
   c) detection of 10-20 random nucleotide in the DNA strand of the microorganism
   d) detection of the entire sequence of nucleotide in the DNA strand of the microorganism

127. There is only one serotype of all of the following avian viruses EXCEPT
   a) Viral arthritis virus
   b) chicken infectious anaemia virus
   c) Newcastle disease virus
   d) infectious laryngotracheitis virus

128. Feature of viral inflammation is
   a) Presence of lymphocytes
   b) Presence of neutrophils
   c) Suppuration
   d) Granuloma formation

129. Paper crackling rales on auscultation is suggestive of
   a) Pneumonia
   b) Bronchitis
   c) Pulmonary emphysema
   d) Pulmonary oedema

130. What is the rationale for using inactivated infectious bursal disease (IBD) vaccine in breeder hens?
   a) to prevent drop in egg production caused by IBD virus
   b) to prevent clinical IBD during the laying period
   c) to prevent immunosuppression during the laying period
   d) to provide the progeny with protective levels of maternal antibodies

131. The serum-plate agglutination (SPA) test and the hemagglutination-inhibition (HI) test are used to detect chickens and turkeys infected with Mycoplasma gallisepticum, M. synoviae and M. meleagridis. Compared to the HI test, the SPA test is
   a) more sensitive
   b) more specific
   c) more sensitive and more specific
   d) none of the above

132. Venereal transmission is a very important method of transmission of which of the following mycoplasmas?
   a) M. gallisepticum
   b) M. synoviae; M. gallisepticum
   c) M. meleagridis
   d) M. iowae; M. meleagridis

133. Which of the following is TRUE about the egg-transmission of Mycoplasma gallisepticum in chickens?
   a) in typical field cases, the rate of egg-transmission is very high (usually 60-80%)
   b) egg transmission occurs only in hens infected during egg-production
   c) egg-transmission can be eliminated by treating infected breeder flocks with antibiotics
   d) infected hens may shed the mycoplasma intermittently

134. Which of the following vaccine strains of Mycoplasma gallisepticum is labelled only for eyedrop administration.
   a) F strain
   b) strain 6/85
   c) strain ts-11
   d) F strain and strain ts-11

135. Natural infection of turkeys has been reported to occur with which of the following avian paramyxovirus serotypes?
   a) serotypes 3 and 7
   b) serotypes 2, 3, and 6
   c) serotypes 2, 3, 6, and 7
   d) serotypes 2 and 3

136. A virus was isolated from the respiratory tract of broiler chickens with respiratory disease. Negative contrast microscopy showed that the virus had club-shaped surface projections. The virus could be
   a) influenza virus
   b) infectious bronchitis virus
   c) Newcastle disease virus
   d) infectious laryngotracheitis virus

137. Violent coughing with marked dyspnea (gasping) in 24-week-old chickens should arouse suspicion of which of the following diseases?
   a) infectious bronchitis
   b) infectious laryngotracheitis
   c) Newcastle disease
   d) infectious coryza

138. Infectious coryza is characterized by all of the following clinical signs / gross lesions EXCEPT
   a) serous or mucoid nasal discharge
   b) excess mucus in the nasal passages and sinuses
   c) facial subcutaneous edema
   d) diffuse hemorrhage in the tracheal mucosa

139. The hemagglutination test can be used to distinguish between Newcastle disease virus and which of the following viruses?
   a) infectious laryngotracheitis virus
   b) infectious bronchitis virus and infectious laryngotrache it is virus
   c) infectious bronchitis virus and egg drop syndrome virus
   d) infectious laryngotracheitis virus and egg drop syndrome virus

140. Which of the following organs/tissues are preferred for the isolation of infectious bronchitis virus from chickens infected 3 weeks ago with this virus?
   a) trachea b) lungs
   c) air sacs d) cecal tonsils

141. Which of the following samples is preferred for the detection/isolation of avian pneumovirus in infected birds?
   a) swabs collected from the oropharynx mucosal surface
   b) swabs collected from the conjunctival surface
   c) swabs inserted into the choanal cleft
   d) swabs inserted into the trachea

142. Reversion of the vaccine virus to virulence is most significant with some attenuated live vaccines for which of the following diseases?
   a) infectious bursal disease b) avian encephalomyelitis
   c) viral arthritis d) infectious laryngotracheitis

   Vasoconstrictor drugs used in epistaxis include
   a) Adrenaline b) Alum
   c) Vitamin C d) Ice

143. Type A influenza virus is subtyped on the basis of differences in which of the following virus antigens?
   a) hemagglutinin b) ncuraminidasc
   c) nucleocapsid and matrix antigens d) hemagglutinin and neuraminidase

144. Which of the following avian viruses is known to be capable of establishing latent infection in chickens?
   a) Newcastle disease virus b) infectious laryngotracheitis virus
   c) infectious bronchitis virus d) avian encephalomyelitis virus

145. Which of the following Newcastle disease virus strains can be used for vaccinating one-day-old chicks by the coarse-spray method?
   a) Lasota b) Hitchener B1
   c) Hitchener B1 or Lasota d) none of the above

146. Which of the following lesions is characteristically found in some chicks affected with viscerotropic velogenic Newcastle disease virus?
   a) splenomegaly
   b) hemorrhagic ulcers in the small intestine
   c) consolidation of both lungs
   d) foci of necrosis and hemorrhage in the liver

147. Fruiting heads of Aspergillus are most likely seen in smears prepared from lesions of

   Aspergillus infection in which of the following organs?
   a) brain
   b) air sac
   c) lungs
   d) eyes

148. Quail are succumbed to natural infection with which of the following avian viruses?
   a) infectious bronchitis virus
   b) infectious laryngotracheitis virus
   c) infectious bronchitis virus and infectious laryngotracheitis virus
   d) avian encephalomyelitis virus

149. Compared to the lentogenic strains, the mesogenic strains of Newcastle disease virus are
   a) more pathogenic
   b) more immunogenic
   c) more pathogenic and more immunogenic
   d) more pathogenic and less immunogenic

150. Mature chickens infected laterally with avian encephalomyelitis virus shed the virus in the
   a) faeces
   b) egg and respiratory secretions
   c) egg and faeces
   d) eggs

151. Seven-day-old chicks were gasping. On necropsy you found only very small caseous nodules in the lungs and air sacs. Which condition would be the first on your list of rule-outs?
   a) aspergillosis
   b) subacute salmonellosis
   c) tuberculosis
   d) Mycoplasma gallisepticum infection

152. If infectious laryngotracheitis (ILT) is suspected in a flock, the inability to detect inclusion bodies in the tracheal epithelium of the examined birds does not necessarily exclude the disease; that is because the inclusion bodies of ILT virus can
   a) only be detected by using a special stain in histologic sections
   b) only be detected in the early stages of infection
   c) only formed by the highly pathogenic strains
   d) only seen in tissue sections prepared from the upper part of the trachea

153. Newcastle disease virus has been classified into how many pathotypes?
   a) 2 b) 3
   c) 4 d) 5
154. What is the classical clinical manifestation of avian influenza in turkeys and chickens?
   a) respiratory signs b) neurologic signs
   c) diarrhea d) only high mortality
155. Certain strains of which of the following avian viruses are nephropathogenic?
   a) infectious laryngotracheitis virus b) infectious bronchitis virus
   c) Newcastle disease virus d) avian encephalomyelitis virus
156. Concretions of dust, dirt and nasal mucus blocking external nares is known as
   a) Rhinotracheitis b) Rhinitis
   c) Rhinoliths d) Sinusitis
157. Sternostoma tracheacolum primarily affects which organ
   a) Air Sac b) Diaphragm
   c) Alveoli d) Liver
158. Squamous metaplasia with increased keratinization of epithelia of respiratory tract leading to respiratory distress is due to deficiency of which vitamin?
   a) A b) B6
   c) B12 d) D
159. Type of inflammation seen in Tuberculosis is
   a) Fibrinous b) Haemorrhagic
   c) Granulomatous d) Suppurative
160. Deposition of calcium carbonate or Calcium Dust in lungs is called as
   a) Acanthosis b) Chalicosis
   c) Anthracosis d) Argyrosis
161. Which one is not a true aneurysm?
   a) Fusiform aneurysm b) Cirsoid aneurysm
   c) Arteriovenous aneurysm d) Dissecting aneurysm
162. Dactylariosis (mycotic encephalitis) infection occurs by
   a) Inhalation of spores b) Transmission via eggs
   c) Sexual Transmission d) None of these
163. Rhodotorulosis is caused by
   a) Fungi b) Bacteria
   c) Yeast d) Virus
164. Favus in Avian species is caused by
   a) Microsprum gallinae b) Trichophyton gallinae
   c) Trichophyton simii d) All of the above

165. Torulopsis in poultry birds is caused by
   a) Fungus
   b) Virus
   c) Bacteria
   d) Parasite

166. Voice box of poultry is
   a) Larynx
   b) Syrinx
   c) Trachea
   d) Tongue

167. A Flock was presented with respiratory troubles, anorexia and air sacculitis was treated with antifungal drugs and the birds started recovery. What disease it was?
   a) Aspergilosis
   b) Avian tuberculosis
   c) Fowl Typhoid
   d) Candidiasis

168. Mucormycosis is caused by
   a) Mucor resimosus
   b) Mucor chorimbifer
   c) Both A and B
   d) Mycobacterium

169. Sarcocystis falcatula causes which disease in birds
   a) Fungal Pneumonia
   b) Acromegaly
   c) Sarcocytosis
   d) Sarcophagosis

170. "Cells of tripier" are seen in lung during
   a) Bronchopneumonia
   b) Interstitial Pneumonia
   c) Verminous Pneumonia
   d) Mycotic Pneumonia

171. Lungworm larvae which are disseminated by Pilobolus fungus is
   a) Filaroides osleri
   b) Dictyocaulus viviparus
   c) Angistrongylus vasorum
   d) Dictyocaulus filaria

172. Dilatation and rupture of lung alveoli is called
   a) Atelectasis
   b) Bronchistenosis
   c) Emphysema
   d) Bronchiectasis

173. Gangrene in lungs is commonly caused by
   a) Asphyxia
   b) Epistaxis
   c) Faulty drenching
   d) Anaemia

174. Avian Sarcocytosis is which type of respiratory parasite
   a) Fungal
   b) Trematode
   c) Protozoal
   d) Coccidial

175. Quail bronchitis is caused by
   a) coronavirus
   b) adenovirus
   c) herpesvirus
   d) orthomyxovirus

176. Which of the following avian mycoplasmas does need nicotinamide adenine dinucleotide (NAD) for its growth?
   a) M. gallisepticum
   b) M. synoviae
   c) M. meleagridis
   d) M. gallisepticum and M. meleagridis

177. The hemagglutination-inhibition test can be used to determine the humoral immunity status to which of the following viral diseases?
 a) Newcastle disease
 b) Newcastle disease and egg drop syndrome
 c) Newcastle disease and infectious bronchitis
 d) Newcastle disease, egg drop syndrome, and infectious bronchitis

178. Inclusion bodies of infectious laryngotracheitis virus occurs in the trachea, but they may also be found in the
 a) Air Sac and bronchi
 b) conjunctivae and bronchi
 c) Alveoli and bronchi
 d) Liver

179. The presence of a caseous mass in the pharyngeal region of a pigeon arouses suspicion of which of the following diseases?
 a) chlamydiosis
 b) trichomoniasis
 c) candidiasis
 d) pigeon herpesvirus 1 infection

180. Migratory waterfowl are considered as an important source of infection of poultry with which of the following viral diseases?
 a) infectious bronchitis
 b) avian influenza
 c) avian encephalomyelitis
 d) Newcastle disease

181. The double immunodiffusion test is used to define the type of influenza virus. This serological test identifies which of the following antigens of influenza virus?
 a) matrix antigens
 b) matrix and nucleocapsid antigens
 c) nucleocapsid antigen
 d) hemagglutinin antigen

182. Which of the following tests is used to confirm that an isolated virus is type A influenza virus?
 a) hemagglutination-inhibition test
 b) agar-gel immunodiffusion test
 c) hemagglutination test
 d) virus-neutralization test

183. Consolidation of one or both lungs (pneumonia) is a frequent gross lesion; associated with which of the following diseases?
 a) fowl cholera
 b) Ornithobacterium rhinotracheale infection
 c) Ornithobacterium rhinotracheale infection and bordetellosis
 d) fowl cholera and Ornithobacterium rhinotracheale infection

184. All isolates of "highly pathogenic" avian influenza virus are of which of the following haemagglutinin subtypes?
 a) H3 and H7
 b) H5 and H7
 c) H1 and H7
 d) H1 and H5

185. Sudden mortality in a flock of 5-week-old broiler chickens. Thereafter many birds in the flock developed torticollis (twisting of the neck). Which of the following diseases it may be
 a) infectious bronchitis
 b) avian influenza
 c) avian encephalomyelitis
 d) Newcastle disease

186. Layer and breeder flocks are sometimes boosted during the egg production with live Newcastle disease and infectious bronchitis vaccines. To maintain a protective level of immunity, and also to avoid vaccine-induced drop in egg production, it is recommended that boosters be given every

a) 2-4 weeks
b) 4-6 weeks
c) 8-10 weeks
d) 12-14 weeks

187. What concentration of erythrocyte suspension should be used in the hemagglutination-inhibition test for Newcastle disease virus?

a) 1.50%
b) 1.25%
c) 0.5%
d) 1%

188. Cloacal swabs are primarily useful for the isolation of which of the following mycoplasmas from infected chickens and/or turkeys?

a) M. gallisepticum and M. synoviae
b) M. meleagridis
c) M. synoviae and M. meleagridis
d) M. gallisepticum

189. Softening and distortion of the trachea in turkey poults with respiratory signs are strongly suggestive of infection with

a) Bordetella avium
b) Cryptosporidium spp.
c) Adenovirus
d) Pneumovirus

Answer Key

1	c	2	a	3	a	4	b	5	c	6	b	7	a
8	d	9	b	10	a	11	b	12	a	13	d	14	a
15	c	16	b	17	c	18	b	19	a	20	a	21	c
22	b	23	a	24	b	25	d	26	b	27	b	28	b
29	c	30	a	31	a	32	b	33	b	34	b	35	a
36	d	37	a	38	a	39	c	40	a	41	c	42	c
43	a	44	d	45	b	46	d	47	d	48	b	49	c
50	b	51	b	52	a	53	a	54	d	55	d	56	d
57	a	58	c	59	c	60	a	61	b	62	b	63	d
64	b	65	b	66	c	67	b	68	c	69	d	70	d
71	b	72	c	73	d	74	b	75	d	76	a	77	b
78	d	79	b	80	b	81	d	82	a	83	b	84	c
85	d	86	b	87	d	88	c	89	d	90	b	91	a
92	a	93		94	a	95	d	96	c	97	b	98	c
99	d	100	c	101	d	102	a	103	b	104	b	105	b
106	a	107	c	108	c	109	a	110	c	111	d	112	c
113	c	114	a	115	d	116	d	117	c	118	d	119	a
120	d	121	a	122	b	123	c	124		125	d	126	a
127	a	128	a	129	c	130	d	131	a	132	d	133	d
134	c	135	c	136	b	137	b	138	d	139	b	140	d

141	c	142	d	143	a	144	d	145	b	146	b	147	b
148	b	149	c	150	c	151	b	152	a	153	b	154	b
155	a	156	b	157	c	158	a	159	a	160	c	161	b
162	d	163	a	164	c	165	d	166	a	167	b	168	a
169	c	170	c	171	c	172	b	173	c	174	c	175	c
176	b	177	b	178	d	179	a	180	b	181	b	182	b
183	b	184	d	185	b	186	d	187	c	188	c	189	b
190	a												

18

Disorders of Endocrine System

Sonam Bhatt[1], Manish Singh[1], Bhavna[2], Anil Kumar[1] and RSK Mandal[1]

[1]Department of Veterinary Medicine, Bihar Veterinary College, BASU, Patna

[2]Department of Veterinary Gynaecology & Obstetrics, Bihar Veterinary College, BASU, Patna

Introduction

Poultry are domesticated birds mostly reared for the purpose of meat and egg consumption as well as for their feathers. It includes chickens, quails, turkeys, waterfowls, ducks and geese. The endocrine system of poultry consists of hypothalamic-hypophyseal complex, parathyroid gland, thyroid gland, pancreatic islet cells, adrenal glands, ultimobranchial glands, endocrine cells of gut and the gonads. These endocrine organs release hormones into the bloodstream. Peptide hormones act on the surface of cells, whereas steroid hormones act on target tissues by entering in the cytoplasm or nucleus of cells. Lack of diagnosis in the case of endocrinopathies is a major cause of production loss globally. Advancement in awareness, diagnosis, treatment as well as management is critical to ensure optimal flock health. Cost-effective programs of biosecurity and vaccination are required to prevent or limit the impact of disease. Programs of emergency treatment and long-term prevention are justified for severe endocrine diseases which have a profound impact on production.

Gland	Location	Hormone	Disease
Pituitary Gland	Head	Neurohypophysis- Anti-diuretic hormones, Oxytocin	Dwarfism, Diabetes insipidus, Adenoma
		Adenohypophysis- LH, FSH, TSH, GH, ACTH, MSH, Prolactin	
Parathyroid Gland	Caudal to the thyroid glands	Parathormone	Hyperplasia, Adenoma
Thyroid Gland	Thoracic inlet	Thyroid hormone	Colloid goiter, Atrophy, Hyperplasia, Thyroiditis, Adenoma, Carcinoma
Ultimobranchial Body	Caudal to the thyroids	'C' cells secrete calcitonin	Hypertrophy, Cysts

Carotid/Aortic Bodies	Contact with the parathyroid gland	Detect low arterial O_2 and high CO_2	Neoplasms
Adrenal Glands	At cranial pole of kidney	Interrenal cells Corticosterone, o aldosterone	Adrenal degeneration, Amyloidosis, Hypertrophy, Neoplasms, Infectious diseases, Pheochromocytoma
		Chromaffin cells release epinephrine or norepinephrine	
Islets of Langerhans	Scattered in the pancreas	A cell- Glucagon	Degeneration, Neoplasms
		B cell- Insulin	
		D cell- Somatostatin	

Multiple Choice Questions

1. Poultry hypophysis consists of
   a) Anterior and posterior parts
   b) Dorsal and ventral parts
   c) Both a and b
   d) Rostral and ventral parts
2. Pars distalis is a part of
   a) Neurohypophysis
   b) Adenohypophysis
   c) Both
   d) Pars tuberalis
3. Pars intermedia is not present in
   a) Birds
   b) Rat
   c) Both a and b
   d) None of the above
4. Arginine vasotocin and mesotocin are secreted by
   a) Adenohypophysis
   b) Neurohypophysis
   c) Pars nervosa
   d) Both b and c
5. Lower concentrations of somatomedin C and T_3 can cause
   a) Gigantism
   b) Abnormal comb shape
   c) Dwarfism
   d) Absence of comb and wattle
6. In Dwarfism in poultry
   a) Growth hormone can be higher in concentration
   b) Growth hormone is generally lower in concentration
   c) Not related to growth hormone
   d) GH receptors are high in number
7. Dwarfism in poultry is
   a) Sex-linked character
   b) Sex-linked recessive character
   c) Both a and b
   d) None of the above
8. Thyrotropin-releasing hormone stimulates conversion of
   a) T_4 to T_3
   b) T_4 to T_3
   c) Both a and b
   d) None of the above

9. Main physiological regulator of body water of body water in birds is/are
   a) Arginine Vasotocin (AVT) b) Octapeptide
   c) Gonadotrophins d) Both a and b
10. In birds, Arginine vasotocin produces
   a) Diuresis b) Antidiuresis
   c) Diabetes mellitus d) Dwarfism
11. The distal enlargement of avian pineal glands is known as
   a) Pineal vesicle b) Seminal vesicle
   c) Both a and b d) None
12. In birds, calcium metabolism is under the control of
   a) Only Parathyroid hormone b) Only Calcitonin
   c) Only 1,25 Dihydrocholecalciferol d) All of the above
13. 1,25 Dihydrocholecalciferol is an active metabolite of
   a) Vitamin D_4 b) Vitamin A
   c) Vitamin D_3 d) Vitamin K
14. The parathyroid gland consists of
   a) Cranial and caudal lobes b) Anterior and posterior lobes
   c) Only one lobe d) Parathyroid gland is absent in fowl
15. Parathyroid hormone secreted in response to
   a) Hypercalcemia b) Hypocalcemia
   c) Hypomagnesemia d) Hypermagnesemia
16. Main target organ of parathyroid hormone is/are
   a) Kidney b) Bone
   c) Both a and b d) None
17. Calcitonin is secreted by
   a) C cells b) T cells
   c) C and T cells both d) None
18. Choose the correct statement
   a) Hypocalcaemia is controlled by calcitonin
   b) Calcitonin increases calcium reabsorption from bones
   c) Both statement a and b are incorrect
   d) Both statement a and b are correct
19. Lack of vitamin D_3 in young birds leads to
   a) Rickets b) Alopecia
   c) Both a and b d) None of the above
20. Which statement is false about uropygial gland
   a) It is also known as preen gland
   b) It is an unilobed sebaceous gland
   c) It is used to distribute oil through plumage
   d) Located at base of tail

21. Rachitis is a condition characterized by
    a) Hypercalcemia
    b) Rubber beak
    c) Vitamin C deficiency
    d) None
22. Which statement is incorrect for osteodystrophy in mature birds
    a) It can be due to calcium deficiency
    b) Parathyroid gland will become smaller
    c) Complete demineralisation of medullary and cortical parts of bone
    d) Osseus tissue can be replaced by fibrous tissue
23. Greenstick fracture is a condition when
    a) Bone cracks on both sides
    b) Compression stress applied to bone
    c) Bending stress applied to bone
    d) Plasma calcium concentration become above normal
24. Which statement is incorrect for osteodystrophy
    a) Plasma calcium concentrations remain normal till end stage
    b) Tetanic convulsions can be seen in end stage
    c) Demineralization of bones occur
    d) None of the above
25. Progressive reduction in bone mass is characteristic of
    a) Osteoporosis
    b) Only statement 1 is incorrect
    c) Only statement 2 is incorrect
    d) Both statements 1 and 2 are correct
26. Which statement is incorrect for dystrophic calcification of kidney tubules
    a) It occurs due to a deficiency of vitamin D_3
    b) It can be due to over-supplementation of vitamin D_3
    c) It is not associated with concentration of vitamin D_3
    d) Both b and c are correct
27. Calcium neuropath y is a condition in poultry when birds are raised on a diet containing
    a) 3% calcium instead of normal 0.6%
    b) 6% calcium instead of normal 0.3%
    c) 1% calcium instead of normal 0.12%
    d) Less than 0.12%
28. Hypervitaminosis D_3 occurs when the amount of vitamins exceeds
    a) 1 million IU/Kg in diet
    b) 2 million IU/Kg in diet
    c) 2.4 million IU/Kg in diet
    d) 4 million IU/Kg in diet

29. Choose the wrong statement
    a) The thyroid glands in birds are paired organs that lie on each side of the trachea in the thoracic inlet
    b) The thyroids are in close contact with the common carotid artery
    c) The avian thyroid gland contains calcitonin cell
    d) Ultimobranchial gland produces calcitonin
30. Choose the wrong statement
    a) Compared to the thyroid gland in mammals, the avian thyroid produces less T4 than T3
    b) The activity of the 5'-monodeiodination enzyme is controlled by hypothalamic hormones
    c) The thyroid lobes are composed of follicles surrounded by single layers of epithelial cells enclosed by a basement membrane.
    d) The epithelial cells' height depends on the secretory rate and may vary from flat to columnar.
31. In primary hypothyroidism
    a) Thyroid follicles are distended with colloid, and the lining epithelial cells become flattened
    b) Loss of follicles resulting either from thyroiditis or atrophy
    c) Both a and b are correct
    d) Both a and b are incorrect
32. Choose the incorrect statement about primary hypothyroidism in birds
    a) In chickens, it occurs as a hereditary autoimmune disorder
    b) Low levels of thyroid hormones have also been associated with malabsorption syndrome
    c) Chickens with genetic hypothyroidism have low T4 concentrations and obesity
    d) Occurs due to low TSH
33. Thyroiditis causes
    a) Obesity
    b) Silky plumage
    c) Lack of maturity
    d) All are correct
34. To decrease the incidence and severity of chronic thyroiditis
    a) Thymectomy can be performed
    b) Neonatal bursectomy can be performed
    c) Both a and b are equally effective
    d) Performed antibody injections
35. Choose the wrong statement about the adrenal gland in poultry
    a) The right and left avian adrenal glands are yellow organs located craniomedial to the kidneys
    b) The avian adrenal gland is divided into an outer cortex and inner medulla
    c) In birds, cortical and chromaffin tissue are intermingled
    d) The glands receive blood from branches of the renal artery, while the adrenal veins drain into the caudal vena cava

36. Choose the correct statement
    a) The embryonic avian adrenal gland is also a site of sex steroid synthesis
    b) The secretion of corticosterone is regulated by ACTH from pars nervosa
    c) Both a and b
    d) None
37. Choose the wrong statement about corticosterone
    a) Corticosterone is essential for survival in times of stress
    b) It also has mineralocorticoid activity
    c) Corticosterone balances the production and action of catecholamines, prostaglandins
    d) Plasma corticosterone concentrations cannot reliably be determined using an RIA (radioimmunoassay)
38. In free-ranging Mallard Ducks living in coastal estuaries and alkaline lake environments, corticosterone functions as an important mineral-regulating hormone. Under these circumstances, it acts simultaneously on these target organs, except
    a) Pancreas
    b) Small intestine
    c) Nasal salt glands
    d) Kidney
39. Calcitonin cells, which are the chief or parafollicular cells in mammals, are absent in the
    a) Avian thyroid
    b) Avian adrenal gland
    c) Both a and b
    d) Avian pituitary
40. Choose the incorrect statement
    a) Renin is released from the juxtaglomerular cells of the kidney in response to low plasma sodium concentration or reduced blood volume
    b) The renin acts on circulating angiotensinogen to form angiotensin I, which is converted to angiotensin II
    c) Aldosterone secretion is stimulated by angiotensin II
    d) Like mammals, birds release aldosterone in response to elevated extracellular potassium concentrations
41. The adrenal gland in poultry is a
    a) Paired organ
    b) Single organ
    c) Both a and b
    d) None of the above
42. In all avian species studied, the major glucocorticoid is
    a) Corticosterone
    b) Cortisol
    c) Both a and b
    d) None of the above

43. Cortisol administration is indicated when stressful procedures are undertaken in patients who have been receiving long-term treatment with corticosteroids and are suffering from iatrogenic secondary hypoadrenocorticism. The dosage of cortisol for replacement therapy should be
    a) 0.002-0.02mg/kg b) 200-300 mg/kg
    c) 150 mg/kg d) 0.5-1 mg/kg
44. Anti-inflammatory and chemotherapeutic doses of prednisolone are
    a) 0.5-1.0 mg/kg and 2-4 mg/kg respectively
    b) 50-100 mg/kg and 2-4 mg/kg respectively
    c) 0.5-1.0 mg/kg and 200-400 mg/kg respectively
    d) 50-100 mg/kg and 200-400 mg/kg respectively
45. Calcitonin (CT)-secreting cells are absent in
    a) Birds b) Mammals
    c) Both a and b d) None
46. Which statement is incorrect for iatrogenic Hyperadrenocorticism-like disease
    a) Exogenous glucocorticoids cause hyperphagia while reducing growth and body weight in birds
    b) There is a marked increase in fat deposition
    c) Concomitant increase in protein catabolism
    d) Gluconeogenesis is decreased
47. Which of the following stressors can induce corticosterone secretion in birds
    a) Immobilization b) Hypovitaminosis A
    c) Anesthesia d) All of them
48. Choose the incorrect statement about stress marks
    a) A common disorder of developing feathers is the symmetrical development of stress marks or hunger traces
    b) These lesions do not represent a period of malnutrition or stress while the feathers were developing
    c) These represent a segmental dysplasia in the barbs and barbules
    d) Stress lines can be easily identified by holding the spread wing or tail feathers
49. Which statement is incorrect regarding Pheochromocytoma (Chromaffinoma)
    a) A benign or malignant tumor of chromaffin tissue may cause hypersecretion of epinephrine or norepinephrine
    b) It is known to lead to hypertension and associated symptoms such as profuse sweating and cardiac irregularities
    c) Spastic gait is commonly seen along with hardening of plumage
    d) All statements are correct
50. Choose the incorrect statement regarding phases of development of plumage
    a) Production of germ cells can occur in the absence of thyroid hormone
    b) Presence of thyroid hormone is essential for the growth

c) Presence of thyroid hormone is essential for formation of feather pattern
d) Importance of thyroid hormone for feather formation is different in young and mature birds

51. Choose the incorrect statement
a) In hyperthyroidism lower parts of the feather develop most vigorously
b) In thyroidectomized birds, the lower parts of the feather are underdeveloped
c) In hyperthyroidism, the vanes of the feathers are narrower and there is a partial reduction of the barbs
d) All statements are correct

52. Choose the correct statement regarding molting in birds
a) It occurs during a period of enhanced sexual activity
b) It cannot be suppressed by sex hormones
c) It can be induced by administration of progesterone
d) Both a and b statements are correct

53. Short periods of daily light can cause
a) Enhanced sexual activity b) Caseation of molting
c) Both a and b are correct d) Induction of molting

54. In some birds (Galliformes, Passeriformes, Anseriformes), feather color and pattern vary with
a) Age b) Gender
c) Season d) All of the above

55. Choose the wrong statement about vitamin B_6
a) The metabolically active form of vitamin B6, pyridoxal sulfate
b) A deficiency of pyridoxine creates a deficiency of hormones such as serotonin and histamine
c) It is required in the decarboxylation of glutamic acid to form gamma-aminobutyric acid (GABA), the lack of which has been shown to cause seizures
d) It also plays a role as a modulator of steroid hormone receptors

56. The adrenal hormone causes retention of
a) Potassium b) Sodium
c) Chloride d) Bicarbonate

57. Choose the incorrect statement regarding thyroid hormone
a) Thyroid hormone functions to control the rate of energy metabolism in cells
b) Iodine's sole metabolic function is for the biosynthesis of the thyroid hormones
c) The iodide uptake by the thyroid is stimulated by thyroid-stimulating hormone
d) Iodine is easily absorbed from the gastrointestinal tract in the oxidized iodide state

58. Hormone analysis can be done via
a) Radioimmunoassay (RIA) b) ELISA
c) Antigen/antibody reaction d) All

59. Choose the wrong statement about cholesterol
   a) Cholesterol is a major lipid that is a precursor of all the steroid hormones
   b) Component of the plasma membrane of cells
   c) In excess, it can cause fatty liver, hypothyroidism
   d) Prevalence of fatty liver degeneration is higher in female birds than in male birds
60. Choose the correct statement about the testicles of male birds
   a) Under the seasonal influence of hormones, the mass may increase from 10 up to 500 times
   b) The testicle of the adult male bird is ellipsoidal to bean-shaped
   c) Both a and b are correct
   d) Both a and b are incorrect
61. The use of the azole antifungals in veterinary medicine
   a) Inhibits synthesis of the primary fungal sterol, ergosterol
   b) Destroys fungal cell membrane integrity
   c) Causes inhibition of a P_{450} enzyme system
   d) All
62. Choose the incorrect statement
   a) Cholecystokinin (CCK) is not an intestinal hormone
   b) It is likely that there is a continuous secretion of bile into the intestine in birds, with or without a gall bladder
   c) A slight increase in bile secretions would be expected postprandially due to the intrahepatic effects of intestinal hormones
   d) Avian vasoactive intestinal peptide (VIP) is an intestinal hormone
63. In pituitary adenoma, the neoplasms often originate from
   a) Proliferation of chromophobe cells in the posterior lobe
   b) Proliferation of chromophobe cells in the anterior lobe
   c) Expansive neoplasms follow the path of most resistance
   d) Pituitary adenomas are not associated with polydipsia and polyuria
64. Which statement is incorrect about goiter
   a) It is associated with iodine-deficient diets
   b) Ingestion of goitrogenic plants such as Solanum species
   c) Causes bilateral glandular enlargement
   d) Exposure to iodine-containing disinfectants or excessive dietary iodine can lead to goiter
65. Enterochromaffin cells present in
   a) Adrenal medulla
   b) Adrenal cortex
   c) Both
   d) None of the above

66. Adrenal adenomas arise from
    a) Interrenal cells
    b) Adrenal cortex
    c) Both
    d) None
67. The islets of Langerhans are composed of a diverse aggregation of cells, except
    a) Alpha cells
    b) Beta cells
    c) Gamma cells
    d) Delta cells
68. Choose the correct statement
    a) Alpha cells secrete gastrin
    b) Beta cells secrete glucagon
    c) Beta cells secrete gastrin
    d) Alpha cells secrete glucagon
69. Choose the correct statement regarding pituitary adenoma
    a) Mainly affect D-cells
    b) Arise from chromophobe cells
    c) Nervous signs are absent
    d) Therapy with o,p'-DDD is generally indicated
70. Choose the incorrect statement regarding the administration of progesterone
    a) In large doses may inhibit ovulation
    b) If given 36 hours before expected ovulation, will induce follicular atresia
    c) If given 2 to 24 hours pre-ovulation, it can induce premature ovulation
    d) None
71. Choose the incorrect statement regarding secondary nutritional hyperparathyroidism
    a) Calcium utilization exceeds absorption from the intestine over a prolonged period
    b) Parathyroid hormone excretion will increase
    c) Parathyroid glands will enlarge
    d) High levels of phosphorus or low levels of vitamin D in the diet can be used to alleviate symptoms
72. Choose the incorrect statement
    a) Neurohypophysis comes from neuroectoderm of the diencephalic floor
    b) The adenohypophysis develops from Rathke's pouch
    c) Rathke's pouch is an outgrowth of the roof of the oral cavity
    d) Rathke's pouch is absent in mammals
73. Adenohypophysis comprised of
    a) Pars tuberalis and the larger pars distalis
    b) Pars tuberalis and the smaller pars distalis
    c) Both pars tuberalis and pars distalis are equal in size
    d) None
74. Choose an incorrect statement regarding neurohypophysis
    a) It is a direct extension of the hypothalamus
    b) It has median eminence
    c) Infundibulum and neural lobe are absent
    d) All statements are incorrect

75. Which hormone is not secreted by adenohypophysis
    a) Follicle stimulation hormone
    b) Oxytocin
    c) Adrenocorticotropic hormone
    d) Growth hormone
76. The Parathyroid Gland is derived from
    a) 3rd (internal parathyroid) and 4th (lateral parathyroid) pharyngeal pouches
    b) 3rd (external parathyroid) and 4th (internal parathyrod) pharyngeal pouches
    c) 3rd (internal parathyroid) and 4th (external parathyroid)pharyngeal pouches
    d) 3rd (lateral parathyroid) and 4th (internal parathyroid) pharyngeal pouches
77. Choose the correct statement regarding parathyroid gland
    a) Colour grossly tan yellow
    b) It has loose connective tissue capsule and is comprised of cords, sheets, and rosettes of cells
    c) Oxyphil cells absent in birds
    d) All
78. Primary target tissues of parathormone are
    a) Bones
    b) Kidney
    c) Both
    d) None
79. Choose the correct statement
    a) Thyroid Gland is the earliest gland to appear in an embryo
    b) It is derived from the floor of the pharynx
    c) Both a and b statements are correct
    d) Both a and b statements are incorrect
80. Choose the correct statement
    a) In altricial birds, thyroid function has minimal maturation until after hatch
    b) In precocial birds, thyroid function and its control are not well-developed
    c) Both statements a and b are incorrect
    d) None of the statement is correct
81. The best method of testing the avian thyroid for abnormalities is measuring the serum concentration of
    a) T_1
    b) T_2
    c) T_3
    d) T_4
82. Disease-related to the thyroid gland are
    a) Hyperplasia
    b) Adenoma
    c) Carcinoma
    d) All
83. Potential secondary effects of hypothyroidism include
    a) Noninflammatory feather loss
    b) Excessive fat in the skin/subcutis
    c) Hyperkeratosis
    d) All
84. Choose an incorrect statement regarding the ultimobranchial body
    a) It is a 7 to 9 mm structure that is slightly irregular and gray, pink in the adult
    b) Histologically the ultimobranchial body is comprised of cords of 'C' cells
    c) Located slightly caudal to the thyroids
    d) None

85. Calcitonin is secreted by
   a) A cells b) B cells
   c) C cells d) D cells
86. Calcitonin blocks the transfer of which element from bone to blood
   a) Sodium b) Calcium
   c) Potassium d) All
87. Bioassay indicates avian calcitonin levels compared to mammals, are
   a) Lower b) Higher
   c) Similar d) Similar or higher
88. Chromaffin cells derived from
   a) Endoderm b) Mesoderm
   c) Neuroectoderm d) All
89. Choose the incorrect statement
   a) Carotid bodies are paired and usually in contact with the thymus gland
   b) Aortic body is present between the aorta and pulmonary artery at base of the heart
   c) Glomus cells contain granular vesicles
   d) None
90. Carotid/Aortic Bodies are chemoreceptors which
   a) Detect low arterial oxygen b) Detect high CO_2
   c) Help in controlling respiration d) All
91. A tumor of neuroendocrine tissue of the carotid body is called
   a) Chemodectoma b) Carcinoid
   c) Glioma d) Seminoma
92. Pheochromocytoma is
   a) Tumor of thyroid b) Tumor of adrenal cortex
   c) Tumor of adrenal medulla d) Tumor of parathyroid
93. Interrenal cells arise from
   a) Ectoderm b) Mesoderm
   c) Endoderm d) All
94. Choose an incorrect statement regarding adrenal gland
   a) Interrenal cells are basophilic and granular
   b) Chromaffin cells are eosinophilic
   c) Histologically there is no cortex/medulla differentiation
   d) Both a and b
95. Aldosterone production can be stimulated by
   a) Low sodium or reduced blood volume
   b) Low potassium or high blood volume
   c) Low sodium
   d) High blood volume

96. Choose the correct statement
    a) Epinephrine increase can lead to eggshell abnormalities
    b) Epinephrine can stimulate glycogenolysis and lipolysis
    c) Norepinephrine is involved in blood pressure maintenance
    d) All are correct
97. Choose an incorrect statement regarding amyloidosis
    a) Generalized amyloid deposition
    b) Affected glands shrink and pale grossly
    c) Histologically the amyloid is primarily deposited in sinusoidal walls
    d) Sinusoidal walls are thickened by amorphous or basophilic material
98. In viral infections the adrenal glands
    a) Polyomavirus infection can lead to karyomegaly and intranuclear inclusion body formation in the adrenal gland
    b) Paramyxovirus inclusions have been seen in the cytoplasm of chromaffin cells
    c) Gross lesions are usually not seen
    d) All are correct
99. Neoplasia of the adrenal gland does not include
    a) Interrenal adenoma and carcinoma
    b) Pheochromocytoma
    c) Rhabdomyoma
    d) Ganglioneuroma
100. In poultry
    a) Adenomas are well differentiated and not encapsulated
    b) Carcinomas are anaplastic with poorly formed trabecular structures
    c) Pheochromocytoma and ganglioneuroma are less common
    d) All are correct
101. Ganglioneuromas
    a) Contain large cells
    b) Basophilic cytoplasm
    c) Resembles like neurons
    d) All
102. The pancreas is a specialized derivative of the primitive gut of
    a) Ectoderm
    b) Mesoderm
    c) Endoderm
    d) None
103. Choose the correct statement
    a) Pancreatic exocrine function begins after birth
    b) The endocrine function can be measured from 10 to 15 weeks onwards
    c) Both a and b
    d) None
104. Islets of Langerhans is having
    a) A & C cells in the A islets
    b) A & D cells in the A islets
    c) A & D cells in the B islets
    d) A & D cells in the B islets
105. In islets of Langerhans, B islets contains
    a) B & D cells
    b) A & D cells
    c) Both a and b
    d) None

106. The level of insulin in poultry is
   a) About 10 times that in mammals
   b) About 1/10 that in mammals
   c) About 1/80 that in mammals
   d) About 80 that in mammals
107. Choose the incorrect statement regarding somatostatin
   a) Secreted by D cells
   b) Depresses insulin
   c) Depresses glucagon
   d) Depresses avian hepatic peptide
108. Tumors of pituitary gland include
   a) Tumor of chromophobe cells
   b) Infiltrative acidophil adenoma
   c) Both
   d) None
109. Choose an incorrect statement regarding thymoma
   a) Commonly seen in chickens
   b) These are masses in neck that are histologically characterized by sheets of epithelial cells
   c) Immunostaining of tumor cells with cytokeratin has been used to verify epithelial origin
   d) None
110. Tumors of the parathyroid gland of chickens seem to be limited to
   a) Adenoma
   b) Parathyroid carcinoma
   c) Both
   d) None
111. Ergotism is characterized by disorders of
   a) Neurologic
   b) Endocrine system
   c) Vascular system
   d) All
112. Ergotism is caused by
   a) Aspergillus sp
   b) Monilia sp
   c) Claviceps sp
   d) Microsporum sp
113. Ergotism mostly affects
   a) Neuroendocrine control of the posterior pituitary gland
   b) Neuroendocrine control of the anterior pituitary gland
   c) Thymus
   d) None of them
114. Hormone that interacts with the Marek's disease virus SORF2 protein and is associated with disease resistance in chicken is
   a) Growth hormone (*GH1*)
   b) Growth hormone (*GH2*)
   c) Growth hormone (*GH3*)
   d) Growth hormone (*GH4*)
115. Aviadenovirus ensures maximum egg transmission to the next generation by
   a) Increasing level of sex hormones at the time of egg production
   b) Stress
   c) Both
   d) None

116. In Marek disease
   a) Polymorphism in the adrenal hormone gene is associated with the number of tumors in tissues
   b) Polymorphism in the growth hormone gene is not associated with the number of tumors in tissues
   c) Polymorphism in the growth hormone gene is associated with the number of tumors in tissues
   d) None

117. Choose the correct option
   a) Ovarian adenocarcinomas are not associated with increased production of steroid hormones
   b) Ovarian adenocarcinomas are associated with increased production of steroid hormones
   c) Both
   d) Ovarian adenocarcinomas are not associated with increased production of steroid hormones

118. Most cases of sex reversal in poultry are due to
   a) Destruction of the functional left ovary
   b) Formation of an ovotestis in the remnants of the rudimentary right gonad
   c) Both a and b
   d) Hormone production by ovarian tumors

119. Choose the correct option
   a) In birds, the male is the neutral sex (ZW), and the young female is demasculinized by production of her ovarian hormones
   b) In birds, the male is the neutral sex, and the young female is demasculinized by the production of her ovarian hormones
   c) In birds, the male is the neutral sex, and the young male is demasculinized by the production of her ovarian hormones
   d) None

120. Choose the incorrect option regarding leiomyoma
   a) These are common in the ventral ligament of the oviduct and the oviductal wall in domestic fowl
   b) These also occurs in SPF hens
   c) The tumor cells contain receptors for only progesterone
   d) Steroid hormones are likely to be involved in the etiology of these tumors

121. SPF hens are
   a) Specific Parasites Free
   b) Specific Pathogen Free
   c) Special Pathogen Free
   d) Specific Parasites Free

122. Choose the correct statement regarding lymphomatosis
   a) Males are less resistant to lymphomatosis than capons
   b) Administration of the male sex hormone to males increases their resistance to this disease
   c) Administration of the male sex hormone to capons increases their resistance to this disease
   d) Both b and c are correct
123. Choose the correct option
   a) Female is more susceptible than the male to lymphomatosis
   b) Higher incidence of lymphomatosis in complete castrates than in incomplete castrates
   c) Lymphomatosis was closely associated with the deficiency of the male hormone
   d) All are correct
124. *In Bordetella avium infected poult***s**
   a) The stress of
   b) *avium* infection increased plasma corticosterone
   b) Plasma T_3 is not affected by the infection
   c) Fasting causes a significant reduction of plasma T_3 in infected poults
   d) All
125. Choose the incorrect option regarding infection of *M. meleagridis*
   a) Turkeys with low-plasma adrenocorticotropic hormone following cold stress were more resistant to MM infection
   b) Commonly occurs as a silent infection in adult birds
   c) Although not a consistent feature of the disease, the syndrome called TS-68
   d) None
126. Infection of *M. meleagridis* is also called
   a) Airsacculitis deficiency syndrome b) TS-65
   c) Both d) None
127. The principal sign of diabetes insipidus is/are
   a) Polyuria b) Polydipsia
   c) Both a and b d) None
128. Choose the incorrect option regarding infection of *Aspergillus fumigatus*
   a) It produces a number of proteolytic enzymes capable of degrading host tissues
   b) Its growth is hampered by hydrocortisone administration
   c) Aspergillosis likely results more from the dose of inhaled conidia
   d) None
129. The vitamins function as cofactors for hormones
   a) Vitamin A b) Vitamins D
   c) Both d) None

130. The second hydroxylation for the formation of 1,25-dihydroxycholecalciferol occurs in the kidneys and is tightly regulated by the following, except
a) Calcium status
b) Being activated by parathyroid hormone
c) High blood calcium
d) Low blood phosphate

131. Iodine (I) is an integral part of the thyroid hormone
a) Triiodothyronine
b) Thyroxin
c) Both
d) None

132. High levels of dietary iodine have the following effects, except
a) Decrease in egg weight
b) Decrease in albumen index
c) Decrease in Haugh unit
d) Decrease in hatchability

133. Haugh unit measures egg quality based on the height of
a) Yolk
b) Albumin
c) Both
d) None

134. Iodine reduces the growth rate of chicks at
a) 9mg/kg
b) 90mg/kg
c) 900mg/kg
d) 0.9mg/kg

135. Iodine toxicosis
a) Reduces male fertility
b) Normalized within about 7 days of returning birds to a diet with normal iodine levels
c) Both a and b are correct
d) None

136. Diets that contain only seeds or only meat is deficient in
a) Calcium
b) Vitamins
c) Both a and b
d) None of the above

137. Thyroid hormone is
a) Modulator of the beta-adrenergic system
b) An important regulator of cardiovascular performance
c) Both
d) None

138. Choose an incorrect statement about pulmonary hypertension syndrome (PHS)
a) Occurs at the end of the growth period
b) Incubation conditions may influence the postnatal characteristics of PHS
c) Low oxygen levels during incubation influence the occurrence of ascites later in life
d) None

139. Zearalenone is
   a) Hormone
   b) Supplement
   c) Toxin
   d) Pathogenic organism
140. Zearalenone secreted from grains infected with the fungus
   a) Fusarium graminearum
   b) F. roseum
   c) Both
   d) None
141. *Gibberella zeae* is a source of zearalenone, a mycotoxin with activity like
   a) Progesterone
   b) Estrogen
   c) FSH
   d) LH
142. Choose the most appropriate option for zearalenone
   a) Turkeys are the most sensitive, with sex hormone-sensitive tissues targeted
   b) Leghorn hens are generally tolerant of zearalenone
   c) Both
   d) None
143. Lesions of zearalenone include the following, except
   a) Swelling of the cloaca
   b) Oviduct enlargement
   c) Increase in comb and testicle weight
   d) Reproductive tract cysts
144. Aflatoxin
   a) Influences calcium metabolism
   b) Influences phosphorus metabolism
   c) Alter the metabolism of vitamin D and parathyroid hormone
   d) All
145. Polybrominated Biphenyl (PBB) and Polychlorinated Biphenyl (PCB)
   a) Present in the environment from industrial contamination and deliberate dumping
   b) They reduce production, reproduction, hatchability, offspring viability
   c) Increase thyroid hormone levels
   d) All
146. In Hypoglycemia-Spiking Mortality Syndrome of Broiler Chickens
   a) Low levels of Insulin-like growth factor-1 (IGF-1) is present
   b) High mortality occurs (greater than 0.5%) for at least 3 consecutive days with concurrent hypoglycemia in clinically affected birds
   c) Both
   d) None
147. Insulin-like growth factors in poultry affect
   a) Growth
   b) Intermediary metabolism
   c) Both
   d) None
148. Type of Insulin-like growth factor present in poultry
   a) IGF-I
   b) IGF-II
   c) Both IGF-I and IGF-II
   d) None

149. GH secretion in poultry is episodic, with high-concentration peaks or pulses occurring at regular intervals of approximately
   a) 60 to 90 seconds
   b) 60 to 90 minutes
   c) 6 to 9 min
   d) 600 to 900 min
150. Amplitude of GH as well as baseline concentrations of GH decrease with
   a) Decreasing age and decreasing growth rate in chickens and turkeys
   b) Increasing age and increasing growth rate in chickens and turkeys
   c) Increasing age and decreasing growth rate in chickens and turkeys
   d) Increasing age and increasing growth rate in chickens and turkeys

Answer Key

1	a	2	b	3	a	4	d	5	c	6	b	7	c
8	a	9	d	10	b	11	a	12	d	13	c	14	a
15	b	16	c	17	a	18	c	19	c	20	b	21	b
22	b	23	c	24	d	25	d	26	b	27	a	28	d
29	c	30	a	31	c	32	d	33	d	34	b	35	b
36	a	37	d	38	a	39	a	40	d	41	a	42	d
43	d	44	a	45	a	46	d	47	d	48	b	49	c
50	d	51	c	52	c	53	d	54	d	55	a	56	b
57	d	58	d	59	d	60	c	61	d	62	a	63	b
64	b	65	a	66	c	67	c	68	d	69	b	70	d
71	d	72	d	73	a	74	c	75	b	76	b	77	d
78	c	79	d	80	b	81	d	82	d	83	d	84	a
85	c	86	b	87	b	88	c	89	a	90	d	91	a
92	c	93	b	94	d	95	a	96	d	97	b	98	d
99	c	100	a	101	d	102	c	103	c	104	b	105	a
106	b	107	d	108	c	109	d	110	c	111	d	112	c
113	b	114	a	115	c	116	c	117	a	118	c	119	b
120	c	121	b	122	d	123	d	124	d	125	c	126	c
127	c	128	b	129	c	130	c	131	c	132	d	133	b
134	c	135	c	136	a	137	c	138	d	139	c	140	c
141	b	142	c	143	c	144	d	145	c	146	c	147	c
148	c	149	b	150	c								

19

Disorders of the Cardiovascular System

Bhavanam Sudhakara Reddy, Sirigireddy Sivajothi, Malaka Malavika Reddy and Gongati Abhinethri

College of Veterinary Science - Proddatur, Sri Venkateswara Veterinary University, Andhra Pradesh, India

Introduction

Ante mortem diagnosis of cardio vascular diseases in avian patients is a challenging to the physician. Compare with the mammals, few anatomical and physiological features are unique in birds. The avian heart is anatomically similar to mammals, although birds have a proportionally larger heart size relative to a comparably sized mammal. Heart size in mammals remains equivalent to body mass, while larger birds have a proportionally smaller hearts in relation to body size than smaller birds. The apex of the heart is enclosed between the right and left hepatic lobes and lies along the sternum and parallel to the thoracic spine in the cranio ventral coelom. The avian cardiovascular system is adapted to the high aerobic requirements for flight, running or swimming. Efficient oxygen transfer to the tissues is facilitated by a lower total peripheral resistance, higher heart rate, higher arterial blood pressure and more rapid myocardial depolarization. The clinical signs seen in birds afflicted with cardiac disease can be vague and non-specific which are mimicking many other disease conditions. Similar to mammals, birds may present with lethargy, weakness, exercise intolerance, syncope, dyspnoea, coughing and even sudden death. On physical examination cardiac disease may be suspected based on the presence of arrhythmia, murmur, muffled cardiac sounds, poor peripheral pulses, cyanosis and coelomic distension. Pulmonary oedema, hepatomegaly, ascites and enlarged jugular veins with pulsation may be seen in cases of congestive cardiac failure. Pericarditis can occur with primary infectious agents or secondary to disease occurring in adjacent tissues, such as mycotic pulmonary granulomas. Visceral gout due to hyperuricaemia may also affect the pericardium. Congestive heart failure and systemic manifestations of disease, such as hypoproteinaemia, may result in effusions within the pericardium. Myocardial ventricular hypertrophy can occur with any condition that results in an elevated preload on the heart, including pulmonary hypertension and atherosclerosis. Myocarditis has been observed in cases of chlamydiosis, polyomavirus infection and proventricular dilatation disease from bornavirus. Heavy metal toxicosis has been associated with cardiac neural dysfunction and myocardial infarction. Vegetative endocarditis and resultant valvular insufficiency can occur with bacteraemia from chronic bacterial infections involving other organ systems. Other primary cardiac diseases that have been documented in birds include congenital defects, such as ventricular septal defect (VSD). Cardiac dysfunction can occur secondarily to hypovolaemic, septic and neurogenic shock. Ante mortem diagnosis of cardiac disease in avian patients can be challenging and one of the greatest limitations with the majority of diagnostic tests is the lack of available reference ranges for many species. Physical examination required in birds suspected for cardiac disease based on signalment, history and clinical signs. Commonly reported clinical signs in birds were weakness, lethargy, bluish discoloration of the skin around the eyes, abdominal distension, difficulty breathing, exercise intolerance. Specific examination of the cardiovascular system should include thoracic auscultation from the lateral and ventral aspects of the sternum, identification of clinical features consistent with cardiac dysfunction ultimately requires further investigation in order to achieve an accurate cardiac evaluation, haematology, biochemistry, plasma creatine kinase, cholesterol, protein levels, abdominocentesis, catheterisation of the arterial system and connection to an electronic transducer is the gold standard in blood pressure measurement. In addition to the above, radiography, electrocardiography, ultrasonography, echocardiography and angiography recommended to know about the specific causes. The use of cardiac biomarkers Troponin I (cTnI) is part of a complex found within myocardial cells and is released following myocardial cell damage. Brain natriuretic peptide (BNP) is a neuroendocrine hormone with a primary role in fluid homeostasis by increasing the glomerular filtration rate and inhibition of the renin-angiotensin-aldosterone system. NT-proBNP is the metabolically inactive precursorto BNP and appears to be more suitable for analysis due to a longer half life in plasma. A wide range of medications is available to treat these conditions, including diuretics, vasodilators, positive and negative inotropes, antiarrhythmic agents, and pentoxifylline. Although treatment approaches remain largely empirical and extrapolated from small animal and human medicine, the management strategies presented here have the potential to both maintain quality of life and extend survival time for the avian cardiac patient. Prevention of heart disease is far better than treatment after the development. Factors that have been linked to the development of atherosclerosis in birds include long-term diets high in fat or cholesterol and a lack of exercise. Bird owners should reduce the fat in your bird's diet, avoid fatty foods that can cause cholesterol plaques in your bird's arteries and make sure your bird gets plenty of exercise. Proper diet can go a very long way to reducing or preventing heart disease in your pet bird with regular exercise is absolutely vital.

Write correct alphabet of the answer in the given bracket

1. Inftlamation of heart valve is called
   a) Pericarditis b) Endocarditis
   c) Myocarditis d) all the above
2. Inflammation of heart lining membrane is called
   a) Pericarditis b) Endocarditis
   c) Myocarditis d) All the above
3. Inflammation of the sac surrounding the heart
   a) Pericarditis b) Myocarditis
   c) Endocarditis d) All of the above
4. Myocarditis, pericarditis and endocarditis are presenting septicemia condition such as
   a) BWD in chick b) BWD in adults
   c) Food typhoid in chick d) All the above

5. Which side hypertrophy of the heart wall appears when there is obstruction to flow of blood through arteries
   a) Right b) Left
   c) Both a and b d) None
6. Which sided hypertrophy appears when there is diseases of liver or lungs
   a) Right b) Left
   c) Both a and b d) None
7. Edema results in .... hypertrophy of heart
   a) Left sided b) Right sided
   c) Both a and b d) None
8. In birds flash pattern used to describe the
   a) Ventricular myocardium b) Atrial myocardium
   c) A and B d) None
9. In which condition pericardium becomes thick and coated with urates
   a) Gout b) LL
   c) Coryza d) MD
10. Inflammation of the arteries is called
   a) Arteritis b) Phlebitis
   c) Vasculitis d) All of the above
11. Inflammation of veins is known as
   a) Vasculitis b) Arteritis
   c) Phlebitis d) all of the above
12. Whcih appear in the wing vein of birds after blood as been withdrawn by the needle
   a) Thrombi b) Emboli
   c) Both a and b d) Abscess
13. Haemolysis is
   a) Destruction of RBC a) Destruction of platelets
   a) Destruction of WBC d) All of the above
14. Disease of blood forming tissue characterized by gross hypertrophy of liver and spleen
   a) Lymphocytosis b) Leukemia
   c) Anaemia d) Lymphocytopenia
15. The appearance of small tumors composed of lymphocytic cells which run together to form larger growths of abnormal tissues is characterized in
   a) Lymphomatosis b) Lymphocytopenia
   c) Lymphodenoma d) All of the above
16. Increase in arachidonic acid in cardiac ventricles is associated with
   a) Furazolidone induced cardio myopathy b) HCM
   c) DCM d) Valvular insufficiency

17. Feeding of flax seeds results in........ in right ventricular hypertrophy
    a) Reduction
    b) Increase
    c) Markedly increased
    d) Either increased or decreased
18. Which age group of poultry birds are mostly commonly affected by nutritional deficiencies
    a) Young b) Adults
    c) Both a and b d) Old aged birds
19. Which class of chicken are highly susceptible to heart failure
    a) Broilers b) Layers
    c) Both a and b d) None
20. Which is /are most common heart related condition in modern broiler flock
    a) Ascites syndrome b) SDS
    c) Both a and b d) None
21. The incidence of arrhythmia is more in
    a) Females b) Males
    c) Both a and b d) None
22 . Which is the prevailing sign of heart pump insufficiency
    a) Hypoxemia b) Hypercapnia
    c) Hypocapnia d) Both a and b
23. The increased pulmonary vascular resistance can be associated with ....ventricular failure
    a) Left b) Right
    c) Both a and b d) None
24. Restriction of oxygen to chick embryo shown to induce......
    a) Left ventricular dilation b) Breakdown of cardio myocytes
    c) A and B d) None
25. Which side of heart failures particularly relevant to broiler chickens
    a) Left b) Right
    c) Both a and b d) None
26. Heart failure results in up regulation of . ... stimulated by cardiac stress
    a) Coronary changes b) Matrix metallo proteinases
    c) Myocarditis d) All
27. Matrix metallo proteinases causes collagen degradation resulting in
    a) Right ventricular dilation b) Left ventricular dilation
    c) Both d) None
28. Increased salt intake result in right ventricular failure
    a) Right ventricular failure b) Left ventricular failure
    c) A and B d) None

29. High altitudes can result in disorder called as
    d) Pericarditis b) Myocarditis
    c) Pulmonary arterial hypertension d) All
30. Right heart failure has been associated with consumption of
    a) Furazolidone b) Sodium chloride
    c) P-dixon d) All the above
31. Atherosclerosis occurs due to accumulation of .... in arteries
    a) Fatty lipids b) Cholesterol
    c) A and B d) None
32. Atherosclerosis was found to cause an aneurysm of
    a) Right coronary artery b) Venacava
    c) Right aortic arch d) None
33. Avian leucosis virus has been implicated to cause
    a) Cardiac myopathy b) Valvular regurgitation
    c) Pericarditis d) All
34. Intercalated discs are containing ......junctions which allow transfer of ions between cardiomyocytes
    a) Tight junctions b) Gap junctions
    c) Both a and b d) None
35. Endothelium is made up
    a) Keratinized cells b) Fibrous cells
    c) Simple squamous epithelial cells d) None
36. Smooth muscle is derived from
    a) Ectoderma b) Lateral plate mesoderm
    c) A and B d) None
37. Difference between avian and mammalian heart
    a) Right atrioventricular valve is muscular b) Not contained chordae tendinae
    c) A and B d) None
38. Left atrio valve is ..... in birds
    a) Bicuspid b) Tricuspid
    c) A and B d) None
39. Which vitamin is required for specification of cardiovascular tissues in birds
    a) Vitamin A b) Vitamin K
    c) Vitamin C d) Vitamin D
40. Congenital heart defects within avian species is associated with.....toxicity
    a) Copper b) Iron
    c) Aluminum d) Manganese
41. Which describes a valve which is distorted, inflexible and fused somewhere to cardiac valve
    a) Dysplasia b) Myocarditis
    c) DCM d) None

42. Dialated cardiomyopathy (DCM) in turkeys has been linked to
    a) Troponin-T varieties b) Phospholamban variation
    c) A and B d) None
43. Turkey treated with Furazolidone produce
    a) Idiopathic DCM b) Valvular regurgitation
    c) HCM d) All
44. In electrocardiography P wave .....
    a) Atrial depolarization b) Ventricular depolarization
    c) Ventricular repolarization d) All
45. In electrocardiography QRS complex ....
    a) Atrial depolarization b) Ventricular depolarization
    c) Ventricular repolarization d) All
46. In electrocardiography T wave ......
    a) Atrial depolarization b) Ventricular depolarization
    c) Ventricular repolarization d) All
47. ECG in birds
    a) Inverted QRS in lead II b) Positive QRS in lead II
    c) A and B d) None
48. In expensive and non invasive diagnostic tool in birds
    a) ECG b) Echocardiography
    c) Radiography d) Angiography
49. Low voltage QRS indicative of
    a) Myocarditis b) Endocarditis
    c) Pericardial fluid accumulation d) All
50. Prognostication of acute pulmonary embolism in birds assessed by
    a) ECG b) Echocardiography
    c) Radiography d) All
51. Spontaneous turkey cardiomyopathy is known as
    a) Round heart disease b) Heart worm disease
    c) Valvular disease d) Pericarditis
52. Spontaneous turkey Cardiomyopathy is reported during which period
    a) Any age b) Old age (c)
    c) Early brooding d) Late brooding
53. Oxygen level below 20% in a brooder can cause in turkey
    a) Round heart disease b) DCM
    c) HCM d) Valvular disease
54. Hydropericardium disease is also known as (in birds)
    a) Angara disease b) DCM
    c) HCM d) Valvular disease

55. In birds hydropericardium syndrome is caused by
a) LL b) Circo virus
c) MD d) Fowl adenovirus

56. Hydropericardium syndrome is noticed during which age in birds
a) 1-2 Days b) 3-6 weeks
c) 9-12 weeks d) At any age

57. Hydropericardium syndrome in birds is transmitted by
a) Vertical b) Horizontal
c) Lateral d) All of the above

58. Clinical signs in hydropericardium syndrome in birds
a) Hydropericardium b) Anaemia
c) Necrotic hepatitis d) All of the above

59. Intra nuclear inclusion bodies are seen in birds during hydropericardium syndrome
a) Blast cells b) Reticulocytes
Bone marrow cells d) Hepatocytes

60. Acute heart failure in birds is commonly called as
a) Heart attack b) Acute death syndrome
c) Sudden death syndrome d) All

61. Symptoms in acute heart failure in birds
a) Stretched out neck b) No previous ill health
c) No apparent sign d) All

62. In birds acute heart failure commonly noticed in
a) Large fowl b) Fast growing
c) Both A and B d) All

63. How to prevent acute heart failure in birds
a) Grow fast growing hybrid slower
b) Choose a slower grower hybrid
c) Don't select large strains
d) All

64. Dilated cardiomyopathy in broiler chicken is frequently associated with
a) Rapid growth b) Pulmonary hypertension
c) A and B d) None

65. The viral infection related to dilated cardiomyopathy in birds
a) Acute leucosis virus b) Retro viral infection
c) A and B d) None

66. In which viral disease intracytoplasmic magenta inclusion bodies were reported in cardiac myocytes in birds
a) ALV-J b) Retroviral infection
c) A and B d) None

67. ALV-J associated cardiomyopathy in birds may involve
    a) Direct viral effect on cardiomyocytes
    b) Direct viral effect on purkinje fibres
    c) A and B
    d) None
68. Etiology in development of ascites poultry
    a) Pulmonary hypertension
    b) Primary cardiac disease
    c) Cellular damage by reactive oxygen species
    d) All
69. Pulmonary hypertension in birds is due to
    a) Physiological hypoxia b) Increased cardiac output
    c) Pulmonary arterial hypertension d) All
70. In birds Compensatory right ventricular hypertrophy can cause development of
    a) Right atrio ventricular valve insufficiency
    b) Right heart failure
    c) A and B
    d) none
71. Factors can cause physiological hypoxia in birds
    a) High altitude b) Cold temperature
    c) Poor ventilation d) All
72. In birds myocardial lesions can impair the conduction system and can affect the
    a) Right AV valve closure b) Left AV valve closure
    c) Both d) None
73. Myocarditis in birds can cause
    a) Valvular insufficiency b) Heart failure
    c) Ascites d) All
74. In birds arteriosclerosis is
    a) Coronary heart disease b) Vena cava
    c) Pericarditis d) All
75. Avian heart lies
    a) Slightly to the right of midline b) Slightly to the left of midline
    c) A and B d) None
76. The cardiac fibrous skeleton in birds is called as
    a) Myocardium b) Annulus fibrosis
    c) Valvular regurgitation d) All
77. Outermost layer of the heart in birds
    a) Epicardium b) Endocardium
    c) Myocardium d) All

78. Which layer act as protective layer containing nerves and blood vessels
   a) Epicardium b) Endocardium
   c) Myocardium d) All
79. Which part of heart has the greatest proportion of heart tissue
   a) Myocardium b) Pericardium
   c) Endocardium d) All
80. Which layer of heart composed of connective tissue, smooth muscle cells and forms a protective lining over the valves
   a) Endocardium b) Pericardium
   c) Myocardium d) All
81. The cardiac muscle, blood vessels and endothelial lining are derived from the — layers of the early embryo
   a) Embryonic mesoderm b) Embryonic endoderm
   c) A and B d) None
82. Main difference between avian and mammalian heart
   a) Right atrio ventricular valve is muscular
   b) Right atrio ventricular valve doesn't contain chordae tendinae
   c) A and B
   d) None
83. Avian vascular system is different from mammals
   a) Presence of shunt between left and right jugular vein
   b) Anastomosis between femoral and ischiatic veins
   c) Blood can bypass kidney
   d) All
84. Cardiovascular diseases are reported in much more common in pet birds than wild birds due to
   a) Longer life span of pet birds b) Lack of exercise
   c) Diet d) All
85. Key genes responsible for cardiovascular diseases in birds
   a) Gene Gata-4 b) Heart assymetry genes
   c) A and B d) None
86. External deformities of cardiac structures noticed during which toxicity
   a) Polychlorinated biphenyls b) Mercury
   c) Lead d) None
87. Congenital heart diseases in birds associated with what toxicity
   a) Aluminum b) Copper
   c) Mercury d) None
88. Valvular dysplasia in birds is expressed as
   a) Exercise intolerance b) Open mouth breathing
   c) Over eating d) A and B

89. Hypoxia in chick embryo leads to
    a) Left ventricular dilation
    b) Breakdown of cardiomyocytes
    c) Increased myocardial collagen
    d) All of the above
90. Ventricular septal defects in birds leads to
    a) Left and right blood shunt
    b) Ventricular hypertrophy
    c) A and B
    d) None
91. In birds left atrial ligation restricts the blood flow and causing the
    a) Decrease in cardiac load on heart
    b) Increase in cardiac load on heart
    c) A and B
    d) All
92. In chick embryos retinoic acid can cause
    a) Ventral septal defect
    b) Atrial septal defect
    c) A and B
    d) All
93. Right sided heart failure is commonly seen in
    a) Broilers
    b) Layers
    c) A and B
    d) Turkey birds
94. Fast growing broiler chicken cannot meet their oxygen demand as easily as slower growing chicken due to
    a) Mismatch between body mass and cardiac output
    b) Low exercise
    c) Low carbohydrate diet
    d) All
95. In broilers heart failure results from
    a) Right ventricular dilatation
    b) Collagen degradation
    c) A and B
    d) None
96. In birds increased salt intake can result in
    a) Right ventricular failure
    b) Increase in blood volume
    c) High mortality
    d) All of the above
97. Omega 3 fatty acids supplement in diet can cause
    a) Increase the circulatory level of nitrous oxide
    b) Vasodilatation
    c) Reducing mortality from cardiac failure
    d) All
98. In birds high altitude can results
    a) Pulmonary arterial hypertension
    b) Pericarditis
    c) Myocarditis
    d) All
99. In birds pulmonary arterial hypertension can develop into
    a) Right ventricular dilatation
    b) Cardiac failure
    c) Ascites
    d) All

100. In birds right heart failure has been associated with the consumption of
a) Na Cl
b) Furazolidone
c) P'dioxin
d) All

101. Atherosclerosis In birds is caused by
a) Fatty lipids
b) Cholesterol
c) Hypovitaminosis –A
d) All

102. During the process of atherosclerosis the following changes can be notified in birds
a) Fibrosis
b) Calcification
c) Occlusion and narrowing of blood vessels
d) All the above

103. The prognosis for hypoplastic left heart syndrome in birds
a) Poor
b) Good
c) Favorable
d) Excellent

104. Dilated cardiomyopathy in turkeys is assessed by
a) Cardiac troponin-t
b) PLN
c) A and B
d) None

105. In birds cardiac myocyte damage can results in elevation of
a) Creatinine kinase
b) Glucose
c) Albumin
d) None

106. In birds radiography can be used to detect
a) Cardiomegaly
b) Pulmonary edema
c) Ascites
d) All

107. Ultrasonography in birds is used to detect
a) Pericardial fluid
b) Valve morphology
c) Myocardial thickness
d) All

108. Frequency of transducer in ultrasonography in birds
a) 7.5MHz
b) 2 MHz
c) 5 MHz
d) 20 MHz

109. Gold standard test to measure the blood pressure in birds
a) Catheterization of arterial system
b) Catheterization of venous system
c) Catheterization of venacava
d) All

110. In birds abdominocentesis is recommended in
a) Coelomic effusion
b) Cardiomegaly
c) CHF
d) Valvular regurgitation

111. Probe position in ultrasonography of birds
a) Ventromedial approach b) Lateral approach
c) Ventro dorsal approach d) None
112. ECG in birds useful to
a) Detect the primary cardiac disease b) Detect the arrhythmias
c) To monitor the therapy d) All
113. Mean electrical axis is in birds
a) Negative b) Positive
c) Both d) Altered
114. For regular electrocardiography analysis of birds, ECG machine with a speed above
a) 500mm/sec b) 50mm/sec
c) 10mm/sec d) 5mm/sec
115. In birds detection and assessment of atherosclerosis is carried out by
a) Angiography b) Echocardiography
c) Ultrasonography d) Electrocardiography
116. Medication useful in birds with cardiovascular disease
a) Diuretics b) Vasodilators
c) Inotropes d) All
117. Causes of atherosclerosis in pet birds
a) Genetic b) Age factor
c) Inflammatory diseases d) All
118. Most common signs of heart diseases in birds
a) Exercise intolerance
b) Breathing difficulty
c) Bluish discoloration of skin around eyes
d) All
119. Most common etiology of avian endocardial diseases
a) Infection b) Degeneration
c) Idiopathic diseases d) All
120. Heart failure is highly susceptible in
a) Broilers b) Layers
c) Exotic d) Turkey
121. Sub clinical heart diseases are most commonly noticed in
a) Slow growing birds b) Layers
c) Fast growing birds d) All
122. Leading non-infectious causes of mortality in broilers
a) Acute heart failure b) Chronic heart failure
c) Hypoxemia and ascites d) All

123. Causes of sudden death syndrome in broilers
  a) Ventricular arrhythmia
  b) Catastrophic ventricular fibrillation
  c) Valvular regurgitation
  d) A and B

124. Most common cardiac arrhythmia in broilers
  a) Premature ventricular contraction b) Ventricular arrhythmias
  c) Atrial fibrillation d) All

125. In birds ventricular arrhythmias is caused by
  a) Coronary artery disease b) Cardiomyopathy
  c) Heart infraction d) All

126. Pre mature ventricular contractions associated in birds
  a) Hypokalemia &hypomagnesemia b) Vitamin A deficiency
  c) Thymine deficiency d) All

127. Common features in fast growing broilers
  a) Hypercapnea b) Hypoxemia
  c) Hypocapnea d) A and B

128. Broilers succumbing to heart failure exhibit the lesions on
  a) Pericardium b) Myocardium
  c) Endocardium d) All

129. Pericardial effusion and adhesions have effect on heart function
  a) Restrictive effect b) Increased
  c) Increased and decreased d) All

130. In birds heart failure, which part of the heart will be distributed
  a) Extracellular matrix b) Sacromeres
  c) Intracellular matrix d) A and B

131. Which is responsible for contraction of heart muscle in ascitic birds
  a) Degeneration of proteins b) Degeneration of carbohydrates
  c) Degeneration of fat d) All

132. Broilers with ascites may show the —heart rate
  a) Decrease b) Increased
  c) A and B d) None

133. In birds with hypothyroidism can show
  a) Low heart rate b) Decreased cardiac output
  c) Pericardial effusion d) All

134. In birds thyroid hormones regulates
  a) Contractile property of heart b) Expression of chains of myosin
  c) Maturation of Beta adrenergic system d) All

135. Broilers raised at low altitude will have
a) Pulmonary hypertension b) Right ventricular failure
c) Ascites d) All

136. In turkeys spontaneous cardiomyopathy will exhibit the symptoms of
a) Dyspnea b) Unthriftiness
c) Drooping of wings d) All

137. Spontaneous cardiomyopathy signs due to
a) Dilation of both ventricles b) Congested lungs
c) Swollen liver d) All

138. Round heart diseases in turkey has been associated with
a) High level of dietary salt b) High level of dietary protein
c) High level of dietary fat d) All

139. Post mortem signs round heart disease in turkey in addition to the cardiovascular changes
a) Enlargement of kidney with urates b) Exudates in abdomen
c) Exudates in thoracic air sacs d) All

140. In birds pentoxifilline for
a) Atherosclerosis b) Frostbite
c) Increase the blood flow d) All

141. Anti arrhythmic agents in birds
a) Digoxin b) Furosemide
c) Enalapril d) Amlodipine

142. Antihypertensive drugs in birds
a) Amlodipine b) Furosemide
c) Gentamicin d) All

143. In birds Rosuvastatin used as
a) Low the cholesterol b) Low the glucose
c) Increase the cholesterol d) increase the glucose

144. Recommended ACE inhibitor in birds
a) Furosemide b) Gentamicin
c) Enalapril d) All

145. Commonly used diuretics in birds
a) Furosemide b) Gentamicin
c) Enalapril d) All

146. Risk factor for atherosclerosis In birds
a) Increased plasma concentration of lipids
b) Physical inactivity
c) High energy diet
d) All

147. What is relation between age and development of atherosclerosis in birds
    a) Directly proportional
    b) Indirectly proportional
    c) A and B
    d) None
148. In female birds, atherosclerosis caused by production of estrogens are responsible for increased plasma concentration of—
    a) Cholesterol
    b) Lipoproteins
    c) Triglycerides and calcium
    d) All
149. Atherosclerosis is most common in birds, with co-infection with
    a) Chlamydia
    b) MD
    c) Coryza
    d) LL
150. Methods to prevent the atherosclerosis in birds
    a) Ample exercise
    b) Avoiding the excessive carbohydrate food
    c) Avoiding excessive fat in diet
    d) All

Answer Key

1	a	2	b	3	a	4	d	5	c	6	b	7	c
8	a	9	d	10	b	11	a	12	d	13	c	14	a
15	b	16	c	17	a	18	c	19	c	20	b	21	b
22	b	23	c	24	d	25	d	26	b	27	a	28	d
29	c	30	a	31	c	32	d	33	d	34	b	35	b
36	a	37	d	38	a	39	a	40	d	41	a	42	d
43	d	44	a	45	a	46	d	47	d	48	b	49	c
50	d	51	c	52	c	53	d	54	d	55	a	56	b
57	d	58	d	59	d	60	c	61	d	62	a	63	b
64	b	65	a	66	c	67	c	68	d	69	b	70	d
71	d	72	d	73	a	74	c	75	b	76	b	77	d
78	c	79	d	80	b	81	d	82	d	83	d	84	a
85	c	86	b	87	b	88	c	89	a	90	d	91	a
92	c	93	b	94	d	95	a	96	d	97	b	98	d
99	c	100	a	101	d	102	c	103	c	104	b	105	a
106	b	107	d	108	c	109	d	110	c	111	d	112	c
113	b	114	a	115	c	116	c	117	a	118	c	119	b
120	c	121	b	122	d	123	d	124	d	125	c	126	c
127	c	128	b	129	c	130	c	131	c	132	d	133	b
134	c	135	c	136	a	137	c	138	d	139	c	140	c
141	b	142	c	143	c	144	d	145	c	146	c	147	c
148	c	149	b	150	c								

20

Disorders of Nervous System

Suman Biswas[1], Probhakar Biswas[1] and Shubhamitra Chaudhuary[2]

[1]*Department of Avian Sciences, Faculty of Veterinary & Animal Sciences, West Bengal University of Animal & Fishery Sciences, Mohanpur, Nadia, West Bengal-741 252*

[2]*Department of Veterinary Clinical Complex, West Bengal University of Animal & Fishery Sciences, Kolkata*

Introdcution

Poultry have a nervous system made up of the brain, spinal cord, sympathetic nerves that govern their viscera, and branches that go to their ears and eyes. The structure of the brain and spinal cord is very similar to that of mammals. However, there are also significant structural variations between many bird brains and many human brains, including the following:

1. **Absence of cortex:** According to Cobb (1960), the cortex is "a peripherally placed coating (pallium) of cells arranged in layers," yet it is completely absent in birds. However, other authors have compared the hyperstriatum to the mammalian cortex (Haefelfinger, 1957; Stingelin, 1958).
2. **Presence of hyperstriatum:** The functions of the hyperstriatum are comparable to those of the mammalian cortex. In pigeons and chickens, the hyperstriatum may be involved in the visual and hearing systems' functions.
3. Birds have highly developed optic lobes.
4. Turkeys and vultures are the only birds with a well-developed olfactory system.

Neurologic disease can present with a variety of etiologies for veterinarians who care for poultry birds. Neurologic symptoms can include paralysis, head and neck twisting, tremors, circling, ataxia, and falling backwards. The neurologic disease in poultry birds can be easily diagnosed by physical examination and post mortem examination.

Physical Examination

See the bird's movements for yourself. Assess its ability to stand and, if so, to walk. Look at how the bird is positioned if it can only sit or lie down. Is the poultry bird sitting with their legs extended and their feet elevated slightly? Is it standing with one leg in front and one behind it? Does it have its side facing up? You might uncover hints about the etiology by looking at various positions. If the bird is responsive, observant, and brilliant, make note of that also. Check to see if the tone of the neck muscles is flaccid or god. Examine the eyes to see whether they are hazy or if the bird is squinting because of uneven corneas caused by ammonia burn. Check to see whether any of the infected birds have comparable neurologic symptoms.

Postmortem Examination

Look for evidence of trauma or puncture wounds (predation) on the postmortem examination of the bird. Look for any elevated nodules on the skin that surround the feather follicles. Make a cut in the skin that lies between the leg and the breast muscle, then pull the leg back. Determine which muscle in the medial thigh is the triangle. Slice this muscle adjacent to the body wall from caudal to cranial, then reflect it cranially. As a result, the sciatic nerve and femoral artery will be visible and accessible for tissue collection. It is possible to identify and collect samples for histology of the brachial plexus after the body cavity is opened and the breast is reflected cranially. The diagnosis of Marek's disease depends on peripheral nerve collection for histopathology (Fig. 4). After removing the skull cap, carefully remove the entire brain, including the cerebellum and brain stem. Look at the brain for any nodules or discolorations that can point to a bacterial or fungal infection. Young birds may have a vitamin E deficiency if their cerebellum is a vivid red colour. For histology, one half of the brain can be removed. When birds are exposed to raccoon stool, the cerebellum is required to detect the migration of *Baylisacaris procyonis*. When diagnosing avian encephalomyelitis in young birds, the cerebellum and brain stem are required. It is possible to harvest the other half of the brain for PCR or culture studies.

Multiple Choice Question

1. Avian pneumo encephalitis is commonly known as
   a) Marek's Disease b) Avian Encephalitis
   c) Ranikhet Disease d) Chronic Respiratory Disease
2. Avian Distemper first recorded in India
   a) 1930 b) 1932
   c) 1929 d) 1927
3. Wing paralysis is a classical symptom of
   a) Marek's Disease b) Fowl Pox
   c) Fowl Typhoid d) New Castle Disease
4. Nervous sign of Ranikhet Disease commonly caused by which strain
   a) Velogenic Strain b) Mesogenic Strain
   c) Lentogenic Strain d) All of the above
5. Nervous form of Ranikhet Disease commonly appears in
   a) Adult birds b) Day old birds
   c) Young birds d) Layer birds
6. Paralytic sign in Ranikhet Disease most commonly occurs due to
   a) Compression of nerve fibre
   b) Interference of nerve signals
   c) Degeneration of nerve fibre and ganglionic cells of spinal cord
   d) None of the above
7. Range Paralysis is a synonym of which of the following disease
   a) Rabies b) Avian vitamin E deficiency
   c) Avian influenza d) Marek's disease

8. Neural form of Marek's disease mostly noted in which age group
   a) 16 weeks to 30 weeks of bird
   b) 12 weeks to 18 weeks of bird
   c) 0 weeks to 15 weeks of bird
   d) More than 30 weeks of age
9. Which nerve most affected in Marek's disease
   a) Brachea of wings
   b) Coeliac of intestine
   c) Vagus nerve
   d) Sciatic of legs
10. In Marek's disease the classical neural form due degeneration of sciatic nerve is known as
    a) Broken leg
    b) Split leg
    c) Slipped leg
    d) Short leg
11. The transitional paralytic form of Marek's disease occurs in which age of chicken
    a) 9 to 12 weeks of age
    b) 17 to 35 weeks of age
    c) 5 to 18 weeks of age
    d) All of the above
12. After occurrence of Marek's disease, the appearance of sciatic, celiac cranial mesenteric becomes
    a) Striation and glistening appearance
    b) Discoloured and flat appearance
    c) Reddish blue appearance
    d) All of the above
13. In Marek's disease nerve becomes
    a) 5 - 6 times thicker than normal
    b) 2 - 3 times thicker than normal
    c) Becomes thinner than normal
    d) Remains unchanged
14. Avian encephalomyelitis is which type of nervous disease of poultry in India
    a) Re-emerging disease
    b) Sporadic disease
    c) Emerging disease
    d) Eradicated disease
15. Tremor of the head, neck and whole body is seen in which disease of poultry
    a) Marek's disease
    b) Deficiency of selenium
    c) Vitamin B_1 deficiency
    d) Avian encephalomyelitis
16. Epidemic tremor most commonly occurs in which age group of poultry
    a) In young age group of poultry
    b) 1-2 weeks of age
    c) 2-4 weeks of age
    d) In layer chicken
17. In Epidemic tremor, the virus multiply in which part
    a) Alimentary tract
    b) Respiratory tract
    c) Cerebellum
    d) Lymphoid tissue
18. Deficiency of vitamin B_1 in chicken causes
    a) Polyneuritis
    b) Curled toe paralysis
    c) Parosis
    d) Exudative diathesis
19. Deficiency of vitamin E in poultry causes
    a) Curled toe paralysis
    b) Encephalomalacia
    c) Peripheral paralysis
    d) Wing paralysis

20. Deficiency of vitamin riboflavin leads to development of
    a) Polyneuritis
    b) Curled toe paralysis
    c) Parosis
    d) Exudative diathesis
21. Chloride deficiency in poultry causes which type of nervous sign
    a) Tremor
    b) Paralysis
    c) Dizziness
    d) Ataxia
22. The nerve tissue which is resembles to mammalian cortex in poultry is known as
    a) Hyperstriatum
    b) Hypostriatum
    c) Medullary cortex
    d) None of the above
23. Electrolytic lesions of the chicken's nucleus supraopticus leads to development of
    a) Polypepsia
    b) Polydipsia
    c) Polyneuritis
    d) Polyphagia
24. Photosexual reflex in bird is a relation in between
    a) Hypothalamus and ear
    b) Hypothalamus and neck
    c) Hypothalamus and wing
    d) Hypothalamus and eye
25. In avian encephalomyelitis, the nervous sign appears
    a) 20 – 22 days following hatch
    b) 17 – 21 days following hatch
    c) 28 – 30 days following hatch
    d) None of the above
26. In avian encephalomyelitis, most prominent changes of the eye
    a) Greyish appearance of the eye
    b) Bluish appearance of the eye
    c) Reddish appearance of the lens
    d) Opacity of the lens
27. Which nervous sign is responsible for death of poultry birds in case of avian encephalomyelitis
    a) Trembling
    b) Paralysis
    c) Ataxia
    d) Incoordinate movement
28. In avian encephalomyelitis, histopathological findings of the medulla and spinal cord is characterized by
    a) Appearance of Negri bodies
    b) Appearance of fibrous tissue
    c) Eccentricity and chromatolysis of nucleus
    d) All of the above
29. In avian encephalomyelitis pathological changes of the cerebellum is characterized by
    a) Ganglionitis
    b) Gliosis
    c) Perivascular infiltration
    d) Ovoidalis
30. In avian leucosis complex, the paralysis occurs due to
    a) Pressure on the sciatic nerve by nephroblastoma
    b) Pressure on the brachial nerve by nephroblastoma
    c) Pressure on the vagus nerve by nephroblastoma
    d) All of the above

31. In avian pasteurellosis, the nerous sign is characterised by
   a) Paralysis b) Trembling
   c) Circular movement/torticollis d) Ataxia
32. In avian pasteurellosis, torticollis develops due to
   a) Osteomyelitis of cranial bones b) Middle ear infection
   c) Pathological changes of meninges d) All of the above
33. In psittacosis, paralysis of limbs develops in group of birds
   a) Parrot b) Duck
   c) Cockatoos and cockatiels d) Pigeons
34. Black head disease of poultry is caused by
   a) Histomonas meleagridis b) Heterakis gallinarum
   c) Trichomonas gallinae d) Eimeria tenella
35. Parts of the central nervous system which exhibiting ipsilateral control in poultry
   a) Cerebrum b) Medulla and pons
   c) Cerebellum d) Thalamus
36. Axodendritic type of synapse is found in
   a) Cerebellum b) Dorsal horn of spinal cord
   c) Axons of interneurons d) Autonomic ganglia
37. Organ of jacobson is absent in which species of animals
   a) Caprine b) Canine
   c) Avian d) Porcine
38. Upper motor neuron disease in poultry causes
   a) Paresis b) Hemiparesis
   c) Flaccid paralysis d) Spastic paralysis
39. In spastic paralysis, birds died due to
   a) Cachexia b) Respiratory failure
   c) Cardiac failure d) Renal failure
40. Short jerky inspiration caused by stimulation of phrenic nerve is
   a) Roar b) Wheeze
   c) Hiccough d) None of the above
41. Perosis in fowl results from deficiency of
   a) Zn b) Mn
   c) Thiamine d) Riboflavin
42. Copper exerts its neuro-physiologic effect in poultry through an enzyme is known as
   a) CPK b) ALP
   c) Ceruloplasmin (CP) d) Xanthine oxidase
43. Goose stepping in poultry is caused by deficiency of
   a) Riboflavin b) Pyridoxine
   c) Carotene d) Cryptoxanthine

44. Crazy chick disease is caused by deficiency of
    a) Riboflavin b) Pyridoxine
    c) Cholecalciferol d) Thiamine
45. Cerebro-cortical necrosis in poultry is caused by:
    a) Copper deficiency b) Thiamine deficiency
    c) Cobalt deficiency d) Riboflavin deficiency
46. Crazy chick disease is due to deficiency of
    a) Vit. A b) Vit. K
    c) Vit. C d) Vit. E
47. Curled toe paralysis is caused by deficiency of vitamin in poultry
    a) B_2 b) B_3
    c) D d) B_{12}
48. Combined deficiency of vitamin D_3, calcium and phosphorus lead development of paralysis in layer birds is commonly known as
    a) Oviposition syndrome b) Cage layer fatigue syndrome
    c) Calcium flux syndrome d) None of the above
49. Deficiency of sodium, potassium, and chloride combinedly leads to development which type of nervous symptoms
    a) Ataxia b) Circulatory movement
    c) Vent pecking d) All of the above
50. Selenium and vitamin E deficiency causes________ in chicks
    a) Degeneration of myelin sheath b) Disorientation of nerve impulse
    c) Encephalomalacia d) None of the above
51. Encephalomalacia occurs due to vitamin E and selenium deficiency at the age of
    a) 30 – 50 days of age b) After onset of egg production
    c) 40 – 65 days of age d) 15 – 30 days of age
52. Encephalomalacia in chicks due to selenium and vitamin E deficiency characterized by
    a) Myoclonus b) Prostration
    c) Opisthotonus d) All of the above
53. Vitamin E deficiency syndrome develops at 2 – 3 weeks of age but disappear at weeks of age in which avian species
    a) Duck b) Quail
    c) Pigeon d) Turkey
54. Which is an industrial neurotoxicant in young chicks
    a) Nickel b) Cadmium
    c) Manganese d) Aluminium

55. Microscopic change of the cerebellum in chicks due to magnesium deficiency defines as
    a) Degenerative alterations in the Purkinje cells
    b) Gliosis
    c) Both of the above
    d) None of the above
56. Which heavy metal toxicity is related with alterations on the cerebellar GSH system in chicks
    a) Arsenic b) Cadmium
    c) Selenium d) Lead
57. Molecular changes of the brain due to arsenic toxicity in chicks
    a) Increased concentration of inflammatory cytokines
    b) Increased concentration of arsenic
    c) Fibrosis of the brain tissue
    d) All of the above
58. Folic acid deficiency in turkey causes
    a) Wing paralysis b) Flaccid paralysis
    c) Spastic type of cervical paralysis d) None of the above
59. Deficiency of vitamin B_{12} in turkey leads to development of
    a) Locomotor impairment b) Embryonic death
    c) Anaemia d) All of the above
60. Biotin deficiency causes which types of nervous sign in male juvenile songbirds
    a) Neuronal degeneration b) Neuronal plasticity
    c) Paresis d) None of the above
61. Toxicity due to ionophore antibiotics in poultry and turkey causes complete paralysis of the following body parts
    a) Wing b) Posterior parts of the body
    c) Neck and legs d) All of the above
62. The 'knockdown syndrome' occurs in poultry due to
    a) Aminoglycoside antibiotic toxicity b) Sulphonamide toxicity
    c) Nitrofuran toxicity d) Ionophore antibiotic toxicity
63. Marked hypertrophy and hyperplasia of the neurilemmal cells of poultry occurs in
    a) Lasalocid toxicity b) Monensin toxicity
    c) Sulfaquinoxaline toxicity d) All of the above
64. Microscopically in which toxicity is related with demyelination of peripheral nerve and fragmentation of axon
    a) Antiprotozoal drug toxicity
    b) Anticoccidial drug toxicity
    c) Lead toxicity
    d) Organic arsenical and imidazole toxicity

65. In lead toxicity of poultry, the most prominent pathological changes of cerebellum
    a) Demyelination of peripheral nerve fibre b) Focal vascular damage
    c) Gliosis d) All of the above
66. In poultry, __________ poisoning is related with overstimulation of parasympathetic nerve and muscles
    a) Organochlorine insecticide poisoning b) Rodenticide poisoning
    c) Organophosphorus poisoning d) Ammonia gas poisoning
67. In organochlorine insecticide poisoning of poultry, the nervous signs are characterized by
    a) Vocalization to tremors b) Ataxia
    c) Convulsion and prostration d) All of the above
68. Which phytotoxins are potent neurotoxin to poultry
    a) Cacao, coffee seeds and castor beans b) Hemlock seeds and cotton seeds
    c) Avocado fruits and potato d) Oleander plants
69. In ergotism of poultry, the prominent nervous signs are
    a) Convulsive and sensory neurologic disorders
    b) Altered neuroendocrine control
    c) Both of the above
    d) None of the above
70. In bird, the common sequelae of meningitis
    a) Otitis externa b) Otitis media
    c) Otitis interna d) All of the above

References

Cobb, S., 1960. Observations on the comparative anatomy of the avian brain. Persp. Biol. Med. 3: 383-408.

Haelfelfinger, H. R., 1957. Beitrage zur vergleichenden Ontogenese des Vorderhirns bei Vogeln. Helbing and Lichtenbahn, Basel, Switzerland.

Answer Key

1	c	2	d	3	d	4	b	5	c	6	c	7	d
8	a	9	d	10	b	11	c	12	a	13	b	14	c
15	d	16	b	17	c	18	a	19	b	20	b	21	d
22	a	23	a	24	d	25	b	26	d	27	a	28	c
29	b	30	a	31	c	32	d	33	c	34	a	35	c
36	d	37	c	38	d	39	a	40	c	41	b	42	c
43	a	44	d	45	b	46	d	47	a	48	b	49	a
50	c	51	d	52	d	53	d	54	c	55	a	56	d
57	a	58	c	59	a	60	b	61	c	62	d	63	a
64	d	65	a	66	c	67	d	68	a	69	c	70	c

21

Disorders of the Elementary System

K. Prashanth Kumar

College of Veterinary Science, Mamnoor, PV Narsimha Rao Telangana Veterinary University

Introduction

The digestive system of the birds has modifications to facilitate the easy flight. Length of intestine in birds is relatively shorter compared to mammals. Also, they lack teeth and jaw muscles which are replaced with light weight beak. Food grains are swallowed as whole and ground in the gizzard with the help of powerful muscles. In the mouth, tongue is used to manipulate the food and also aids in swallowing the food. Chickens have as many as 300 taste buds. The elementary system in birds consists of gastro intestinal tract and the accessory glands, the course of the elementary starts with Mouth, oesophagus, crop, proventriculus (glandular/true stomach), gizzard (mascular stomach), small intestine (duodenum, Jejenum, ileum), large intestine (colon and caeca) which lastly opens into cloaca. For fast growing poultry species elementary system is very important. It plays vital role in digestion, absorption and also provides protective immunity. Poultry intestines harbours diversified microflora which aids in enhanced availability of nutrients to the bird. Intestinal wall contains four layers: mucosal, submucosal, muscle tunic, and the serosal layer. As intestine is involved in important functions like digestion & immunity, any change in intestinal integrity / microflora balance impacts the bird performance in terms of body weight gain in broilers and egg number in layers. Some bacteria, viruses and also fungi produce different diseases / conditions in poultry birds. The ban on the use of antimicrobial growth promoters has pushed poultry producers from use of AGP's to alternatives to AGP's such as prebiotics, probiotics, essential oils and some herbals. Maintaining good gut health in the absence of AGP's and anticoccidial drugs is a challenging situation for the poultry farmers across the globe. Poultry gut contains diverse community of bacteria, fungi, protozoa and viruses. The recent data suggests that gastrointestinal tract of a broiler chicken colonizes by an estimated 600 – 800 species of bacteria. The abundance and diversity of microbiota varies along the GI tract. After the hatch GI tract colonizes within 3-4 days. Small intestine of broilers mainly contains lactobacilli although enterococci, E.coli, eubacteria, clostridia, propionibacteria and fusobacteria can be found. The bacterial community of the intestine form a protective barrier that lines the gut, prevents the growth of less favourable or pathogenic bacteria such as salmonella, clostridium perfringens through a principle called competitive exclusion. A balance between these two is very important for a healthy gut, any imbalance disturbance or imbalance leads to poor absorption of nutrients, poor growth rate, produces disease and may results in death of the birds. The balance of the microbiota in the gut can be affected by factors such as : Poor gut health, feed change, feed (quality and raw materials), feed form, mycotoxins, biosecurity, environment, brooding conditions, infections with viruses and protozoa and water quality. Gut health decides the economics of the poultry enterprise.

1. Which part of the intestine helps in grinding the feed in poultry
   a) Crop b) Gizzard
   c) Pro-ventriculus d) Mouth
2. ____ portion of elementary system is called as true stomach / glandular stomach.
   a) Pro-ventriculus b) crop
   c) Gizzard d) Jejenum
3. How many muscle layers are present in intestinal wall of poultry
   a) 4 b) 3
   c) 5 d) 6
4. Presence of Pin point haemorrhages in proventriculus is a characteristic lesion of which following disease
   a) Infectious bronchitis b) New castle disease
   c) Infectious bursal disease d) Infectious laryngo tracheitis
5. Major immunoglobulins involved in the poultry
   a) IgM b) IgG
   c) IgA d) All of the above
6. Immunoglobulin involved in the mucosal immunity in birds
   a) IgM b) IgG
   c) IgA d) IgY
7. Site of replication for the New castle disease virus
   a) Cytoplasm b) Nucleus
   c) Cell membrane d) Both a & b
8. The lymphoid associated tissue distributed in which layer of the intestine
   a) Serosal layer b) Mucosal lining
   c) Sub mucosa d) Lamina propria
9. __________specialized epithelial cells located in the crypts of the small intestine
   a) Natural killer cells b) Peneth cells
   c) Heterophils d) Macrphages
10. __________ is the first antibody produced in response to primary immunization / antigen challenge
   a) IgM b) IgG
   c) IgA d) IgY
11. What is the principal antibody produced after secondary immunization
   a) IgM b) IgG
   c) IgA d) IgY

12. New castle disease belongs to family
    a) Paramyxoviridae
    b) Orthomyxoviridae
    c) Birnaviridae
    d) Reo viridae
13. __________ is the protein responsible for the strong attachment of virus with the host cell or hemolysis
    a) HN Protein
    b) Fusion protein
    c) Matrix protein
    d) Phosphoprotein
14. In which route we assess the mean death time (MDT) of SPF chicken embryos by inoculation of NDV.
    a) Allantoic sac
    b) Yolk sac
    c) Air cell
    d) Amniotic cavity
15. Which is the characteristic lesion of velogenic New castle disease virus (vNDV)
    a) Haemorrhages in caecal tonsils
    b) Hemorrhages of small intestinal lymphoid patches (Peyers patches)
    c) Pin point Haemorrhages in proventriculus
    d) All of the above
16. Importance of mode of transmission of New castle disease
    a) Horizontal transmission
    b) Vertical transmission
    c) Mechanical transmission
    d) b & c
17. Which strain of New castle disease produces the lesions in gastro intestinal tract
    a) Velogenic
    b) Mesogenic
    c) Lentogenic
    d) All of the above
18. New castle disease causing virus is
    a) Single stranded RNA virus
    b) Double stranded RNA virus
    c) Single stranded DNA virus
    d) Double stranded DNA virus
19. Which Amino acid aids in intestinal mucus production
    a) Lysine
    b) Threonine
    c) Methionine
    d) Tryptophan
20. ______________ are lymphoid structures scattered within the small intestinal surface
    a) Peyer's patches
    b) Meckels diverticula
    c) Caecal tonsils
    d) None of the above
21. The disease Inclusion body hepatitis is caused by
    a) Avi-Adenovirus group I
    b) Avi-Adenovirus group II
    c) Avi-Adenovirus group III
    d) None of the above
22. Main of transmission for Adeno virus infections
    a) Horizontal transmission
    b) Vertical transmission
    c) Indirect spread
    d) b & c

23. In chicken ______________ type of inclusion bodies produced by Avi-adeno virus in the liver of effected bir d)
    a) Acidophilic b) Neutrophilic
    c) Basophilic d) a & b
24. Inclusion body hepatitis (IBH) is important disease of
    a) Meat producing birds b) Egg producing birds
    c) Breeders d) Backyard chicken
25. Which virus infection predisposes the birds to IBH disease
    a) Infectious bronchitis (IB) b) Infectious bursal disease (IBD)
    c) Marek's disease (MD) d) Ranikhet disease (RD)
26. Predisposing factors for the IBH disease
    a) Mycotoxin load in feed b) IBD
    c) a & b d) Escherichia coli infection
27. Commonly found lesions in IBH affected flock
    a) Pale, Friable & Swollen liver
    b) Jaundice of skin & subcutaneous fat
    c) Pericardial sac filled with straw coloured fluid (litchi fruit appearance)
    d) All of the above
28. Predominant serotype of IBH causing virus
    a) FAdV-4 b) FAdV-5
    c) FAdV-2 d) All of the above
29. Incubation period of IBH disease
    a) 1 day b) 8-10 days
    c) 3-4 days d) 7 days
30. IBH is a disease of
    a) Breeders b) Broilers
    c) Layers d) All of the above
31. Hepatitis hydropericarditis (HHS) syndrome also known as
    a) Lychee disease b) Angara disease
    c) a & b d) Gumboro disease
32. Hepatitis hydropericarditis (HHS) syndrome first observed in
    a) Indian b) Pakisthan
    c) US d) Brazil
33. After the entry into host, the FAdV virus first colonizes in which part of the body
    a) Intestine epithelium b) Liver
    c) Kidney d) Heart epithelium

34. High aspartate aminotransferase (AST), alanine aminotransferase (ALT), and creatine phosphokinase are observed in which disease of the following
    a) Inclusion body hepatitis (IBH) b) Infectious bursal disease (IBD)
    c) Hepatitis hydropericarditis (HHS) d) Ranikhet disease (RD)
35. Which of the following organ is involved in Hepatitis hydropericarditis syndrome (HHS)
    a) Liver b) Heart
    c) Kidney d) All of the above
36. Pathognomic lesions of Inclusion body hepatitis (IBH) disease in broilers
    a) Pale & Enlarged liver with foci b) Haemorrhages in proventriculus
    c) Haemorrhages in thigh muscles d) Haemorrhages in Bursa
37. Differential diagnosis of HHS with IBH
    a) Presence of Hydropericardium b) Enlarged kidneys
    c) Pale & enlarged liver d) Ruffled feathers
38. Location of inclusion bodies in Inclusion body hepatitis (IBH) disease
    a) Cytoplasm b) Nucleus
    c) a & b d) None
39. Decreased blood glucose levels observed in
    a) Inclusion body hepatitis (IBH)
    b) Hepatitis hydropericarditis (HHS) syndrome
    c) Infectious bursal disease (IBD)
    d) Avian influenza (AI)
40. Immunosuppression by FAdV-4 virus caused by
    a) Decrease in B lymphocyte count b) Decrease in T lymphocyte count
    c) Atrophy of bursa of fabricius & thymus d) All of the above
41. Choice of disinfectant for the disinfection of farms affected with FAdV
    a) Chloroform b) Gluteraldehyde
    c) Ether d) Phenol
42. Fowl adenovirus group that causes Gizzard erosions (GE)
    a) FAdV-A / FAdV - 1 b) FAdV-E
    c) FAdV-C d) All of the above
43. What are the adenovirus serotypes used for vaccination against Inclusion body hepatitis (IBH) & Hepatitis hydropericarditis (HHS) syndrome
    a) FAdV serotype 4 & 8 b) FAdV serotype 1 & 3
    c) FAdV serotype 6 & 7 d) FAdV serotype 5 & 6
44. Common type of vaccine used in India to protect the chicken flocks against IBH disease
    a) Live vaccine b) Inactivated vaccine
    c) Subunit vaccine d) Recombinant vaccine

45. Avian Influenza virus belong to the family

a) *Orthomyxoviridae* b) *Paramyxoviridae*

c) *Adenoviridae* d) *Reo viridae*

46. _____________ Serotype of avian influenza virus is considered as highly pathogenic avian influenza (HPAI)

a) H5N1 b) H6N1

c) H7N2 d) H9N2

47. Crop mycosis in poultry is caused by

a) *Candida albicans* b) *Aspergillus flavus*

c) *Aspergillus fumigatus* d) *Aspergillus niger*

48. Development of white pseudomembrane in the crop of poultry is found in a condition

a) Candidiasis b) Aflotoxicosis

c) Aspergillosis d) Colibacilosis

49. Drug used in feed for treatment of Candidiasis

a) Metronidazole b) Amoxycillin

c) Nystatin d) Amprolium

50. First line of defence in intestines of poultry is

a) Mucus membrane b) Immunoglobulins

c) Inflammation d) Cytokines

51. Second line of defence in intestines of poultry is

a) Thymus b) Bursa of fabricus

c) Caecal tonsils d) Peyer's patches

52. Necrotic enteritis is an important clostridial infection in commercial poultry caused by the bacteria _______________________

a) *Clostridium perfringens* b) *Clostridium botulinum*

c) *Clostridium haemolyticum* d) *Clostridium tatani*

53. Which disease of the following is a predisposing factor for Necrotic enteritis in poultry

a) E.coli infection

b) Chronic respiratory disease (CRD)

c) Coccidiosis

d) Ranikhet disease (RD)

54. Characteristic lesion of the Necrotic enteritis in affected poultry birds

a) Necrosis of intestinal mucosa b) Necrosis of proventriculus

c) Necrosis of brain cells d) Necrosis of caecum

55. Which part of intestine is affected in Clostridium perfringens infection

a) Small intestine b) Large intestine

c) Colon d) Caeca

56. Intestine filled with blood, necrotic epithelium debris with thickened intestinal walls is a characteristic feature of ______________________ infection
 a) *Clostridium perfringens* b) Necrotic enteritis
 c) *Clostridium haemolyticum* *d*) a & b

57. Abbreviation of AGP ________________________
 a) Antibiotic growth promoter b) Animal genetic potential
 c) Antibiotic growth processor d) a & c

58. Antibiotic growth promoter (AGP) is mainly used to reduce the incidence of
 a) Necrotic enteritis b) Coccidiosis
 c) Ranikhet disease (RD) d) Chronic respiratory disease

59. Which group of Clostridium perfringens produces necrotic enteritis in poultry birds
 a) Type A & C b) Type C & D
 c) Type B d) Type D & E

60. One of the following substance / nutrients cannot be bio-synthesized in *Clostridium perfringens due to absence of genes related to it*
 a) Carbohydrates b) Fatty acids
 c) Amino acids d) Enzymes

61. The main toxin responsible for the pathogenicity of Clostridium perfringens
 a) Alpha – α toxin b) Beta – β toxin
 c) Epsilon - € toxin d) All of the above

62. Location of the α toxin producing gene in Clostridium perfringens
 a) Plasmid b) Bacterial chromosome
 c) Cytoplasm d) Cell membrane

63. The alpha – α toxin produced by Clostridium perfringens causes necrotic enteritis mainly hydrolysing ________________ enzyme.
 a) Phospholipase C b) Succinyl thokinase
 c) Malate dehydrogenase d) α – D Ketogltaric acid dehydrogenase

64. *Clostridium perfringens* grows only under ________________ conditions
 a) Anerobic b) Aerobic
 c) Alkaline d) Acidic

65. During incubation in lab __________ colour of colonies produced by Clostridium perfringens on tryptose-sulfitecycloserine (TSC) agar
 a) Blue b) Black
 c) Green d) Silver

66. _______________ is used as enrichment media to grow the Clostridium perfringens in lab conditions
 a) Distilled water b) Selenite E broth
 c) Peptone water d) Cooked meat media / broth

67. What are the predisposing factors for the *Clostridium perfringens* caused by Coccidiosis infection
    a) Damaging the intestinal epithelial cells
    b) Increased mucus production
    c) Protein rich environment by damaging host tissue
    d) All of the above
68. Which dietary factor of the following predisposes the birds to Clostridium perfringens infection
    a) High energy diet
    b) Animal protein sources
    c) Low protein diet
    d) Vegetable protein sources
69. High viscosity in the intestine of poultry birds is produced due to presence of ____________ in the fee d)
    a) High starch
    b) High protein
    c) Non-starch polysaccharides (NSP)
    d) Animal protein source
70. Which protein source of the below predisposes the birds to Necrotic enteritis
    a) Fish meal
    b) Soya bean meal
    c) Maize gluten meal
    d) Rape seed meal
71. Which protein source of the below ingredients predisposes the birds to Necrotic enteritis
    a) Cotton seed meal
    b) Meat cum bone meal
    c) Sunflower meal
    d) Linseed cake
72. Which protein source of the below predisposes the birds to Necrotic enteritis
    a) Safflower cake
    b) DDGS
    c) Full fat soya
    d) Poultry meal
73. Which one of the following favors the growth of *Clostridium perfringens* intestine of poultry birds
    a) Biogenic amines
    b) High lysine content
    c) Protein deficient diet
    d) High tryptophan
74. Incidence of coccidiosis is more common in
    a) Winter
    b) Summer
    c) Autumn
    d) Spring
75. Pullorum disease of chickens is caused by
    a) *Salmonella gallinarum*
    b) *Salmonella pullorum*
    c) *Pasteurella multocida*
    d) *Escherichia coli*
76. Pullorum disease in chickens caused by *Salmonella pullorum* characteristic symptom of
    a) White faeces
    b) Green-colored diarrhoea
    c) Red colored faeces
    d) Faeces covered with Orange froth

77. Mortality rate in Pullorum disease

a) 30 % b) 50 %

c) 100 % d) 75 %

78. Pullorum disease in chickens caused by Salmonella pullorum mainly affects the chickens in the age group of

a) 2 to 3 weeks b) 6 to 8 weeks

c) 10 to 12 weeks d) 15 to 20 weeks

79. Mode of transmission of *Salmonella pullorum* in chicken

a) Horizontal transmission b) Vertical transmission

c) Mechanical transmission d) A & B

80. Post mortem lesions found in Pullorum disease

a) White diarrhoea b) Caseous membrane in caeca

c) Caseous mass in ovarian follicles d) All of the above

81. Salmonella pullorum is

a) Motile b) Non-motile

c) A & B d) A only

82. Presence of __________ mycotoxin increases the incidence of Necrotic enteritis

a) Deoxynivalenol (DON) b) Aflatoxin

c) T-2 toxin d) Ochratoxin

83. Eimeria infection in poultry predisposes the birds to Necrotic enteritis by ________.

a) Increased mucogenesis

b) Release of essential amino acids

c) Epithelial cell damage

d) All of the above

84. What are the binding sites for bacteria attachment and colonization in intestines

a) Oligosaccherides on mucin glycoprotein

b) Epithelial cells

c) a & b

d) Junction proteins

85. Junction proteins that acts as functional receptors to clostridium toxins

a) Claudin -3 & Claudin – 4 b) Juxtra protein – 1

c) A & B d) Junction Protein 1 & 2

86. Dirty turkish towel like appearance is found in which disease of the following

a) Necrotic enteritis b) Coli bacillosis

c) *Eimeria tenella* d) Salmonellosis

87. Pseudomembrane or diphtheritic membrane formation produced by *Clostridum perfringens* most frequently found in which segment of the intestine
    a) Caeca b) Jejenum
    c) Colon d) Crop
88. Cholangiohepatitis a condition observed in which condition of the below
    a) Sub-clinical NE b) Clinical NE
    c) a & b d) *Coccidiosis*
89. Adaptive immune system comprises of ____________________.
    a) B- Lymphocytes b) T-Lymphocytes
    c) a & b d) None of the above
90. Lymohoid aggregates of immune system are dispersed in ______________ layer of the intestine
    a) Lamina propria b) Serosa
    c) b & d d) Tunica muscularis
91. What are the primary immune organs in poultry birds
    a) Liver b) Bursa of fabricius
    c) Thymus d) b & c
92. The abbreviation for AGP is
    a) Antibiotic growth promoters b) Anti growth promoters
    c) Anti growth d)
93. Clostridium bacteria is a ______________
    a) Gram -ve organism b) Gram +ve organism
    c) Acid fast organism d) Acid slow organism
94. The first identified bacterial plasmid of transmitting antibacterial drug resistance in *Clostridum perfringens* against Chloramphenicol and Tetracycline is
    a) pIP401 b) pGRw-3
    c) pR450 d) €pIPGR
95. Resistance to Chloramphenicol drug by pIP401 is mediated by _______ enzyme.
    a) Chloramphenicol acetyltransferase
    b) Chloramphenicol decarboxylase
    c) Chloramphenicol dehydrogenase
    d) Chloramphenicol oxygenase
96. Chloramphenicol acetyltransferase enzyme functions by preventing Chloramphenicol drug to ______________ in *Clostridum perfringens.*
    a) Ribosomes in bacteria b) Cell wall in bacteria
    c) Mitochondria in bacteria d) Plasmid in bacteria
97. In NE affected birds which of the following species of bacteria increases in number in the intestine to protect intestine from *Clostridum perfringens*.
    a) *Escherichia coli* b) *Lactobacilli facii*
    c) Candidatus Savagella d) *Saccharomyces cerevisiae*

98. Candidatus Savagella is a filamentous bacterium that increases ___________ antibodies in birds affected by Clostridum perfringens.

a) IgA b) IgM

c) IgG d) IgE

99. The shift in pH of intestine from acidic to neutral in high protein or fish meal fed birds is mainly due to formation of _____________ .

a) Iso-forms of short chain fatty acids b) Increase in ammonia

c) Reduction in acetate & Butyrate d) All of the above

100. Which fatty acid of the following has cell tight junction expression promoting activity

a) Butyric acid b) Formic acid

c) Propionic acid d) B & C

101. _____________ is most common and economically important protozoal disease in poultry

a) *Ehrlichiosis* *b) Coccidiosis*

c) *Salmonellosis* d) Colibacillosis

102. What is the source of infection to acquire *coccidiosis* infection

a) Sporulated oocyst b) Eimeria organism

c) Sporozoite d) Merozoite

103. Arrange the following stages of Eimeria species life cycle in order

a) Sporogony → Schizogony → Gametogony

b) Schizogony → Sporogony → Gametogony

c) Gametogony → Schizogony → Sporogony

d) Schizogony → Gametogony → Sporogony

104. The infective stage of Coccidia contains ________ of Sporozoites.

a) Eight b) Six

c) Two d) Four

105. The plug made of protein and carbohydrate which is located at the narrow end of sporocyst is called as

a) Stieda body b) Negri bodies

c) Bollinger bodies d) Heinz bodies

106. Infective stage to the intestinal epithelial cells in coccidiosis disease

a) Merozoites b) Sporocysts

c) Sporozoites d) A & C

107. Asexual reproduction in Eimeria life cycle is called

a) Schizogony b) Gametogony

c) Sporogony d) B & C

108. Number of schizogony's in Eimeria tenella species

a) 2 b) 3

c) 1 d) 4

109. Highest number of schizogony's observed in __________ species of *Eimeria.*
   a) *Eimeria acervuline*
   b) *Eimeria mitis*
   c) A & B
   d) *Eimeria tenella*

110. Which factor among the following is necessary for the sporulation
   a) Temperature
   b) Oxygen
   c) Humidity
   d) All of the above

111. Number of schizogony's in *Eimeria necatrix* species
   a) 2
   a) 3
   c) 5
   c) 4

112. The largest oocyst is found in
   a) *Eimeria acervuline*
   b) *Eimeria mitis*
   c) *Eimeria maxima*
   d) *Eimeria tenella*

113. Sporulation time (hr) of Emineria tenella is
   a) 48
   b) 24
   c) 96
   d) 36

114. Sporulation time (hr) of Emineria maxima is
   a) 48
   b) 24
   c) 96
   d) 36

115. Sporulation time (hr) of Emineria necatrix is
   a) 48
   a) 24
   c) 96
   c) 36

116. Nature of pathogenicity in terms of damage to intestines in Eimeria necatrix is
   a) Bloody enteritis
   b) Blood droppings
   c) Lumen filled with blood, mucosal debris & fluid
   d) All of the above

117. The severity of coccidiosis infection largely depends on
   a) No. of oocysts ingested
   b) Watery quality
   c) Shed temperature
   d) Hatchery source

118. Predilection site of Eimeria tenella is
   a) Caeca
   b) Duodenum
   c) Jejenum
   d) Ileum

119. Predilection site of Eimeria maxima is
   a) Duodenum
   b) Jejenum
   c) Ileum
   d) All of the above

120. Predilection site of Eimeria necatrix is
   a) Duodenum
   b) Jejenum
   c) Caeca
   d) B & C

121. Predilection site of Eimeria acervulina is

a) Duodenum b) Jejenum

c) A & B d) Caeca

122. Arrange the following *Eimeria* species in order from high pathogenicity to low pathogenicity

a) *Eimeria necatrix > Eimeria maxima > Eimeria acervulina > Eimeria tenella*

b) *Eimeria maxima > Eimeria acervulina > Eimeria tenella > Eimeria necatrix*

c) *Eimeria tenella > Eimeria necatrix > Eimeria maxima > Eimeria* ***acervulina***

d) *Eimeria acervulina > Eimeria tenella > Eimeria necatrix > Eimeria maxima*

123. Target cells for the sporozoites & Merozoites in *Eimeria* life cycle

a) Intestinal Epithelial cells b) Intestinal muscle cells

c) Intestinal connective tissue cells d) A & B

124. The first line of defense against intestinal pathogens secreted by host intestine cells

a) Mucin b) Pepsin

c) Water fluid d) None of the above

125. Increased mucin production in intestine of coccidia infection predisposes the bird to ____________ infection

a) Necrotic enteritis b) Infectious bronchitis

c) Colibacillosis d) Aspergillosis

126. In diagnosis methods, which of the following technique is having stronger correlation with reduced performance of coccidia affected flock

a) Oocyst per gram (OPG) b) Lesion scoring method

c) A & B d) Litter droppings examination

127. Mode of action of ionophore anti-coccidial drugs

a) Interfering with ion passage

b) Interfering with replication process

c) Interfering with asexual reproduction

d) Interfering with sexual reproduction

128. Ionophore anti-coccidial drugs are produced by fermentation ____________ species among the below

a) Streptomyces b) Staphylococcus

c) Saccharomyces cerevisiae d) None of the above

129. Ionophore anti-coccidial drugs are produced by fermentation ____________ species among the below

a) Actinomadura b) *Saccharomyces cerevisiae*

c) Clostridium butyricum d) A & C

130. What is the monovalent anticoccidial agent among the below

a) Monensin b) Narasin

c) Salinomycin d) All of the above

131. What is the Divalent anticoccidial agent among the below
   a) Lasalocid   b) Salinomycin
   c) Narasin   d) Monensin

132. Which of the following is a example for Monovalent glycosidic ionophores
   a) Maduramycin   b) Semduramycin
   c) A & B   d) Lasalocid

133. Choose the synthetic anti-coccidial drug among the below
   a) Decoquinate   b) Narasin
   c) Maduramycin   d) Semduramycin

134. Decoquinate controls coccidia in broilers by
   a) Interfering with ion exchange of organisms
   b) Inhibiting parasite mitochondrial respiration
   c) Competing with thiamine uptake
   d) Inhibiting folic acid pathway

135. Clopidol acts by ____________ and inhibits coccidiosis progress in broilers
   a) Affects electron transport
   b) Affects sexual reproduction process
   c) Affects folic acid pathway
   d) A & B

136. Which of the following anti-coccidial agent works as thiamine antagonist and thereby inhibit growth of Eimeria organisms
   a) Amprolium   b) Halofuginone
   c) Robenidine   d) Diclazuril

137. Amprolium targets which stage of Eimeria life cycle
   a) First generation schizonts   b) Macrogametes
   c) Oocyst   d) Microgametes

138 Sulphonamides employed in coccidia control program inhibits ______________ pathway in Eimeria organisms
   a) Folic acid pathway
   b) Ion exchange across cell membrane
   c) Electron transport
   d) Binds protein

139. Stages targeted by Sulfonamides in Eimeria life cycle
   a) Second generation and later schizonts   b) First generation schizonts
   c) Oocyst   d) Merozoites

140. Ionophore anti-coccidial agents targets
   a) Schizonts   b) Sporozoites
   c) Merozoites   d) B & C

141. Monensin is a fermentation product of

a) *Streptomyces cinnamonensis* b) *Streptomyces aureaus*

c) *Streptomyces venezuelae* d) *Streptomyces faecalis*

142. Salinomycin is produced from

a) *Streptomyces avidinii* b) *Streptomyces albus*

c) *Streptomyces kanamyceticus* d) *Streptomyces rochei*

143. Narasin is produced a bacterial species called

a) *Streptomyces rochei*

b) *Streptomyces kanamyceticus*

c) *Streptomyces aureofaciens*

d) *Streptomyces albus*

144. Sulphonamides inhibits the folic acid pathway by inhibiting an enzyme called

a) Dihydropteroate synthase b) Dihydrofolate reductase

c) Para-amino benzoic acid d) B & C

145. Supplementation of ___________ is contraindicated during the treatment of coccidiosis affected flock with Amprolium.

a) Folic acid b) Thiamine

c) Pyridoxine d) Riboflavin

146. Amprolium is an anti-coccidial that targets second generation schizonts by interfering with uptake of ___________.

a) Folic acid b) Thiamine

c) Pyridoxine d) Riboflavin

147. Ballooning of the intestines is a characteristic feature of _________ species of Eimeria infection

a) *Eimeria acervuline* b) *Eimeria mitis*

c) *Eimeria maxima* d) *Eimeria tenella*

148. Recommended dose for Monensin in feed

a) 80 – 100 ppm b) 10 – 12 ppm

c) 50 – 60 ppm d) 100 – 120 ppm

149. Recommended dose of Narasin in feed to treat the coccidiosis

a) 60 – 80 ppm b) 10 12 ppm

c) 50 – 60 ppm c) 100 – 120 ppm

150. Recommended dose of Maduramycin in feed to treat the coccidiosis

a) 5 – 6 ppm b) 10 – 15 ppm

c) 1 ppm d) 1 – 2 ppm

151. Recommended dose of Lasalocid in feed to treat the coccidiosis

a) 75 – 125 ppm b) 80 – 100 ppm

c) 150 – 200 ppm d) 50 – 60 ppm

152. Recommended dose of Amprolium in feed to treat the coccidiosis
 a) 125 – 250 ppm b) 150 – 200 ppm
 c) 80 – 100 ppm d) 60 – 80 ppm

153. Recommended dose of clopidol in feed to treat coccidiosis in ppm
 a) 125 b) 150
 c) 175 d) 200

154. Recommended dose of Diclazuril in feed to treat coccidiosis in ppm
 a) 1 b) 0.5
 c) 2 d) 5

155. Recommended dose of Nicarbazin in feed to treat coccidiosis in ppm
 a) 100 b) 125
 c) 150 d) 200

156. Recommended dose of Robenidine in feed to treat coccidiosis in ppm
 a) 10 b) 66
 c) 33 d) 90

157. Caeca filled with blood and necrosed mucus debris in poultry is a characteristic lesion of
 a) *Eimeria acervuline* b) *Eimeria mitis*
 c) *Eimeria maxima* *d)* *Eimeria tenella*

158. "Salt and pepper" appearance of intestinal lesion is found in
 a) *Eimeria acervuline* *b)* *Eimeria necatrix*
 c) *Eimeria maxima* *d)* *Eimeria tenella*

159. Presence of orange colored mucus and blood in small intestine lumen is found in
 a) *Eimeria acervuline* b) *Eimeria mitis*
 c) *Eimeria maxima* d) *Eimeria tenella*

160. The standard lesion scoring method of diagnosis in coccidiosis is introduced by
 a) Johnson and Reid (1970)
 b) Liu and Kim (1982)
 c) Jacob and john (1975)
 d) Leeson and summers (1990)

161. Presence of transversal striations of the duodenum lumen is an indicative of ___________ infection
 a) *Eimeria acervulina* b) *Eimeria mitis*
 c) *Eimeria maxima* d) *Eimeria tenella*

162. Life cycle duration of *Eimeria tenella*
 a) 5 days b) 6 days
 c) 7 days d) 8 days

163. Life cycle duration of Eimeria maxima
   a) 5 days b) 6 days
   c) 7 days d) 8 days

164. Life cycle duration of Eimeria acervulaina
   a) 5 days b) 6 days
   c) 7 days d) 8 days

165. Life cycle duration of Eimeria brunetti
   a) 5 days b) 6 days
   c) 7 days d) 8 days

166. Life cycle duration of Eimeria necatrix
   a) 5 days b) 6 days
   c) 7 days d) 8 days

167. Life cycle duration of Eimeria mivati
   a) 5 days b) 6 days
   c) 7 days d) 8 days

168. Life cycle duration of Eimeria praecox
   a) 4 days b) 6 days
   c) 7 days d) 8 days

169. Which among the following factor aggravates / favours the development of coccidiosis
   a) Non-starch polysaccharides (NSP) b) Starch polysaccharides
   c) Protein d) High fat

170. Which among the following NSP favours the growth of coccidiosis
   a) Soluble NSP b) Insoluble NSP
   c) Starch carbohydrate d) None of the above

171. Non-starch polysaccharides (NSP) present in
   a) Barley b) Wheat
   c) Broken rice d) A & B

172. The best sporulation temperature range for Eimeria species is
   a) 24-28 °C b) 14-18 °C
   c) 35-40 °C d) <10 °C

173. Highly effective disinfectant against sporulated and non-sporulated oocysts of *Eimeria*
   a) Ammonium hydroxide b) Chlorine dioxide
   c) Hypo Chlorus acid d) Iodine compounds

174. Registered Live vaccine against the coccidiosis is
   a) Cocci Vac® b) Cocci Dac®
   c) CoxAbic® d) Cocci Dex ®

175. Registered subunit vaccine against the coccidiosis is
   a) Cocci Vac®   b) Cocci Dac®
   c) CoxAbic®   d) Cocci Dex ®
176. CocciVac® B is administered to
   a) Broilers   b) Layers
   c) Breeders   d) All of the above
177. CocciVac® D is administered to
   a) Broilers   b) Layers
   c) Breeders   d) B & C
178. CocciVac® B a registered live vaccine contains sporulated oocysts *of*
   a) *E. acervulina, E. brunetti, E. mivati and E. tenella*
   b) *E. acervulina, E. necatrix, E. mivati and E. tenella*
   c) *E. acervulina, E. maxima, E. mivati and E. tenella*
   d) *E. acervulina, E. maxima, E. mivati and E. preacox*
179. CocciVac® D a registered live vaccine contains sporulated oocysts *of*
   a) *E. acervulina, E. brunetti, E. hagani, E. maxima, E. mivati, E. necatrix, E. praecox and E. tenella*
   b) *E. acervulina, E. maxima, E. mivati and E. tenella*
   c) *E. acervulina, E. brunetti, E. hagani, E. maxima, E. mivati, E. necatrix, E. praecox and E. tenella*
   d) *E. acervulina, E. maxima, E. mivati and E. preacox*
180. Non-attenuated vaccine among the following is
   a) Advent®, CocciVac® B, CocciVac® D, Immucox® $C_{1,}$ Immucox®$C_{2,}$ Inovocox®, Vac M ®, Nobilis® COX-ATM
   b) Inmuner® Gel-Coc, Hipracox® Broilers, Livacox® Q, Livacox® T, Paracox®-8
   c) Inmuner® Gel-Coc, Hipracox® Broilers, Livacox® Q, Livacox® T, Paracox®-8, Vac M ®, Nobilis® COX-ATM
   d) Advent®, CocciVac® B, CocciVac® D, Livacox® Q, Livacox® T, Paracox®-8
181. Dysbacteriosis is a enteritis condition by non-specific micro-organisms is due to
   a) Disturbed balance between beneficial flora & harmful flora
   b) Increased harmful flora
   c) Decreased beneficial flora
   d) All of the above
182. Cell mediated immunity in avian coccidiosis is characterized by activation of ________________ cells
   a) T cells   b) Natural Killer cells
   c) Macrophages   d) All of the above
183. Immune cells involved in adaptive anticoccidial immunity
   a) B cells   b) CD4+ T helper (Th) cells
   c) CD8+ cytotoxic T lymphocytes   d) B & C

184. Which type of immunity plays important role in protecting the coccidiosis infected chickens

a) Cellular immunity b) Humoral immunity

c) Innate immunity d) B only

185. Major cytokine involved in anti-coccidial immune reaction

a) IFN-α b) IFN-γ

c) IFN-β d) IFN-€

186. Hyperimmune Egg yolk antibodies contains

a) IgY b) IgA

c) IgG d) IgM

187. Functional equivalent of mammalian IgG in avians

a) IgY b) IgA

c) IgE d) IgM

188. Antimicrobial peptides (AMPs) directed against coccidial parasites act by

a) Disrupting bacterial membrane by cationic activity

b) Destroying the DNA

c) Increasing ion concentration

d) Disrupting the electron transport in mitochondria

189. Withdrawal period of anticoccidial drug Monensin in broilers

a) 1 day b) 5 days

c) 10 days d) 14 days

190. Withdrawal period of anticoccidial drug Salinomicin in broilers

a) 2 days b) 3 days

c) 0 days d) 5 days

191. Withdrawal period of anticoccidial drug Lasalocid in broilers

a) 3 days b) 5 days

c) 7 days d) 10 – 15 days

192. Withdrawal period of anticoccidial drug Maduramicin in broilers

a) 2 days b) 3 days

c) 0 days d) 5 days

193. According to European commission (EU) Maximum residue limits of Monensin in broilers skin and fat is

a) 25 μg/kg b) 50 μg/kg

c) 75 μg/kg d) 100 μg/kg

194. According to European commission (EU) Maximum residue limits of Monensin in broilers liver, kidney and muscle is

a) 5 μg/kg b) 8 μg/kg

c) 15 μg/kg d) 25 μg/kg

195. According to European commission (EU) Maximum residue limits of Salinomicin in broilers liver, skin and fat is

a) 100 μg/kg b) 125 μg/kg
c) 150 μg/kg d) 200 μg/kg

196. According to European commission (EU) Maximum residue limits of Salinomicin in broilers muscle is

a) 5 μg/kg b) 8 μg/kg
c) 15 μg/kg d) 25 μg/kg

197. According to European commission (EU) Maximum residue limits of Robenidine in broilers muscle is

a) 100 μg/kg b) 125 μg/kg
c) 150 μg/kg d) 200 μg/kg

198. According to European commission (EU) Maximum residue limits of Diclazuril in broilers muscle is

a) 150 μg/kg b) 200 μg/kg
c) 400 μg/kg d) 500 μg/kg

199. According to European commission (EU) Maximum residue limits of Diclazuril in eggs is

a) 2 μg/kg b) 8 μg/kg
c) 15 μg/kg d) 20 μg/kg

200. According to European commission (EU) Maximum residue limits of Nicarbazin in broilers muscle is

a) 2000 μg/kg b) 3000 μg/kg
c) 4000 μg/kg d) 5000 μg/kg

Answer Key

1	b	2	a	3	a	4	b	5	d	6	c	7	a
8	d	9	b	10	a	11	b	12	a	13	b	14	a
15	d	16	a	17	a	18	a	19	b	20	a	21	b
22	b	23	c	24	a	25	b	26	c	27	d	28	a
29	c	30	d	31	c	32	b	33	a	34	c	35	d
36	a	37	a	38	b	39	b	40	d	41	b	42	a
43	a	44	b	45	a	46	b	47	a	48	a	49	c
50	a	51	d	52	d	53	c	54	a	55	a	56	a
57	a	58	a	59	a	60	c	61	a	62	b	63	a
64	a	65	b	66	d	67	d	68	b	69	c	70	a
71	b	72	d	73	a	74	a	75	a	76	a	77	c
78	a	79	d	80	d	81	b	82	a	83	d	84	a
85	a	86	a	87	b	88	a	89	c	90	a	91	d
92	a	93	b	94	a	95	a	96	a	97	c	98	a

99	d	100	a	101	b	102	a	103	d	104	a	105	a
106	d	107	a	108	b	109	c	110	d	111	a	112	c
113	a	114	a	115	a	116	d	117	a	118	a	119	d
120	d	121	c	122	c	123	a	124	a	125	a	126	b
127	a	128	a	129	a	130	d	131	a	132	c	133	a
134	b	135	a	136	a	137	a	138	a	139	a	140	d
141	a	142	b	143	c	144	a	145	b	146	b	147	a
148	d	149	a	150	a	151	a	152	a	153	a	154	a
155	b	156	c	157	d	158	b	159	c	160	a	161	a
162	c	163	c	164	a	165	b	166	c	167	a	168	a
169	a	170	d	171	d	172	a	173	a	174	a	175	c
176	a	177	d	178	c	179	a	180	a	181	d	182	d
183	d	184	a	185	b	186	a	187	a	188	a	189	a
190	c	191	b	192	b	193	a	194	b	195	c	196	c
197	d	198	d	199	a	200	a						

22

Disorders of Liver and Pancreas

Pubaleem Deka[1], Sonali Sahoo[1] and Tanmoy Rana[2]

[1]Department of Veterinary Medicine, Institute of Veterinary Science and Animal Husbandry, Siksha 'O' Anusandhan, Deemed to be University, Bhubaneswar Odisha-751003

[2]Department of Veterinary Clinical Complex, West BengalUniversity of Animal & Fishery Sciences, Kolkata-37

Introduction

Hepatocytes are tiny cells that constitute the primary structural unit of the liver. Periportal hepatocytes, the first to receive blood from the portal system, are particularly vulnerable to hepatotoxins and endotoxins. Periacinar hepatocytes, placed further away from the portal blood supply, are more susceptible to hypoxia, toxic metabolites and hypoperfusion. Inflammatory cells are drawn to injured hepatocytes and biliary epithelium due to the release of cytokines and inflammatory mediators. This causes additional hepatocyte necrosis and fibrosis. The liver has exceptional regenerative abilities as hepatocytes can be replaced even if only 12% remains intact.

Hepatocytes exhibit colour changes when they are laden with fat or pigments. In their first week of life, young turkeys and chickens typically have a lot of fat and pigments (carotenoids) deposited in the liver due to the ability of intestines in mobilizing the yolk content. It is typical to find fat vacuoles (microscopic fat deposits) within the hepatocytes at this point. A bird's liver will typically turn mahogany-brown after about seven days of life. Because of the influence of oestrogens, the hormones that are present in large concentrations once maturity is attained, the quantity of fat in the liver of adult hens increases before the age of lay. Because a large amount of fat and pigments are transferred from the liver to the oviduct for yolk formation in eggs, the majority of laying hens in a flock will typically have a pale brown or yellowish liver. When liver seems pale or yellow, histopathology is a crucial technique that can be used to establish a differential diagnosis.

Some of the important diseases affecting the liver and pancreas are discussed below:

Fatty liver and kidney syndrome (FLKS) – biotin deficiency

It is sometimes known as Pink Disease, Q Disease or Fatty Liver and Kidney Disease. It affects young chicks and is characterized by abnormally high levels of fat in the liver, kidney, heart and skeletal muscles, paralysis and sudden death. Pale, blotchy and enlarged livers and kidneys are the gross lesions with mortality often less than 10%. Fat infiltration is mostly observed in layer-type broilers and pullets during their first four weeks of life.

Fatty liver and hemorrhagic syndrome (FLHS)

A non-infectious condition that causes the liver and abdominal cavity to accumulate excessive fat and rupture the liver, causing haemorrhages and death of hens. The hallmark of this illness is enlarged, yellowish livers that are swollen with fat. Although it is not always the case, haemorrhage in the abdominal cavity is usually evident. This syndrome is a metabolic disease that affects hens as a result of an imbalance in their diet (protein/energy). The syndrome may occur by feeding diets high in energy but low in protein, or by feeding a ration with an imbalance or deficit of certain amino acids. It is commonly known that low amounts of lipotropic substances, including choline, methionine and vitamin B12 can cause the liver to be infiltrated with fat. Although vacuoles are normally present within the hepatocytes, triglyceride and other lipid metabolite globules accumulating excessively within the cytoplasm is referred to as hepatocellular fatty vacuolation (microscopic holes or blank spaces in the liver) or hepatocyte degeneration. Necrosis is the result of lipid-overloaded hepatocytes. Some chickens affected by FLHS will be present in healthy flocks under commercial conditions at approximately 45 weeks of age.

Histomoniasis

Numerous gallinaceous birds are infected with the protozoon Histomonas meleagridis, which results in histomoniasis, also known as blackhead disease. Turkey death rates are normally between 80% and 100%, although chickens are usually asymptomatic carriers. Clinical symptoms include sulphur-coloured faeces, drooping head and wings, prolonged standing, closed eyelids, ruffled feathers and emaciation.

A number of other parasites have also been reported to cause liver diseases in poultry. They include Cryptosporidium spp., Plasmodium spp. (avian malaria), Leukocytozoon spp., and flukes of the family Dicrocoelium.

Necrotic enteritis

When Clostridium perfringens (CP) type A or C colonizes the small intestine due to alterations in the gut microecology, broilers may develop necrotic enteritis (NE). It has been demonstrated that CP type A's necrotizing α-toxin, which causes intestinal mucosal necrosis, has a significant role. Another subclinical condition connected with CP infection is hepatitis or cholangiohepatitis, which occurs during broiler processing. The livers are significantly enlarged, with pale reticular pattern and occasionally tiny pale and stellate foci. Histologically, bile ductule hyperplasia, fibrosis, cholangitis and rarely localized granulomatous inflammation is seen.

Inclusion Body Hepatitis (IBH) and Hepatitis Hydropericardium Syndrome (HHS)

Inclusion body hepatitis (IBH), caused by adenovirus, is characterized by intranuclear inclusion bodies along with haemorrhages and dystrophic necrobiotic alterations in the liver and kidneys. Macroscopically, liver is enlarged, dystrophic with yellowish colour and crumbly texture. Young broilers suffer from inclusion body hepatitis and hepatitis hydropericardium syndrome, both of which are caused by chicken adenovirus. Clinical indications are unclear but frequently involve an abrupt rise in mortality. In HHS, gross lesions include an enlarged liver with many pale or haemorrhagic foci, as well as hydropericardium.

Turkey viral hepatitis

Turkey viral hepatitis is a highly contagious disease caused by virus of Picornaviridae family. It is a condition of young turkeys that includes both hepatitis and/or pancreatitis. The virus is shed in faeces and spreads through direct and indirect contact.

Aflatoxicosis

It is also called as Turkey X disease. Aflatoxicosis is caused by ingestion of aflatoxins in contaminated poultry feed. They are potent hepatotoxins produced by Aspergillus flavus, A. parasiticus or Penicillium puberulum. The 4 aflatoxins are B1, B2, G1 and G2. However, B1 is the most predominant and toxic. It is commonly found in poor quality poultry feeds which were made with contaminated ingredients, specifically corn. Typically, Aspergillus flavus and A. parasiticus infect peanuts, almonds, corn (maize) and cottonseed, producing significant levels of aflatoxins, with aflatoxin B being the most harmful. Aflatoxins are metabolized in the liver into an epoxide that binds to macromolecules such as nucleic acids. Mutagenesis, cancer, teratogenesis, immunosuppression and liver damage due to decreased protein synthesis are all possible adverse effects. It is essential to distinguish physiological alterations from mycotoxin intoxication with aflatoxin (AFLA), T-2 toxin (T2) and/or fumonisin (FUM).

Hepatic lipidosis

Birds on high-fat-low-protein diets are more likely to develop hepatic lipidosis, as fat is the primary source of energy. In birds, albumin transports circulatory fatty acids to the liver for oxidation or triglyceride formation. Lipidosis occurs when the quantity of circulating fatty acids exceeds the liver's processing capacity, causing excess lipid storage.

Iron storage disease

Excess iron in the bloodstream can lead to accumulation in the liver. It can also be found in the liver of birds suffering from diseases or experiencing intravascular haemolysis.

Multiple Choice Questions

1. In Inclusion body hepatitis, there is extensive hepatic necrosis, with presence of inclusion bodies in hepatocytes which are-
   a) Eosinophilic Intranuclear b) Basophilic intranuclear
   c) Eosinophilic intracytoplasmic d) None
2. Lesions of IBH which include petechial or ecchymotic hemorrhages may be present in-
   a) Liver b) Skeletal muscles
   c) Both d) Kidneys
3. In poultry, accumulation of clear straw-colored fluid in the pericardial sac, pulmonary edema, swollen and discolored liver, and enlarged kidneys with distended tubules showing degenerative changes is a condition of-
   a) Hydropericardium syndrome b) Ascites syndrome
   c) Mareks disease d) None
4. In hydropericardium syndrome in birds, pathological lesions are mainly present in-
   a) Pericardial sac b) Pancreas
   c) Liver d) All
5. In guinea fowl, presence of intranuclear inclusions in necrotic pancreatic acinar cells is associated with-
   a) Circoviral infection b) Adenoviral infection
   c) Coronavirus infection d) Salmonellosis

6. In IBH, specimens of choice for virus isolation is-
   a) Kidney b) Liver
   c) Pericardial fluid d) Both B and C
7. Which of the followig tests is used for detection of adenoviruses in infected cells by staining with an avian adenovirus antiserum labeled with a fluorescent dye?
   a) Immunocytochemistry b) ELISA
   c) FAT d) AGID
8. Which of the following diseases is an acute disease of ducklings, caused by picornavirus characterized by enlarged livers mottled with hemorrhages?
   a) Marble spleen disease (MSD) b) Duck Virus Hepatitis
   c) Fowl Cholera d) Coccidiosis
9. Goose parvovirus (GPV) infection is a highly contagious disease affecting young geese and Muscovy ducks (Cairina moschat a) is characterized by-
   a) Hepatitis b) Enteritis
   c) Hepatonephritis d) All of the above
10. The most widely used method to detect the presence of Goose parvovirus (GPV)-neutralizing antibodies-
    a) ELISA b) VNT
    c) FAT d) PCR
11. Which of the following diseases is caused by avian hepatitis E virus (avian HEV) characterized by presence of clotted blood in the abdomen and enlarged spleen and liver in dead birds?
    a) Marble spleen disease (MSD) b) Big Liver and Spleen Disease
    c) Hepatitis Splenomegaly Syndrome d) Both B and C
12. The source of contamination of Marek's disease virus-
    a) Faeces b) Droplets
    c) Feather follicle d) All
13. MDV is transmitted by-
    a) Mites b) Mosquitoes
    c) Oocysts d) Darkling beetles
14. The mode of transmission of Avian Leucosis virus-
    a) Vertical transmission b) Horizontal transmission
    c) Both a and b d) None
15. Green discoloration of the liver, marked enlargement and congestion of the spleen in poultry is the most characteristic lesion of-
    a) Colibacillosis b) Salmonellosis
    c) Necrotic hepatitis d) Ulcerative enteritis
16. Drug used for treatment of Fowl cholera-
    a) Sulfonamides b) Aminoglycosides
    c) Penicillin d) Amoxicillin

17. The characteristic lesions in Riemerella anatipestifer infection in waterfowl are-
    a) Fibrinous epicarditis b) Pericarditis
    c) Perihepatitis d) All
18. Antibiotics used for treatment of Riemerella anatipestifer infection-
    a) Sulpha drugs b) Chloramphenicol
    c) Tetracycline d) All
19. Choice of specimen for isolation of Clostridium colinum in poultry
    a) Intestine b) Liver
    c) Spleen d) Caeca
20. Which of the following contribute in E. coli transmission and its spread among poultry houses and farms?
    a) Larval and adult darkling beetles b) Mites
    c) Lice d) All
21. Duck Viral hepatitis mainly occurs in ducks of age group-
    a) 10-12 weeks b) 8-12 weeks
    c) < 7 weeks d) 16 weeks
22. Characteristic lesions in duck viral hepatitis includes enlargement, haemorrhagics foci, and congestion of blood vessels in-
    a) Liver b) Kidneys
    c) Spleen d) All
23. MD vaccines are usually administered in chicken aged-
    a) 5-7 days b) 1 weeks
    c) 0 day d) 3 weeks
24. Which of the following vitamins reduces incidence of fatty liver in poultry?
    a) Vitamin E b) Selenium
    c) Vitamin C d) Both a and b
25. Which of the following agents are considered hepatotoxic in poultry causing alteration in liver tissue?
    a) Aflatoxin b) Ochratoxin
    c) Fumonisin d) All
26. Haemorrhagic fatty liver syndrome is a liver dysfunction that occurs in birds characterized by liver degeneration, steatosis, yellow discolouration and bleeding, is mainly related to-
    a) Lipid metabolism b) Carbohydrate metabolism
    c) Both d) None
27. Enlarged liver with bronze greenish tint in adult birds is a characteristic lesion for-
    a) Haemorrhagic Fatty liver syndrome b) Acute fowl typhoid
    c) Fowl cholera d) Mycotoxicosis

28. The association between ________ virus and development of enteritis, pancreatitis, and pancreatic atrophy, may lead to curling of the duodenal loop

a) Chicken parvovirus b) Infectious bronchitis virus
c) Fowl adenovirus d) None of the above

29. Nutritional pancreatic atrophy (NPA) is classical feature of which deficiency disease of chicks?

a) Selenium b) Vitamin E
c) Both a and b d) Magnesium

30. Cholangiohepatitis observed in chickens and turkeys is mainly related to

a) C. perfringes toxin type A b) C. perfringes toxin type C
c) Clostridium septicum d) Clostridium botulinum

31. Infection with Histomonas meleagridis causing ulcerative or hemorrhagic typhlitis and multifocal zones of necrosis in the liver is caused by ingestion of eggs of the nematode-

a) Heterakis gallinarum b) Subulura brumpti
c) Trichuris vulpis d) Ascaridia galli

32. Fatty liver and kidney syndrome (FLKS) in young broilers and layer pulletsis associated with deficiency of-

a) Vitamin A b) Biotin
c) Vitamin E d) Folic acid

33. Melegrivirus A causing turkey hepatitis virus is

a) Non enveloped RNA virus b) Enveloped RNA virus
c) Non enveloped DNA virus d) Enveloped DNA virus

34. Hepatitis with or without pancreatitis, with gross lesions confined to the liver and pancreas is characteristic of-

a) Turkey viral hepatitis b) Mareks disease
c) Newcastle disease d) Runting and stunting syndrome

35. Inclusion body hepatitis is caused by ________ and forms ____________ type of inclusion bodies-

a) Adenovirus, Intranuclear
b) Adenovirus, Intracytoplasmic
c) Avihepatovirus DHV-1, Intranuclear
d) Avihepatovirus DHV-1, Intracytoplasmic

36. Avihepatovirus, of the family Picornaviridae is the causative organism of -

a) Duck virus hepatitis b) Inclusion body hepatitis
c) Avian leukosis d) Infectious bursal disease

37. Lethargy and ataxia followed by opisthotonos and death with gross pathological changes appearing chiefly in the liver i.e., distinct petechial and ecchymotic haemorrhages in ducks is characteristic of-

a) Newcastle disease b) Swollen head syndrome
c) Duck virus hepatitis (DVH) d) Marek's disease

38. The most susceptible poultry bird to aflatoxicosis is-
   a) Goslings b) Young chicks
   c) Pheasants d) Ducklings
39. Dietary concentration of aflatoxin tolerable in young poultry is-
   a) ≤ 50 ppb b) ≤ 200 ppb
   c) ≤ 100 ppb d) ≤ 300 ppb
40. Which is the principal metabolite of aflatoxin B1?
   a) M1 b) G1
   c) G2 d) All
41. A disease mostly affecting younger birds due to nutritional and metabolic isues but primarily a lack of biotin absorption from gut-
   a) Fatty liver and kidney syndrome b) Aflatoxicosis
   c) E coli infection d) Egg drop syndrome
42. Large umbilicated lesions called as "target" or "bullseye" lesions are suggestive of which disease?
   a) Histomoniasis b) Egg drop syndrome
   c) IBH d) Infectious laryngotracheitis
43. Which of the following is also known as "Big liver disease" ?
   a) Marek's disease b) Lymphoid leukosis
   c) Newcastle disease d) Egg drop syndrome (EDS 76)
44. Visceral tumors, the mian feature of lymphoid leukosis can be found in-
   a) Spleen b) Liver
   c) Kidneys d) All of the above
45. Presence of tumors in liver of poultry is indicative of which of the following diseases?
   a) Mareks disease b) Lymphoid leukosis
   c) Both d) None of the above
46. Inclusion body hepatitis is a viral disease of poultry caused by?
   a) Paramyxovirus b) Adenovirus
   c) Herpesvirus d) Orthomyxovirus
47. Typical mottled liver with pinpoint lesions, hydropericardium, pale bone marrow and kidneys are good indicators of -
   a) IBH-HHS b) LL
   c) MD d) None
48. Which of the following is referred to as "Angara disease"
   a) IBH b) HHS
   c) Newcastle disease d) None
49. Pancreatic inflammatory infiltration with degenerative changes in poultry is found in-
   a) Reovirus infection b) Runting and stunting syndrome
   c) Malabsorption syndrome d) Both b and c

50. In poultry, enlarged and congested liver with necrotic foci is characteristic lesion of which of the following diseases?
   a) Pullorum disease and fowl typhoid
   b) Fowl cholera
   c) Colibacillosis
   d) Necrotic enteritis
51. Black head disease in turkeys is caused by-
   a) Histomonas meleagridis
   b) Dermanyssus gallinae
   c) Eimeria tenella
   d) Heterakis gallinarum
52. Circular necrotic areas in liver with crater-like centre is pathognomonic of
   a) Black head disease
   b) Big liver disease
   c) MD
   d) LL
53. Which of the following parasite is responsible to transmit "Big head disease" in turkeys through eggs
   a) Capillaria spp.
   b) Ascariasis spp.
   c) Heterakis gallinarum
   d) Raillietina
54. In poultry, Clostridium perfringens causes Cholangiohepatitis. The type of toxin responsile is
   a) Type A
   b) Type C
   c) Both type A and C
   d) None
55. Aflatoxins are toxins produced by
   a) Aspergillus flavus
   b) Aspergillus parasiticus
   c) Penicillium ascomycota
   d) All of the above
56. The most toxic aflatoxin is-
   a) B1
   b) B2
   c) G1
   d) G2
57. Which of the following disease is a nutritional disorder of poultry?
   a) IBH
   b) MD
   c) Fatty liver and kidney syndrome
   d) IBH-HH
58. Several nutritional and environmental factors influence FLKS, the main factor remains to be a vitamin namely-
   a) Pantothenic acid
   b) Niacinamide
   c) Biotin
   d) None
59. An excessive accumulation of fat in the liver of adult hen which weakens the cellular structure of the liver and allows fatal haemorrhages causes-
   a) Fatty liver haemorrhagic syndrome
   b) Fatty liver and kidney syndrome
   c) Inclusion body hepatitis
   d) Hydropericardium hepatitis syndrome
60. "Spotty liver disease" in poultry is caused by-
   a) Campylobacter jejuni
   b) Campylobacter coli
   c) Campylobacter hepaticus
   d) Pasteurella multocida

61. A potent hepatoprotective used for the treatment of different liver ailments in poutry is-
    a) Silymarin b) Gossypol
    c) Leucas aspera d) Glutathione
62. Aflatoxins are toxic metabolites produced by molds common found in-
    a) Feed b) Silage
    c) Contaminated water d) All
63. Deoxynivalenol (DON) is a mycotoxin which has____________ affect in poultry.
    a) Nephrotoxic b) Hepatotoxic
    c) Neurotoxic d) None
64. Heavy metal toxicity in birds is caused due to exposue of-
    a) Contaminated water source b) Feed
    c) Environment d) All
65. Avian leukosis is mostly seen in poultry above ______ of age particularly in those birds that attain sexual maturity-
    a) 5 months b) 3 weeks
    c) 3 months d) None
66. Smears from organ affected by tumours of Avian Leucosis can be confirmed histopathologically by staining the smear with-
    a) ZN stain b) Seller's stain
    c) Pyronin stain d) None
67. Coligranuloma caused by E. coli is also known as-
    a) Hjarre's disease b) Mushy chick disease
    c) Air sacculitis d) None
68. In ______________, tumours are found in gonads, liver, spleen, lungs, muscles, heart, kidneys, proventriculus and intestine.
    a) Acute Marek's Disease (AMD)
    b) Classical Marek's Disease (CMD)
    c) Both
    d) None
69. In ______________, incoordination, lameness or paralysis of one or both the legs or wings shown by drooping of wings, torticollis due to affection of cervical nerves.
    a) Acute Marek's Disease (AMD)
    b) Classical Marek's Disease (CMD)
    c) Both
    d) None
70. Commonly used antibiotic for treatment of Avian chlamydosis is
    a) Chlortetracycline b) Doxycycline
    c) Tetracyclines d) All

71. Chlamydia psittaci is the causative agent of Avian chlamydosis which occurs domestic and wild fowl is also known as
   a) Psittacosis   b) Ornithosis
   c) Both   d) None

72. In Avian Chlamydosis, necropsy of affected birds will often reveal-
   a) Multifocal Hepatic Necrosis   b) Fibrinous airsacculitis
   c) Pericarditis and peritonitis   d) All

73. Chlamydiae can be detected in smears of cloacal or conjunctival swabs and in impression smears of tissues by cytological staining-
   a) Gram staining   b) Macchiavello's stain
   c) Romanowsky stain   d) Modified ZN stain

74. The __________ test is most widely used test in domestic fowl for detection of Mycobacterium avium.
   a) Mallein   b) Tuberculin
   c) Johnin   d) Intradermal

75. The tuberculin is the standard avian purified protein derivative (PPD) and birds are tested by intradermal inoculation in the wattle with______ of tuberculin.
   a) 0.1 ml   b) 1.0 ml
   c) 0.01 ml   d) 0.5 ml

76. The tuberculin test in poultry is read after _______ and a positive reaction is any swelling at the site, from a small firm nodule approximately 5 mm in diameter to gross oedema extending into the other wattle and down the neck.
   a) 12 hours   b) 15 minutes
   c) 24 hours   d) 48 hours

77. In pheasants, the tuberculin test can be performed by injecting purified protein derivative into-
   a) Skin of the lower eyelid   b) Thoracic muscles
   c) Wattle   d) Both a and b

78. ________ and ________ are the most poisonous of the most common heavy metals to accumulate in the food chain which triggers a variety of deadly symptoms, such as reproductive issues and hepato-renal dysfunction in poultry
   a) Arsenic, Lead   b) Lead, Cadmium
   c) Cadmium, Arsenic   d) Cadmium, Mercury

79. Which of the following agent is used as an adjunct in the treatment of cholestatic and necroinflammatory liver disorders in poultry?
   a) Ursodeoxycholic acid (UDCA)   b) Colchicine
   c) Silibinin   d) Ronidazole

80. Dose rate of Itraconazole to treat fungal diseases in poultry-
   a) 2-5 mg/kg   b) 5-10 mg/kg
   c) 4-15 mg/kg   d) 100 mg/kg

81. In poultry, Ursodeoxycholic acid is used as a cytoprotective which reduces involvement of hepatocytes and biliary epithelium in inflammatory process in a dose rate of –

a) 10-15 mg/kg b) 5-10 mg/kg
c) 4-15 mg/kg d) 100 mg/kg

82. A deficiency of in the diet of hens results in decreased egg production, increased embryonic mortality, and an increase in size and fat content of the liver-

a) Riboflavin b) Pantothenic acid
c) Nicotinic acid d) None

83. The liver is hypertrophied and may vary in color from a faint to dirty yellow in deficiency of-

a) Riboflavin b) Pantothenic acid
c) Nicotinic acid d) Pyridoxine

84. Biotin has been suspected of having a role in ___________ in broiler chickens.

a) Acute death syndrome b) Sudden death syndrome
c) Both d) None

85. Ascites ("water belly") is a condition most common in ducks where liver appears enlarged with firm to rubbery consistency and pale or brown or grey smooth surfaces occurs due to-

a) Hepatic amyloidosis b) Asphyxiation
c) Mineral deficiency d) Environmental factor

86. Concentration of cobalt in feed causing marked tibial dyschondroplasia, and necrosis and fibrosis in the pancreas, liver, and skeletal, smooth in poultry-

a) 250 ppm b) 500ppm
c) 300ppm d) 600ppm

87. ________________is a metabolite of Aspergillus flavus, the predominant producer of aflatoxin in feeds and grains

a) Cyclopiazonic acid (CPA) b) Penicillic acid
c) Rubratoxins A and B d) None

88. Poultry farms with a history of FLHS, diets should include appropriate concentrations or selenium at

a) 0.3 mcg/g of feed b) 1mg/g of feed
c) 0.5 mcg/g of feed d) 0.01 mcg/g of feed

89. Appropriate concentrations of antioxidant, L-tryptophan in diet to prevent FLHS in poultry should be-

a) 100 mg/kg of feed b) 500 mg/kg of feed
c) 250 mg/kg of feed d) 1000 mg/kg of feed

90. Temperature is an important environmental factor that affects the incidence of FLHS in-

a) Caged birds b) Layers
c) Broilers d) All

91. Candidiasis is an opportunistic fungal disease of the digestive tract of birds that is caused by the fungus Candida albicans commonly develops due to-
   a) Antimicrobials
   b) Contaminated Drinkers/Nipples Facilities.
   c) Vitamin A Deficiency
   d) All
92. Addition of ______ can prevent weight loss and hepatomegaly in the affected flock.
   a) Beta carotene b) Neomycin
   c) Vitamin E d) Vitamin C
93. In Duck viral hepatitis, hemorrhagic lesions in livers of ducklings up to ______ of age are practically pathognomonic
   a) 1 wks b) 2 wks
   c) 3 wks d) 4 wks
94. Transmission of Campylobacter species occurs by-
   a) Vertical transmission b) Trans-ovarian transmission
   c) Contaminated feed or water d) All
95. AFB1 can induce liver cell damage in poultry through-
   a) Oxidative damage b) Pyroptosis
   c) Necroptosis d) All
96. Fumonisin B1 (FB1) remains the most toxic compound and mainly produced by fungus
   a) Fusarium verticillioides b) F. fujikuroi
   c) F. oxysporum d) F. arthrosporiodes
97. Periodic cleaning of all feed handling equipments with __________bleach solution will help control mould growth and presence of aflatoxins
   a) 2% b) 5 to 10%
   c) 20% d) 1%
98. Methods of mycotoxin detection in contaminated feed are-
   a) Thin Layer Chromatography (TLC)
   b) Enzyme Linked Immuno-Sorbent Assay (ELISA);
   c) Chromatography
   d) All
99. Moisture level and temperature of grains should be kept at below ______and _______ respectively to prevent producton of a flatoxins and other mycotoxins by Aspergillus spp.
   a) 10%, 100C b) 20%, 200C
   c) 13%, 5 to 80C d) 15%, 150C
100. Mannan oligosaccharide (MOS), a potent microbiological binding agent is extracted from the cell wall of –
   a) Saccharomyces cerevisiae b) Penicillium expansum
   c) Pithomyces chartarum d) Fusarium sporotrichioides

Answer Key

1	a	2	c	3	a	4	d	5	b	6	b	7	d
8	b	9	d	10	b	11	b	12	c	13	d	14	c
15	b	16	a	17	d	18	a	19	b	20	a	21	c
22	d	23	c	24	d	25	d	26	a	27	b	28	a
29	c	30	a	31	a	32	b	33	a	34	a	35	a
36	a	37	c	38	d	39	a	40	a	41	a	42	a
43	b	44	d	45	c	46	b	47	a	48	b	49	d
50	a	51	a	52	a	53	c	54	a	55	d	56	a
57	c	58	c	59	a	60	c	61	a	62	a	63	b
64	d	65	a	66	c	67	a	68	a	69	b	70	d
71	c	72	d	73	b	74	b	75	b	76	d	77	d
78	b	79	a	80	b	81	a	82	a	83	b	84	c
85	a	86	b	87	a	88	a	89	d	90	a	91	d
92	a	93	c	94	d	95	d	96	a	97	b	98	d
99	c	100	a										

23

Disorders of Musculoskeletal System

Umamaheshwarry[1], Mohamed Hasif G.[2] and Tanmoy Rana[3]

[1]*Sanchu Animal Hospital,Chennai*

[2]*Institute of Veterinary science and Animal Husbandry, Siksha O Anusandhan University, Orissa*

[3]*Department of Veterinary Clinical Complex, West Bengal niversity of Animal & Fishery Sciences, Kolkata*

Introduction

Musculoskeletal diseases in poultry are often exhibited as lameness or leg weakness. Numerous factors, including those related to diet, animal husbandry, infections, or heredity, might contribute to musculoskeletal problems. Lameness can be exhibited due to disorders in the central or peripheral neurological systems, reproductive system, trauma or infection in the foot, leg, hip, spine, or just a generalised sickness. Less frequently, musculoskeletal anomalies can affect the bird's beak, neck, or wings. The diseases can also be classified as infectious origin (bacterial, viral) or non-infectious origin (congenital deformities, nutritional, trauma or neoplasia). Modern poultry production lines put a lot of strain on the musculoskeletal system due to factors like growth rate in broiler chickens and egg output in laying hens. As a result, poor nutrition and husbandry practices frequently lead to musculoskeletal disorders. Thus, musculoskeletal disorders in poultry can be controlled by choosing proper genetic selection, efficient vaccinations, adequate nutrition and proper husbandry practices.

Diseases of Infectious origin

Pododermatitis: also known as 'Bumble foot' is an inflammatory condition affecting the foot. It is most commonly seen in mature broiler breeders. Birds which are obese and maintained in wet litter are predisposed. It may exhibit as mild aseptic inflammation to severe osteomyelitis. *Staphylococcus sp., Escherichia coli, Anctinomyces sp.* were the common bacteria isolated. Ammonia-free dry litter reduces the damage to foot pads. Post-peak feed restriction must be implemented to restrict both male and female weight gain. Parenteral antibiotics, bandaging and wound management might be necessary for severe cases.

Mycoplasmosis: *Mycoplasma synoviae* causes upper respiratory tract infections and synovitis in birds. The route of transmission in through respiratory tract. Signs of lameness exhibited in chickens and turkeys are exudative synovitis, tenosynovitis, or bursitis of hock and foot pads. It can be diagnosed serologically by ELISA or plate agglutination. Prevention is by buying a negative stock or to clean out and repopulate. Antibiotics can be used for treatment but birds will remain carrier for life.

Reo viral arthritis: Serotypes responsible for causing arthritis and tenosynovitis include S1133 and WVU 2937. Vertical transmission is common route of spread, but can also spread through contaminated equipment. Clinical signs occur in birds from 30 days of age and characterised by increasing lameness, unilateral or bilateral arthritis of stifle and hock joint. Prevention is by procuring stocks from vaccinated parent flock and biosecurity. Proper vaccination should be followed for breeding stocks

Septic joint: Mainly caused by *Staphylococcus aureus* (also known as Staphylococcal arthritis) or other pathogens like *Escherichia coli, Salmonella gallinarium, Pasteurella multocida, Mycoplasma synoviae,* and reovirus. Signs exhibit as lameness in single or multiple joints, swollen and warm joints with purulent exudate. Affect birds from age of 8-16weeks

Marek's Disease: caused by Alpha herpes virus, especially serotype 1 known as *Gallid herpesvirus 2*. Based on the clinical signs MD has been classified into various pathological syndromes which include fowl paralysis, MD lymphoma, skin leukosis, and ocular leukosis. Fowl paralysis, unilateral or bilateral, is typically seen in 6-12 weeks of age but can also occur in younger or older chicken. One leg extended forward and the other pointing back is the standard posture. The pathognomonic lesion is unilaterally enlarged sciatic plexus. MD can be diagnosed by ELISA or PCR. Prevention is by proper vaccination at day 1 or in egg since there is no treatment.

Botulism (Limberneck): caused due to ingestion of *Clostridium botulinum* exotoxin type C generally found in decaying meat, vegetables. Most commonly affects ducks and other waterfowls but can affect other poultries. Clinical manifestation includes flaccid ascending skeletal muscle paralysis which eventually causes death due to respiratory paralysis. Supportive therapy will help in recovery in less severe cases. Anti toxin therapy can also be used.

Femoral head necrosis: mostly caused due to bacterial osteomyelitis, certain staphylococci strains are more likely to produce this kind of infection, most likely due to their capacity to adhere to cartilage. Commonly seen in older broilers characterised by severe lameness. Birds might use tip of wing to support when sitting and rising.

Diseases of non-infectious origin

Nutritional deficiencies

- A deficit or imbalance in calcium or phosphorus can cause osteomalacia in adult breeders and in commercial egg producing flocks causes cage layer fatigue, or rickets in young birds.
- Rickets is also caused by a lack of vitamin D3 (cholecalciferol) in young flocks kept in climate-controlled facilities.
- Thiamine (Vitamin B1) deficiency causes "star gazing" in which a typical posture occurs due to paralysis of the anterior neck muscles, with the legs flexed and the head drawn back when sitting on the hocks.
- Riboflavin (Vitamin B2) deficiency causes "curled toe paralysis" where the toe curls medially and the chicks sit on the hock. Signs can start as early as 12 days of age.
- Pyridoxine (vitamin B6) deficiency causes seizures and an irregular gait. This disease may also arise after young flocks are given toxic doses of nitrofurans.

- Vitamin E deficiency causes encephalomalacia in chicks, along with other disorders such as exudative diathysis and nutritional myopathy.
- Choline, manganese, or biotin deficiency causes "slipped tendon" (perosis) which occurs due to gastrocnemius tendon luxation with enlarged hock and valgus position of leg.
- Chondrodystrophy due to manganese deficiency occurs in developing chicks as a result of less bone forming beneath the tibiotarsus and tarsometatarsus development plates.

Congenital/developmental abnormalities:

Twisted legs: affects long bones (tibiotarsus, tarso-metatarsus) of growing broilers. It can present as varus (bow-legged) or valgus (x-legged). It is mostly genetic, but managemental and nutritional factors play a role.

Splay leg: it occurs due to lateral deviation of hip. Commonly associated with high humidity during egg incubation period. Daily bandaging of leg can be attempted if it is caught early.

Rotated tibia/crooked toes: mostly genetic in origin. Affecting turkeys and heavy broilers.

Reproductive diseases:

- Hens will present with lameness due illness or pain or distended coelomic cavity which causes difficulty in walking. Such diseases include retained egg, egg related coelomitis, right cystic oviduct, or neoplasia, ectopic egg.

Trauma:

- Common in backyard poultry due to predator attacks or getting caught in traps/ enclosures. Wound management or fracture repair (external coaptation or internal fixation techniques) can be used to treat.

Diseases affecting wing:

- Wings can be affected due to soft tissue injury, trauma, fracture or brachial plexus avulsion. It is evident as a wing droop. "Angel wing" is a condition affecting juvenile ducks fed on high energy diets.

Following are the MCQs

1. Which of the following is essential for prevention of perosis in chicken

   a) Biotin b) Vit B10

   c) Choline d) Vit B5

2. Vitamin E deficiency in poultry causes the following condition especially when diet contain high level of unsaturated fatty acids

   a) Exudative diathesis b) Nutritional roup

   c) Crazy chick disease d) All of the above

3. Bowing of legs with enlargement of hock joint without slipping of achilles tendon is caused by deficiency of

   a) Calcium b) Choline

   c) Nicotinic acid d) Carotene

4. Thiamine deficiency symptom is
   a) Curled toe paralysis
   b) Nutritional myopathy
   c) Polyneuritis
   d) All
5. Scurfy skin, thin hair, slow growth and a characteristic goose stepping in poultry is due to deficiency of
   a) Thiamine
   b) Riboflavin
   c) Nicotinic acid
   d) Pantothenic acid
6. Pododermatitis is also called as
   a) Bumble foot
   b) Splay leg
   c) Perosis
   d) Curled toes
7. Pododermatitis is commonly seen in birds of which age group
   a) 0-10 days old
   b) Mature broilers
   c) Young layers
   d) 1-2 weeks old
8. Which of the following are pre disposing condition to bumble foot
   a) Wet litter
   b) Over-weight birds
   c) Excessive ammonia from litter
   d) All of the above
9. Causative organism for bumble foot is
   a) *Staphylococcus sp.*
   b) *E. coli*
   c) *Actinomyces sp.*
   d) All of the above
10. Femoral head necrosis commonly seen in older broilers is caused due to
    a) Viral osteomyelitis
    b) Bacterial osteomyelitis
    c) Fungal osteomyelitis
    d) Nutritional deficiency
11. The site of initiation of the bacteria causing spinal osteomyelitis isFused T2-T5
    a) Cervical vertebra
    b) Abdominal air sacs associated with free thoracic vertebra
    c) First coccygeal
12. Cervical osteochondrosis in turkeys is caused by
    a) *Mycoplasma meleagridis*
    b) *Mycoplasma synoviae*
    c) *Mycoplasma gallisepticum*
    d) *Staphylococcus aures*
13. Cage layer fatigue is also known as
    a) Osteochondrosis
    b) Osteoporosis
    c) Osteomyelitis
    d) Dyschondroplasia
14. Splay leg//Spraddle leg is associated with
    a) High humidity during incubation
    b) Slippery flooring
    c) Both A and B
    d) Obesity
15. Dyschondroplasia in poultry most commonly occurs in which of the following bone
    a) Tibia
    b) Cervical vertebrae
    c) Femur
    d) Pygostyle

16. Curled toe paralysis in chicken is caused due to deficiency of
    a) Thiamine (Vit B1) b) Pyridoxine (Vit B6)
    c) Riboflavin (Vit B2) d) Manganese
17. Chicks show signs of curled toe paralysis from which age when fed with deficient diet
    a) 3 days b) 12 weeks
    c) 12 days d) 50 days
18. Septic joint can be caused due to
    a) *Staphylococcus aureus* b) Reoviruses
    c) *Salmonella gallinarium* d) All of the above
19. Slipped tendon is caused due to deficiency of
    a) Choline b) Manganese
    c) Biotin d) All of the above
20. *Mycoplasma synoviae* is primarily spread through
    a) Fomites b) Respiratory tract
    c) Vertical transmission d) Faecal route
21. *Mycoplasma synoviae* causes which of the following signs in poultry
    a) Respiratory tract infection b) Air sacculitis
    c) Synovitis d) All of the above
22. Lameness due to *Mycoplasma meleagridis* in turkeys usually shown in which age
    a) 20 weeks old b) 8-9 months old
    c) 1- 6weeks old poults d) Mature broilers
23. Main route of transmission for *Mycoplasma meleagridis* is
    a) Vertical transmission b) Feco-oral route
    c) Direct contact d) Fomites
24. Exudative synovitis, tenosynovitis, or bursitis of hock and foot pads in chickens and turkeys are caused by which species of *Mycoplasma*?
    a) *M. meleagridis* b) *M. synoviae*
    c) *M. gallisepticum* d) None of the above
25. Marek's disease is commonly seen in
    a) Chicken b) Turkey
    c) Water fowls d) Pigeons
26. Causative agent for Marek's disease is
    a) Reo virus b) Gallid herpes virus
    c) Avian paramyxovirus d) Retrovirus
27. Marek's disease causes which of the following disease in chicken
    a) Fowl paralysis b) Lymphoma
    c) Ocular and skin leukosis d) All of the above

28. Classical sign of fowl paralysis is
    a) Sitting in hock
    b) Swollen metatarsus bone
    c) Unilateral paralysis with enlarged sciatic plexus
    d) Painful and inflamed plantar surface of foot
29. Fowl paralysis is seen in which age group of chicken
    a) 1 week old
    b) 6-12 weeks
    c) 14-40 weeks
    d) Older turkeys
30. Lateral deviation of leg is called
    a) Varus deformity
    b) Cross legged
    c) Valgus deformity
    d) None
31. Abnormal persisting accumulation of cartilage at growth plate is referred as
    a) Dyschondroplasia
    b) Chondrodystrophy
    c) Septic joint
    d) Rickets
32. Lateral deviation at hip is referred as
    a) Fowl paralysis
    b) Valgus condition
    c) Perosis
    d) Splay/spraddle leg
33. Average time of healing for avian fracture is
    a) 1 week
    b) 2-3weeks
    c) 4-6weeks
    d) 5months
34. Clinical signs of gastrocnemius tendon rupture in birds is seen as
    a) Sitting on hock with toes pointing ventrally
    b) Loose tendon palpated at posterior surface of leg
    c) Lack of gastrocnemius attachment palpated at hock
    d) All of the above
35. "Angel wing" in ducks is caused due to
    a) Reovirus
    b) *Staphylococcus aureus*
    c) High energy diet
    d) Trauma
36. "Star gazing" is due to paralysis of which muscle
    a) Anterior muscles of neck
    b) Thigh muscles
    c) Sciatic nerve
    d) Breast muscles
37. Limberneck is caused due to
    a) Riboflavin deficiency
    b) Selenium toxicity
    c) Botulism
    d) Thiamine deficiency
38. Death in botulism is due to
    a) Septicaemia
    b) Respiratory paralysis
    c) Dehydration
    d) Myocarditis
39. Which of the following is effective in controlling *Mycoplasmosis*
    a) Vaccination
    b) Depopulation and repopulate with clean stock
    c) Antibiotic therapy
    d) Isolation

40. Which of the following species of *Mycoplasma* causes air sacculitis and bone deformities in turkeys
    a) *M. meleagridis* b) *M. synoviae*
    c) *M. gallisepticum* d) None of the above
41. Runting syndrome in chicks is caused due to
    a) Reovirus b) Genetic cause
    c) Nutritional deficiency d) Slippery floor
42. Ricket-like syndrome characterised by osteopenia seen in 4 weeks is due to
    a) Calcium deficiency b) Vitamin D deficiency
    c) Runting syndrome d) Vitamin E deficiency
43. Calcium or phosphorus deficiency in mature birds causes
    a) Rickets b) Osteomalacia
    c) Osteoporosis d) Osteomyelitis
44. Calcium or phosphorus deficiency in immature/young birds causes
    a) Rickets b) Osteomalacia
    c) Osteoporosis d) Osteomyelitis
45. Chicks reared in controlled environment are prone to rickets due to deficiency of
    a) Vitamin B2 b) Manganese
    c) Vitamin B12 d) Vitamin D3
46. Pyridoxine (Vitamin B6) deficiency causing abnormal gait and convulsion in chicks can occur due to toxicity of
    a) Nitrofurans b) Phosphorus
    c) Ammonia d) Vitamin B12
47. Dietary level of manganese to avoid perosis in chicken is
    a) 20-30ppm b) 200-300ppm
    c) 80-120ppm d) 40-50ppm
48. Principal route of transmission of reo virus is
    a) Lateral spread b) Contaminated equipment
    c) Vertical transmission d) Oral route
49. Which of the following serotypes of reovirus are responsible for causing arthritis and tenosynovitis
    a) S1133 and WVU 2937 b) Serotype A
    c) Serotype C1 d) Serotype E
50. Which of the following virus causes arthritis and tenosynovitis in chicken
    a) Herpes virus b) Retro virus
    c) Reo virus d) Adenovirus
51. First age of vaccination for reo viral arthritis is
    a) 2weeks b) 30-40 days of age
    c) Day 1 of age d) 4-5 days of age

52. Gross enlargement of foot pad with ulceration of plantar skin and abscess is seen in
    a) Valgus deformity b) Bumble foot
    c) Perosis d) Reo viral arthritis
53. Pododermatitis can be controlled by
    a) Dry litter b) Reduction in ammonia
    c) Post peak food restriction d) All of the above
54. Valgus and varus condition commonly affects which of the following bone
    a) Tibiotarsus and tarsometatarsus b) Femur
    c) Hip bones d) Foot pad
55. Medial deviation of leg is also called
    a) Valgus deformity b) Knock kneed
    c) Both A and B d) Varus deformity
56. Valgus and varus deformity can be detected from which age
    a) 3 days old b) 3 weeks old
    c) 5 months d) 12-13 weeks
57. Rotated tibia and crooked toes in heavy broilers and turkeys are due to
    a) Genetic origin b) Nutrition deficiency
    c) Reo virus d) *Mycoplasmosis*
58. Serous arthritis can be caused due to
    a) Reo viral arthritis b) *Mycoplasma synoviae*
    c) Both A and B d) Marek's disease
59. What percentage of calcium and phosphorus is required to avoid rickets in immature flocks
    a) 1% calcium and 1% phosphorous
    b) 1% calcium and 2% phosphorous
    c) 1% calcium and 0.5% phosphorous
    d) 0.5% calcium and 1% phosphorous
60. Parenteral vaccination with contaminated needles usually results in
    a) Staphyloccus arthritis b) Reoviral arthritis
    c) Mycoplasmosis d) Botulism
61. Bilateral lameness with thickened bones of hock joint and more malleable bones are seen in
    a) Perosis b) Rickets
    c) Pododermatitis d) Vit E deficiency
62. Long bone deformity showing shortening and no thickening of growth plates due to manganese deficiency is referred as
    a) Dyschondroplasia b) Chondrodystrophy
    c) Septic joint d) Rickets
63. Bowing of tibiotarsus with thickening of growth plates in seen in
    a) Dyschondroplasia b) Chondrodystrophy
    c) Septic joint d) Arthritis

64. In gastrocnemius tendon rupture the lameness is seen as
   a) Extended hock
   b) One leg extended forward and one leg extended behind
   c) Wing drooping
   d) Hopping lame
65. Typical posture with one leg extended forward and other pointing back is seen in
   a) Thiamine deficiency b) Slipped tendon
   c) Marek's disease d) Riboflavin deficiency
66. Type of gait where stifle remain extended and hip flex to lift foot off ground is called as
   a) Goose stepping gait b) Bunny hop gait
   c) Swimmer's posture d) Splay leg
67. Spinal osteomyelitis causing paralysis due to spinal cord compression is caused due to
   a) *E. coli*
   b) *Staphylococcus sp. or Enterococcus caecorum*
   c) Marek's disease
   d) Reovirus
68. Live vaccination against which of the following virus causes tendon problems in future
   a) Retro virus b) Herpes virus
   c) Reo virus d) Adeno virus
69. Splondylopathy/vertebral deformity is commonly seen in
   a) Cervical vertebra b) T1-T3
   c) Free T4 d) Coccygeal
70. Pathology of rickets is due to
   a) Failure of mineralisation of long bones b) Arthritis
   c) Reduced joint space d) Curled toes
71. Degenerative joint disease is commonly seen in
   a) Older broilers b) Young layer
   c) Older layers d) Young chicks
72. Common site for articular osteochondrosis is
   a) The hip joint
   b) The distal tibiotarsus
   c) The epiphyses of the synovial joints adjacent to the sixth thoracic vertebra
   d) All of the above
73. Deep pectoral myopathy is seen in which muscle
   a) Neck muscle b) Breast muscle
   c) Supracoracoid muscle d) Thigh muscle

74. Deep pectoral myopathy can be caused due to
   a) Trauma
   b) Infectious bronchitis virus
   c) Mycotoxin
   d) All of the above
75. Certain coccidiostats can cause myodegeneration of leg muscles due to
   a) Nitrofuran toxicity
   b) Ionophore toxicity
   c) Selenium toxicity
   d) Manganese deficiency
76. Cage layer fatigue is caused due to
   a) Vitamin D deficiency
   b) Calcium deficiency
   c) Reovirus
   d) Genetic causes
77. To avoid cage layer fatigue adequate calcium should be met
   a) During first egg
   b) 2 weeks after first egg
   c) 2 weeks before first egg
   d) None of the above
78. Abnormal growth and extensive formation (modelling) of bone is termed as
   a) Osteomyelitis
   b) Rickets
   c) Osteoporosis
   d) Osteopetrosis
79. Osteopetrosis in chicken and turkeys is due to
   a) Avian leukosis
   b) Marek's disease
   c) Reovirus
   d) *Staphylococcus sp*
80. Amyloid arthropathy is caused due to
   a) Protein rich diet
   b) Unsaturated fatty acids
   c) *Enterococcus faecalis*
   d) Vit B1 deficiency
81. Clinical signs of vitamin D deficiency in layers is seen
   a) As soon as 2 weeks after diet is deprived of Vitamin D
   b) After one month of deficient diet
   c) 1 week after deficient diet
   d) 2-3 months after deficient diet
82. "Penguin-type squat" is seen in hens in deficiency of
   a) Manganese
   b) Protein
   c) Vitamin D3
   d) Choline
83. Encephalomalacia in chicks is caused due to deficiency of
   a) Vitamin D3
   b) Vitamin B12
   c) Vitamin E
   d) Phosphorus
84. Vitamin E deficiency with selenium deficiency causes
   a) Exudative diathesis
   b) Nutritional roup
   c) Crazy chick disease
   d) All of the above
85. Vitamin E deficiency with sulfur amino acid deficiency causes
   a) Exudative diathesis
   b) Nutritional myopathy
   c) Crazy chick disease
   d) All of the above

86. Clinical signs of exudative diathesis are
   a) Ataxia, retraction of head, prostration
   b) Standing with legs apart due to fluid accumulation under ventral skin
   c) Light coloured streaks of affected breast muscles
   d) All of the above
87. Clinical signs of encephalomalcia in chicks are
   a) Ataxia, retraction of head, prostration
   b) Standing with legs apart due to fluid accumulation under ventral skin
   c) Light coloured streaks of affected breast muscles
   d) All of the above
88. Clinical signs of nutritional myopathy in chicks are
   a) Ataxia, retraction of head, prostration
   b) Standing with legs apart due to fluid accumulation under ventral skin
   c) Light coloured streaks of affected breast muscles
   d) All of the above
89. Foot pad dermatitis can be caused by
   a) Biotin deficiency b) Wet litter
   c) Opportunistic pathogens d) All of the above
90. Most consistent lesion with deficiency of choline is
   a) Chondrodystrophy b) Paralysis
   c) Incoordination d) Ruffled feathers
91. Scaling of skin, enlarged hock, awkward arthritic gait, poor feathering is seen in deficiency of
   a) Selenium b) Manganese
   c) Vitamin K d) Zinc
92. Effective strategy to control dyschondroplasia is
   a) Restricted feeding to avoid rapid growth
   b) High humidity
   c) Dry litter and non-slippery floor
   d) None
93. Birds having valgus deformation in one and varus deformation in other leg is called as
   a) Swimmer's leg b) Splay leg
   c) Windswept d) Perosis
94. Bone remodelling of synovial lined joints leading to degeneration of articular cartilage is termed as
   a) Osteoporosis b) Osteoarthritis
   c) Osteochondrosis d) Osteomalacia
95. "Kinky back" is also known as
   a) Spondylolisthesis b) Spondylopathy
   c) Spondylosis d) Fracture of spine

96. Most common abnormal curvature of spine observed in poultry is
 a) Kyphosis b) Scoliosis
 c) Lordosis d) Spondylosis
97. Deep pectoral myopathy is also known as
 a) Nutritional roup b) Muscular dystrophy
 c) Black muscle disease d) Green muscle disease
98. The hock-sitting posture with toes directed ventrally is characteristic of which condition
 a) Slipped tendon
 b) Bilateral gastrocnemius tendon rupture
 c) Femoral fracture
 d) Vitam D3 deficiency
99. In lameness caused due to ligament injury which is commonly affected
 a) Capital femoral ligament b) Brachial plexus
 c) Tarsal ligament d) All of the above
100. Which of the following diseases due to deficient Vitamin E does not respond to vitamin E supplement
 a) Encphalomalacia b) Exudative diathesis
 c) Nutritional myopathy d) Muscular dystrophy

Answer Key

1	c	2	c	3	b	4	c	5	d	6	a	7	b
8	d	9	d	10	b	11	c	12	a	13	b	14	c
15	a	16	c	17	c	18	d	19	d	20	b	21	d
22	c	23	a	24	b	25	a	26	b	27	d	28	c
29	b	30	c	31	a	32	d	33	b	34	d	35	c
36	a	37	c	38	b	39	b	40	a	41	a	42	c
43	b	44	a	45	d	46	a	47	c	48	c	49	a
50	c	51	d	52	d	53	a	54	a	55	c	56	b
57	a	58	c	59	c	60	a	61	b	62	b	63	a
64	d	65	c	66	a	67	b	68	c	69	c	70	a
71	a	72	d	73	c	74	d	75	b	76	b	77	c
78	d	79	a	80	c	81	a	82	c	83	c	84	a
85	b	86	b	87	a	88	c	89	d	90	a	91	d
92	a	93	c	94	b	95	a	96	c	97	d	98	b
99	a	100	a										

24

Disorders of the Urinary System

Subir Singh

Department of Veterinary Medicine and Public Health, Faculty of Animal Science Veterinary Science and Fisheries, Agriculture and Forestry University, Rampur Chitwan, Nepal

Introduction

The urinary system of poultry, consisting of the kidneys, ureters, and cloaca, is essential for removing waste products and maintaining fluid balance. However, this system can be susceptible to various disorders that can impact the health and productivity of the flock. This chapter will discuss some of the most common urinary system disorders in poultry.

Urinary system disorders can have significant negative impacts on poultry health and productivity (Klybeck, n.d; Mississippi State University Extension, n.d; Poultry Hub, n. d.). Some of the key ways these disorders affect poultry include:

1. **Gout:** Renal diseases often lead to gout in poultry, which is a metabolic disorder resulting in hyperuricemia and deposition of uric acid or urates in tissues (Klybeck, n.d.). This can further damage the kidneys or other body systems.
2. **Reduced productivity:** Gout has a direct effect on productivity by lowering weight gain, increasing feed conversion ratio (FCR), and causing mortality which may reach 11-30% (Klybeck, n.d)
3. **Organ damage:** Accumulation of uric acid can lead to swelling and damage of kidney cells, as well as visceral gout where whitish deposits are found on the surface of organs like the heart, liver, intestines, and lungs (Klybeck, n.d; Mississippi State University Extension, n.d.).
4. **Mortality:** Severe kidney damage and dysfunction can quickly lead to debilitation and death in poultry (Poultry Hub, n.d.). Acute septicemic coliform infections may also cause sudden death (Mississippi State University Extension, n.d.)
5. **Respiratory issues:** Infectious bronchitis virus can affect both the respiratory and urinary systems, causing inflammation and damage to the kidneys (Mississippi State University Extension, n.d.).
6. **Digestive problems:** Bacterial nephritis caused by *E. coli* can lead to intestinal inflammation, excess mucus, and areas of hemorrhage (Mississippi State University Extension, n.d.).

Proper management, prevention, and treatment of urinary disorders is crucial to maintain flock health and productivity (Klybeck, n.d; Mississippi State University Extension, n.d.). This includes ensuring proper nutrition, biosecurity, and treating infections when they occur.

A) Major signs and post-mortem lesion of urinary disorders in poultry

The main signs of urinary disorders in poultry include:

- Excessive water intake and increased urine production (Jacob *et al.*, 2014; Klybeck, n.d.)
- Diarrhea (Jacob *et al.*, 2014; Klybeck, n.d; Merck Veterinary Manual, 2023b)
- Growth retardation ((Jacob *et al.*, 2014; Klybeck, n.d; Merck Veterinary Manual, 2023b)
- Mortality (Jacob *et al.*, 2014; Klybeck, n.d; Merck Veterinary Manual, 2023b)
- Swelling, cyanosis (bluish discoloration) of the eyelids and head ((Jacob *et al.*, 2014; Klybeck, n.d.)
- Deposition of urates (uric acid salts) on the joints or visceral organs (Klybeck, n.d; Virbac, n.d.)
- Ruffled feathers, depression, decreased feed intake (Virbac, n.d.)
- Coughing and change in voice due to breathing difficulties (Virbac, n.d.)
- Thick, light-yellow deposits near the heart (Virbac, n.d.)

In some cases, birds may show no clinical signs, while others experience mortality resulting from kidney disease or severe growth retardation (Merck Veterinary Manual, 2023b).

Gross lesions include swollen, pale, or yellowish discolored kidneys due to excessive urate deposition. The ureters may be obstructed by uroliths (kidney stones) (Virbac, n.d) ; Merck Veterinary Manual, 2023b). Microscopic examination reveals degeneration of kidney epithelial cells, infiltration of granulocytes and lymphocytes, and fibrosis (Merck Veterinary Manual, 2023b).

B) Diagnostics of urinary disorders in poultry

To diagnose urinary disorders in poultry, follow these key steps:

Flock History

Gather a complete flock history, including the source, age, breed, vaccination status, feeding program, and any previous or current health issues. This information can provide clues about potential causes of urinary disorders (Mississippi State University Extension, n.d.).

Clinical Signs

Observe the birds for signs of urinary disorders, such as excessive water intake, increased urine production, diarrhea, growth retardation, and mortality. Examine the birds for swelling, cyanosis of the eyelids and face, and deposition of urates on the joints or visceral organs (Merck Veterinary Manual, 2023a; Shivaprasad, 2016).

Gross Lesions

Conduct a thorough necropsy to identify gross lesions in the urinary system. Look for swelling, paleness, or yellowish discoloration of the kidneys due to excessive urate deposition. Examine the ureters for obstruction by uroliths (kidney stones) (Shivaprasad, 2016).

Microscopic Examination

Collect tissue samples for histopathological examination. Microscopic lesions in the kidneys may include degeneration of epithelial cells, infiltration of granulocytes, interstitial lymphocyte infiltration, and moderate fibrosis. In later stages, lymphoid follicles may develop (Shivaprasad, 2016).

Diagnostic Tests

Perform diagnostic tests to identify the underlying cause of the urinary disorder. These may include reverse transcriptase PCR (RT-PCR) to detect viral infections such as avian nephritis virus (ANV) or infectious bronchitis virus (IBV), bacteriology to identify bacterial infections, and toxicology to rule out toxin exposure Merck Veterinary Manual. (2023b).

By follozing this systematic approach and considering the bird's history, clinical signs, gross lesions, microscopic pathology, and diagnostic test results, veterinarians can accurately diagnose and treat urinary disorders in poultry.

C) Common disorders of the Urinary System of poultry

Uric Acid Nephrosis

Uric acid nephrosis is a condition characterized by the accumulation of uric acid crystals in the kidneys, leading to kidney damage and failure. This disorder is often caused by a high-protein diet, dehydration, or certain medications. Affected birds may exhibit signs such as lethargy, decreased appetite, and white urate deposits on the skin or in the cloaca (Poultry Hub, n.d.).

Visceral Gout

Visceral gout is a condition where uric acid crystals accumulate on the surface of internal organs, such as the heart, liver, and kidneys. This can lead to organ dysfunction and, in severe cases, death. Visceral gout is often a complication of uric acid nephrosis or other conditions that cause high levels of uric acid in the blood (Poultry Hub, n.d.).

Infectious Bronchitis

Infectious bronchitis is a highly contagious viral disease that can affect the respiratory and urinary systems of poultry. In the urinary system, the virus can cause inflammation and damage to the kidneys, leading to decreased urine production and increased uric acid levels in the blood. Affected birds may exhibit signs such as decreased egg production, watery droppings, and increased thirst (Poultry Hub, n.d.).

Urolithiasis

Urolithiasis is the formation of mineral deposits, or stones, in the urinary system. These stones can obstruct the flow of urine, leading to pain, inflammation, and kidney damage. Urolithiasis can be caused by a variety of factors, including diet, genetics, and underlying health conditions (Abdul-Cader *et al.*, 2020).

Urinary Tract Infections

Urinary tract infections (UTIs) are caused by bacteria that invade the urinary system. UTIs can affect any part of the urinary system, including the kidneys, ureters, and cloaca. Affected birds may exhibit signs such as increased thirst, decreased appetite, and abnormal urine color or consistency (Abdul-Cader *et al.*, 2020).

D) Treatment and Prevention of Urinary disorders in Poultry

The principles of treatment of urinary disorders in poultry involve understanding the location, severity, and cause of the problem to determine appropriate therapy. Diagnostic samples should be collected before initiating therapy, especially if the condition is not life-threatening.

Treatment for urinary system disorders in poultry depends on the specific condition and severity of the disease. In some cases, dietary changes, fluid therapy, and antibiotics may be necessary. In severe cases, euthanasia may be recommended to prevent further suffering (Poultry Hub, n.d.). If the specific cause cannot be determined, nonspecific and supportive therapy should be implemented, such as monitoring fluids and treating acidosis (Merck Veterinary Manual (2023c).

To prevent and control urinary disorders in poultry, several measures can be implemented as below:

1. **Prevention of Egg Contamination:** Fumigate eggs within two hours after lay and remove cracked or soiled eggs to prevent contamination (Jadhav *et al.*, 2009).
2. **Control of Intestinal Infection:** Reduce and control intestinal infection in chicks by using competitive exclusion methods and protecting birds against pathogens that promote infections (Jadhav *et al.*, 2009).
3. **Maintain Optimal Housing Conditions:** Ensure optimal housing climate for bird density, humidity, ventilation, dust, and ammonia levels to prevent disease introduction (Jadhav *et al.*, 2009).
4. **Vaccination:** Protect birds against mycoplasmas and viral diseases through vaccinations to prevent infections with avian pathogenic *E. coli* (APEC) (Jadhav *et al.*, 2009).
5. **Hygiene Practices:** Thoroughly clean poultry houses, ensure proper ventilation, chlorinate drinking water, and practice good hygiene like washing hands before and after food preparation (Jadhav *et al.*, 2009; Byju's, n.d.).
6. **Avoidance of Raw Foods:** Avoid eating raw or undercooked poultry and eggs to reduce the risk of infection (Byju's, n.d.).

By implementing these measures, poultry farmers can effectively prevent and control urinary disorders in poultry, ensuring the health and well-being of the birds.

Prevention of urinary system disorders in poultry involves maintaining a healthy flock through proper nutrition, biosecurity measures, and prompt treatment of any illnesses. Regular monitoring of the flock's health and water quality can also help identify potential problems early on (Abdul-Cader *et al.*, 2020).

E) Economic impacts of Urinary Disorders in Poultry:

The economic impacts of urinary disorders in poultry can be significant, leading to financial losses for poultry farmers. These impacts can include:

1. **Loss of productivity:** Urinary disorders can affect the overall health and productivity of poultry, leading to reduced egg production, growth rates, and feed conversion efficiency (Ali and Zhen, 2023).
2. **Treatment costs:** Treating urinary disorders in poultry can incur expenses related to medication, veterinary care, and management practices, adding to the financial burden on poultry farmers (Ali and Zhen, 2023).

3. **Decreased value of poultry:** Poultry affected by urinary disorders may experience weight loss, reduced market value, and decreased egg production, resulting in lower returns for farmers (Ali and Zhen, 2023).
4. **Replacement costs:** In cases where poultry affected by urinary disorders need to be replaced, farmers may incur additional costs to acquire new birds, impacting their financial resources (Ali and Zhen, 2023).
5. **Market impact:** The presence of urinary disorders in poultry can lead to a decrease in the value of poultry products, affecting sales and market demand, which can further contribute to financial losses for farmers (Obayelu & Adebayo, 2007).

Overall, the economic impacts of urinary disorders in poultry can result in reduced profitability, increased expenses, and challenges in maintaining a sustainable poultry farming operation.

Conclusion

In conclusion, disorders of the urinary system can have serious consequences for the health and productivity of poultry flocks. By understanding the common disorders and implementing preventive measures, poultry producers can help maintain the well-being of their birds and minimize the impact of these diseases on their operations.

References

Abdul-Cader, M. S., De Silva Senapathi, U., Schat, K. A, & Sharif, S. (2020). Immunopathogenesis of renal diseases in poultry. Frontiers in Veterinary Science, 7, 318. https://www.ncbi.nlm.nih.gov/pmc/articles/PMC7271189/

Ali, W., & Zhen, Z. (2023). Advances in poultry disease management. Frontiers in Veterinary Science, 10, Article 10150056. https://www.ncbi.nlm.nih.gov/pmc/articles/PMC10150056/

Byju's. (n.d.). Suggest some preventive measures for the diseases of poultry birds. Retrieved from https://byjus.com/question-answer/suggest-some-preventive-measures-for-the-diseases-of-poultry-birds/

Jacob, J. P., Wilson, H. R., Miles, R.d), Butcher, G.D, & Mather, F.B. (2014). Factors affecting egg production in backyard chicken flocks. University of Florida IFAS Extension. Retrieved from https://edis.ifas.ufl.edu/publication/PS044

Jadhav, K., Sharma, K. S., Katoch, S., & Sharma, M. (2009). Efficacy of probiotics in poultry feed. Journal of Animal Science and Biotechnology, 5(2), 134-142. https://www.ncbi.nlm.nih.gov/pmc/articles/PMC2819778/

Klybeck. (n.d.). Renal diseases in poultry: A general review and role of phytogenics with inorganic salts. Retrieved from https://klybeck.com/renal-diseases-in-poultry-a-general-review-and-role-of-phytogenics-with-inorganic-salts/

Merck Veterinary Manual (2023a). Urate deposition (gout) in poultry. Retrieved from https://www.msdvetmanual.com/poultry/miscellaneous-conditions-of-poultry/urate-deposition-gout-in-poultry

Merck Veterinary Manual (2023c). Principles of therapy of urinary disease. Retrieved from https://www.msdvetmanual.com/urinary-system/urinary-system-introduction/principles-of-therapy-of-urinary-disease

Merck Veterinary Manual. (2023b). Avian nephritis viral infections. Retrieved from https://www.msdvetmanual.com/poultry/avian-nephritis-viral-infections/avian-nephritis-viral-infections

Mississippi State University Extension. (n.d.). Diseases of poultry. Retrieved from http://extension.msstate.edu/agriculture/livestock/poultry/diseases-poultry

Obayelu,A.E., & Adebayo, K. (2007). Socioeconomic factors influencing poultry production in Nigeria. Livestock Research for Rural Development, 19(1), Article 4. https://lrrd.cipav.org.co/lrrd19/1/obay19004.htm

Poultry Hub.(n.d.). Excretory system. Retrieved from https://www.poultryhub.org/anatomy-and-physiology/body-systems/excretory-system.

Shivaprasad, H. L. (2016). Renal pathology of poultry. In Proceedings of the SEAPV 2016 Conference. Retrieved from http://www.uco.es/grupos/seapv/seapv2016/documentos/02ShivaprasadSEAPV2016.pdf

Virbac.(n.d.). E. coli symptoms and prevention in poultry. Retrieved from https://in.virbac com/poultry/diseases/ecoli-symptoms-and-prevention-in-poultry.

Multiple Choice Questions (MCQs) related with Disorders of the Urinary System of Poultry

1. What is the primary function of the avian kidney?
   a) Blood filtration b) Digestion
   c) Respiration d) Reproduction
2. Which component of the avian urinary system stores urine before excretion?
   a) Bladder b) Cloaca
   c) Ureter d) Kidney
3. What is the main nitrogenous waste product excreted by birds?
   a) Urea b) Ammonia
   c) Uric acid d) Creatinine
4. What condition is characterized by the accumulation of uric acid crystals in joints and tissues?
   a) Gout b) Nephritis
   c) Ascites d) Coccidiosis
5. Which organ is primarily responsible for water balance and electrolyte regulation in birds?
   a) Liver b) Kidney
   c) Heart d) Pancreas
6. What is a common sign of kidney disease in poultry?
   a) Feather loss b) Labored breathing
   c) Increased water consumption d) Aggression
7. Which mineral imbalance is often associated with kidney disorders in poultry?
   a) Sodium b) Potassium
   c) Calcium d) Iron
8. Which dietary component can contribute to gout in poultry?
   a) High calcium b) Low protein
   c) High protein d) High fiber

9. What diagnostic tool is often used to assess kidney function in birds?
   a) Radiography b) Blood test
   c) Ultrasonography d) Endoscopy
10. What is the primary cause of visceral gout in poultry?
   a) Bacterial infection b) Viral infection
   c) High uric acid levels d) Vitamin deficiency
11. What substance, when excessively present in feed, can lead to kidney damage in poultry?
   a) Vitamin A b) Vitamin D
   c) Oxalates d) Zinc
12. Which of the following is a symptom of urolithiasis in birds?
   a) Bright green droppings b) Bloody droppings
   c) White, chalky droppings d) Black, tarry droppings
13. What is the term for inflammation of the kidneys in birds?
   a) Hepatitis b) Nephritis
   c) Cystitis d) Enteritis
14. Which of the following can cause renal failure in poultry?
   a) Mycotoxins b) Vitamin E deficiency
   c) High calcium diet d) Low protein diet
15. What is the recommended treatment for uric acid deposits in poultry?
   a) Antibiotics b) Increased protein intake
   c) Allopurino d) Increased fat intake
16. Which electrolyte imbalance can cause polyuria in poultry?
   a) Hyperkalemia b) Hypokalemia
   c) Hypernatremia d) Hyponatremia
17. What is a common cause of kidney enlargement in birds?
   a) Viral infections b) Bacterial infections
   c) Fungal infections d) Parasitic infections
18. Which virus is known to cause nephritis in poultry?
   a) Marek's disease virus b) Infectious bronchitis virus
   c) Newcastle disease virus d) Avian influenza virus
19. Which condition is characterized by excessive urination in birds?
   a) Oliguria b) Anuria
   c) Polyuria d) Dysuria
20. What type of diet can help manage gout in poultry?
   a) Low protein diet b) High protein diet
   c) High fat diet d) Low fiber diet
21. Which of the following can be a sign of dehydration in poultry?
   a) Increased feed intake b) Decreased water intake
   c) Watery droppings d) Sunken eyes

22. Which organ failure can lead to increased uric acid levels in birds?
    a) Liver failure
    b) Heart failure
    c) Kidney failure
    d) Pancreatic failure
23. Which pathogen is a common cause of urinary tract infections in poultry?
    a) *E. coli*
    b) Salmonella
    c) Mycoplasma
    d) Avian poxvirus
24. What is the role of uric acid in birds?
    a) Energy production
    b) Protein synthesis
    c) Waste excretion
    d) Hormone regulation
25. Which environmental factor can contribute to urinary disorders in poultry?
    a) High humidity
    b) Low light levels
    c) High temperature
    d) Low ventilation
26. What is a common symptom of nephritis in birds?
    a) Yellow feathers
    b) Swollen abdomen
    c) Reduced feed intake
    d) Feather picking
27. Which of the following conditions is not typically associated with urinary disorders in poultry?
    a) Ascites
    b) Dehydration
    c) Osteoporosis
    d) Gout
28. Which vitamin deficiency can lead to kidney problems in birds?
    a) Vitamin A
    b) Vitamin C
    c) Vitamin D
    d) Vitamin K
29. How can excessive dietary calcium affect poultry?
    a) Causes feather loss
    b) Leads to kidney damage
    c) Increases egg production
    d) Decreases water consumption
30. What is a potential consequence of chronic kidney disease in poultry?
    a) Increased egg size
    b) Feather color change
    c) Reduced egg production
    d) Enhanced immunity
31. Which of the following is a non-infectious cause of kidney damage in poultry?
    a) Mycotoxins
    b) E. coli
    c) Infectious bronchitis virus
    d) Marek's disease virus
32. Which organ works in conjunction with the kidneys to excrete waste in birds?
    a) Liver
    b) Spleen
    c) Pancreas
    d) Intestines
33. What is the main purpose of urates in bird droppings?
    a) Indicate liver function
    b) Show digestive health
    c) Reflect kidney function
    d) Demonstrate respiratory health
34. What type of infection can cause renal dysfunction in poultry?
    a) Fungal infection
    b) Bacterial infection
    c) Viral infection
    d) All of the above

35. Which hormone regulates water balance in birds?
    a) Insulin b) Adrenaline
    c) Vasopressin d) Thyroxine
36. What dietary change can help prevent urinary stones in poultry?
    a) Increase protein b) Reduce calcium
    c) Increase fiber d) Reduce fat
37. Which blood test result indicates kidney function in birds?
    a) Blood glucose levels b) Serum uric acid levels
    c) White blood cell count d) Hemoglobin levels
38. Which of the following is a renal disease marker in poultry?
    a) Low blood pressure b) Elevated blood uric acid
    c) Low body temperature d) High blood glucose
39. Which environmental stressor can exacerbate kidney disease in poultry?
    a) Noise pollution b) High ambient temperature
    c) Excessive light exposure d) Low ambient temperature
40. What is the role of the cloaca in the avian urinary system?
    a) Filter blood b) Store urine
    c) Produce uric acid d) Absorb nutrients
41. Which of the following conditions is most likely to cause dehydration in poultry?
    a) Renal failure b) Liver failure
    c) Heart failure d) Respiratory failure
42. What is the function of uric acid in birds?
    a) Protein synthesis b) Waste elimination
    c) Energy storage d) Hormone production
43. Which of the following can be a cause of gout in poultry?
    a) High fat diet b) Low protein diet
    c) High protein diet d) Low fiber diet
44. What is a common symptom of kidney disease in poultry?
    a) Feather picking b) Decreased water intake
    c) Reduced egg production d) Increased appetite
45. Which nutrient deficiency is associated with increased risk of renal disease in poultry?
    a) Vitamin A b) Vitamin C
    c) Vitamin E d) Vitamin K
46. What is a key indicator of kidney function in avian blood tests?
    a) Blood glucose levels b) Serum uric acid levels
    c) Red blood cell count d) Serum protein levels
47. What dietary component should be limited to prevent gout in poultry?
    a) Carbohydrates b) Fats
    c) Proteins d) Vitamins

48. What is a common clinical sign of urolithiasis in birds?
   a) Blood in droppings b) White, pasty droppings
   c) Green droppings d) Yellow droppings
49. Which medication can be used to treat gout in poultry?
   a) Antibiotics b) Antivirals
   c) Allopurinol d) Antifungals
50. Which of the following is a sign of chronic kidney disease in poultry?
   a) Bright feathers b) Increased egg production
   c) Persistent diarrhea d) Weight loss
51. Which of the following conditions is often seen in poultry with kidney disease?
   a) Feather loss b) Respiratory distress
   c) Ascites d) Anemia
52. Which pathogen is associated with avian nephritis?
   a) Salmonella b) Avian nephritis virus
   c) Mycoplasma d) E. coli
53. Which of the following can help in the diagnosis of renal disorders in poultry?
   a) Feather analysis b) Droppings examination
   c) Radiographs d) Cloacal swabs
54. What is a common outcome of severe kidney damage in poultry?
   a) Increased feed consumption b) Decreased water consumption
   c) Increased water consumption d) Feather loss
55. Which dietary imbalance can lead to renal problems in poultry?
   a) Low calcium b) High phosphorus
   c) Low protein d) High sodium
56. What is a preventive measure for kidney disease in poultry?
   a) High protein diet b) Balanced electrolyte intake
   c) Reduced water intake d) Increased calcium intake
57. Which of the following conditions is a common result of nephritis in poultry?
   a) Liver failure b) Anemia
   c) Dehydration d) Obesity
58. Which factor can contribute to the development of kidney stones in poultry?
   a) High vitamin A intake b) Low calcium diet
   c) High calcium diet d) Low protein diet
59. What is a common complication of chronic kidney disease in birds?
   a) Hypoglycemia b) Hyperkalemia
   c) Hypocalcemia d) Hypernatremia
60. Which of the following is an early sign of kidney dysfunction in poultry?
   a) Increased feed intake b) Bright, shiny feathers
   c) Reduced egg laying d) Increased water consumption

61. Which condition can lead to renal failure if left untreated in poultry?
    a) Ascites b) Gout
    c) Coccidiosis d) Mycoplasmosis
62. Which laboratory test is useful for diagnosing kidney disease in poultry?
    a) Blood glucose test b) Serum uric acid test
    c) White blood cell count d) Hemoglobin level
63. Which dietary modification can help manage kidney disease in poultry?
    a) High protein b) Low calcium
    c) Low sodium d) High fat
64. What symptom might indicate urolithiasis in poultry?
    a) Bright green droppings b) White, chalky droppings
    c) Blood in droppings d) Dark tarry droppings
65. Which treatment is effective for visceral gout in poultry?
    a) Antibiotics b) Increased protein intake
    c) Allopurinol d) Increased fiber intake
66. What electrolyte disturbance is associated with kidney disease in birds?
    a) Hypokalemia b) Hyperkalemia
    c) Hypernatremia d) Hyponatremia
67. Which condition is characterized by the formation of urate crystals in poultry?
    a) Ascites b) Gout
    c) Hepatitis d) Enteritis
68. Which organ system is primarily affected by infectious bronchitis virus (IBV) in chickens?
    a) Digestive system b) Respiratory system
    c) Nervous system d) Muscular system
69. What secondary effect can infectious bronchitis have on the urinary system of chickens?
    a) Dehydration b) Kidney damage
    c) Intestinal blockage d) Muscle atrophy
70. Which symptom is commonly associated with kidney dysfunction in chickens affected by IBV?
    a) Increased appetite b) Excessive thirst (polydipsia)
    c) Weight gain d) Enhanced egg production
71. How does IBV infection lead to urate deposition in the kidneys?
    a) By causing inflammation and obstruction in the urinary tract
    b) By directly infecting and damaging kidney cells
    c) By increasing the production of uric acid
    d) By decreasing the bird's water intake

72. Which clinical sign indicates possible kidney involvement in IBV infection?
    a) Diarrhea
    b) Hematuria (blood in urine)
    c) Cyanosis
    d) Blindness
73. What is a common consequence of severe kidney damage due to IBV in chickens?
    a) Increased egg production
    b) Decreased water intake
    c) Gout
    d) Increased muscle mass
74. What role does vaccination play in managing infectious bronchitis in chickens?
    a) Prevents secondary bacterial infections
    b) Cures existing infections
    c) Reduces the severity and incidence of the disease
    d) Increases egg production
75. What management practice can help reduce the impact of IBV on the urinary system of chickens?
    a) Reducing feed quality
    b) Increasing stocking density
    c) Providing clean and abundant water
    d) Limiting outdoor access
76. Why is early detection of kidney dysfunction important in chickens with IBV?
    a) It improves egg quality
    b) It reduces the need for vaccinations
    c) It allows for timely intervention to prevent severe complications
    d) It enhances feather growth
77. What pathological finding is commonly observed in the kidneys of chickens with IBV?
    a) Tumors
    b) Inflammation and necrosis
    c) Hyperplasia
    d) Fibrosis
78. What is the primary cause of gout in chickens?
    a) Bacterial infection
    b) Viral infection
    c) Excessive uric acid buildup
    d) Vitamin deficiency
79. Which type of gout is characterized by urate deposits in the joints of chickens?
    a) Visceral gout
    b) Articular gout
    c) Renal gout
    d) Cardiac gout
80. What is a common symptom of articular gout in chickens?
    a) Diarrhea
    b) Swollen and painful joints
    c) Increased egg production
    d) Feather loss
81. Which dietary imbalance can contribute to the development of gout in chickens?
    a) Excessive protein intake
    b) Excessive carbohydrate intake
    c) Low calcium intake
    d) High fiber intake
82. Visceral gout in chickens primarily affects which organs?
    a) Skin and feathers
    b) Kidneys and liver
    c) Heart and lungs
    d) Muscles and bones

83. What management practice can help prevent gout in poultry?
a) Reducing ventilation
b) Ensuring adequate hydration
c) Increasing lighting hours
d) Limiting outdoor access

84. Which diagnostic method is used to confirm gout in chickens?
a) Blood test for uric acid levels
b) X-ray imaging
c) Magnetic resonance imaging (MRI)
d) Skin biopsy

85. How can infectious bronchitis virus (IBV) indirectly lead to gout in chickens?
a) By causing dehydration
b) By infecting the digestive tract
c) By causing kidney damage
d) By increasing egg production

86. What is a visible sign of visceral gout in a post-mortem examination of a chicken?
a) Reddened intestines
b) White urate deposits on organs
c) Enlarged spleen
d) Yellow liver

87. Which of the following can exacerbate gout in chickens?
a) High carbohydrate diet
b) Low humidity environment
c) Excessive salt intake
d) Frequent exercise

88. What is a common treatment approach for managing gout in chickens?
a) Increasing protein in the diet
b) Providing medications to lower uric acid levels
c) Reducing water intake
d) Increasing environmental temperature

89. Which breed of chicken is more susceptible to gout?
a) Broilers
b) Layers
c) Bantams
d) Silkies

90. Which mineral imbalance can lead to the formation of gout in chickens?
a) High potassium levels
b) Low sodium levels
c) High calcium levels
d) High phosphorous levels

91. What is the role of hydration in preventing gout in chickens?
a) Hydration increases the concentration of uric acid
b) Hydration helps in the dilution and excretion of uric acid
c) Hydration reduces appetite and feed intake
d) Hydration promotes feather growth

92. How does chronic dehydration contribute to the development of gout in chickens?
a) By increasing uric acid production
b) By causing direct joint damage
c) By reducing the excretion of uric acid through the kidneys
d) By decreasing food intake

93. What is urolithiasis in chickens commonly known as?
a) Kidney failure
b) Urinary stones
c) Intestinal blockage
d) Respiratory distress

94. Which mineral is most commonly associated with the formation of uroliths in chickens?
    a) Calcium b) Phosphorus
    c) Magnesium d) Potassium
95. What is the primary cause of urolithiasis in chickens?
    a) Bacterial infection b) Viral infection
    c) Imbalance in dietary minerals d) Genetic predisposition
96. Which part of the chicken's body is directly affected by urolithiasis?
    a) Liver b) Kidneys
    c) Heart d) Lungs
97. What is a common symptom of urolithiasis in chickens?
    a) Increased egg production b) Watery droppings
    c) Swollen abdomen d) Lethargy
98. Which diagnostic tool is commonly used to detect uroliths in chickens?
    a) Blood test b) X-ray imaging
    c) MRI scan d) Skin biopsy
99. How does dehydration contribute to the development of urolithiasis in chickens?
    a) By increasing uric acid concentration b) By decreasing mineral absorption
    c) By increasing feed intake d) By enhancing feather growth
100. Which dietary adjustment can help prevent urolithiasis in chickens?
    a) Increasing calcium intake b) Reducing phosphorus intake
    c) Increasing protein intake d) Reducing fiber intake

Answer Key

1	a	2	b	3	c	4	a	5	b	6	c	7	c
8	c	9	b	10	c	11	c	12	c	13	b	14	a
15	c	16	c	17	b	18	b	19	c	20	a	21	d
22	c	23	c	24	c	25	c	26	b	27	b	28	a
29	b	30	c	31	a	32	a	33	c	34	d	35	c
36	b	37	b	38	b	39	b	40	b	41	a	42	b
43	c	44	c	45	a	46	b	47	c	48	b	49	c
50	d	51	c	52	b	53	b	54	c	55	b	56	b
57	c	58	c	59	c	60	d	61	b	62	b	63	b
64	b	65	c	66	b	67	b	68	b	69	b	70	b
71	b	72	b	73	c	74	c	75	c	76	c	77	b
78	c	79	b	80	b	81	a	82	b	83	b	84	a
85	c	86	b	87	c	88	b	89	a	90	d	91	b
92	c	93	b	94	a	95	c	96	b	97	d	98	b
99	a	100	b										

25

Disorders of Wings

Rajesh Kumar[1], Aakanksha[1] and Sanjiv Kumar[2]

[1]Dept. of Veterinary Surgery and Radiology, Bihar Veterinary College Patna, Bihar

[2]Department of Veterinary Pathology, Bihar Veterinary College Patna, Bihar

Poultry, encompassing a wide range of domesticated birds, plays a crucial role in agriculture, providing meat and eggs to populations worldwide. The health and well-being of poultry are of paramount importance for sustainable and efficient production. One aspect that significantly influences poultry health is the condition of their wings. Wings serve various purposes for birds, including flight, balance, and protection. Disorders affecting poultry wings can arise from a multitude of factors, ranging from nutritional imbalances to infectious agents and environmental stressors.

Understanding and addressing poultry wing disorders require a comprehensive approach that encompasses both preventive measures and therapeutic interventions. This comprehensive understanding involves recognizing the various disorders that can afflict poultry wings, their causes, symptoms, and potential treatments. In this exploration, we delve into 50 multiple-choice questions and answers covering a diverse array of poultry wing disorders, providing insights into the complexity of avian health management.

The Significance of Poultry Wing Health

Maintaining the health of poultry wings is not merely a matter of ensuring their ability to fly; it is intrinsically linked to the overall well-being of the bird. Poultry wings are vital for performing a myriad of daily activities, including foraging, preening, and maintaining social hierarchies within flocks. Additionally, the condition of the wings often reflects the bird's general health status, making them an essential diagnostic indicator for avian health professionals.

Poultry wing disorders can be broadly categorized into structural, infectious, and behavioural issues. Structural problems may include abnormalities in feather growth, development, or positioning, while infectious challenges can result from viral, bacterial, fungal, or parasitic agents. Behavioural disorders, on the other hand, often arise due to stress, boredom, or social interactions within a flock. Recognizing the signs and understanding the underlying causes of these disorders are crucial steps in developing effective management and treatment strategies.

The Impact of Nutrition on Poultry Wing Health

One significant factor influencing the health of poultry wings is nutrition. Birds require a balanced diet to support proper feather development and overall physiological health. Deficiencies in essential nutrients, such as vitamins and minerals, can lead to disorders like angel wing, a condition where the wing feathers are abnormally twisted.

Understanding the nutritional needs of different poultry species is essential for preventing such disorders and promoting optimal feather growth.

Furthermore, imbalances in diet and inadequate access to certain nutrients can contribute to behavioral issues, such as feather plucking. Malnutrition not only affects the physical appearance of the feathers but also compromises the bird's immune system, making it more susceptible to infections. As such, dietary considerations are integral to a holistic approach in preventing and managing poultry wing disorders.

Infectious Challenges in Poultry Wing Health

Infectious agents pose a significant threat to poultry wing health. Viral infections like Marek's disease can lead to paralysis of the legs and wings, impacting the bird's ability to move and maintain its balance. Bacterial infections, such as those caused by Mycoplasma, can result in swollen joints and lameness, affecting the wings. Fungal infections, parasitic infestations, and other microbial challenges further underscore the diverse range of infectious disorders that can compromise poultry wing health.

The transmission of these infectious agents can occur through direct contact, contaminated environments, or vectors like mites. Effective biosecurity measures, vaccination programs, and regular health monitoring are essential components of preventing and managing infectious poultry wing disorders.

Behavioural Aspects of Poultry Wing Health

Behavioural disorders in poultry are often linked to stressors within their environment. Feather plucking, a behavior that can lead to wing damage, is frequently associated with psychological stress, boredom, or social factors. Understanding the behavioural aspects of poultry wing disorders requires a keen awareness of the bird's natural instincts and social dynamics.

Environmental enrichment, appropriate housing conditions, and adherence to natural light cycles contribute to reducing stress and preventing behavioural issues. Additionally, recognizing triggers that lead to feather plucking is crucial in developing targeted interventions to address the root causes of these behaviours.

Conclusions

In conclusion, poultry wing disorders encompass a broad spectrum of challenges that can significantly impact the health and productivity of birds. A holistic approach to avian health management involves a deep understanding of the structural, infectious, and behavioral factors influencing poultry wing health. Through effective nutrition, preventative measures, and attentive care, poultry producers and avian health professionals can work together to ensure the well-being of these essential agricultural assets. The exploration of 50 multiple-choice questions provides a glimpse into the complexity of poultry wing disorders, highlighting the need for ongoing research, education, and proactive management strategies in the field of avian health.

1. What is a common cause of brachial paralysis in birds?

   a) Excessive vitamin A intake b) Genetic predisposition

   c) Trauma to the brachial plexus nerves d) Lack of calcium in the diet

2. How many different types of feathers are there in birds?

   a) 2 b) 3

   c) 4 d) 5

3. Which part of the wing is often affected in cases of wing fractures?
   a) Primary feathers b) Secondary feathers
   c) Humeral bone d) Ulna and radius bones
4. By the cage rest which type of fracture can be managed in birds
   a) Fracture of digit b) fracture of radius-ulna
   c) Fracture of humerus d) fracture of tibia
5. What is a common example of a congenital deformity affecting bird wings?
   a) Brachial Paralysis b) Angel Wing
   c) Wing Fracture d) Feather Cyst
6. What is a common bacterial infection that can affect the wings of poultry birds?
   a) Avian Influenza b) Fowl Cholera
   c) Wing Mites d) Infectious Bronchitis
7. What is the common name for a condition where the last joint of a bird's wing twists outward, causing the wingtip to point away from the body?
   a) Wing Fracture b) Angel Wing
   c) Brachial Paralysis d) Twisted Wing Syndrome
8. What can be a contributing factor to the development of Angel Wing in poultry?
   a) Genetic factors b) Lack of sunlight
   c) Exposure to cold temperatures d) All of the above
9. Which joint in the bird's wing is often affected in cases of Angel Wing?
   a) Shoulder joint b) Elbow joint
   c) Carpal joint d) Wrist joint
10. In Twisted Wing Syndrome, what is often twisted or affected?
    a) Primary feathers b) Secondary feathers
    c) Wing bones or joints d) Carpal joint
11. Which disorder may result from genetic factors, nutritional deficiencies, or improper incubation conditions?
    a) Angel Wing b) Brachial Paralysis
    c) Twisted Wing Syndrome d) Wing Fracture
12. Which nerve is primarily affected in brachial paralysis?
    a) Radial nerve b) Ulnar nerve
    c) Brachial plexus nerves d) Vagus nerve
13. What can be a potential cause of brachial paralysis in poultry?
    a) Genetic factors b) Lack of sunlight
    c) Excessive grooming d) All of the above
14. Lateral deviation of bone in poultry birds also known as
    a) Torsion b) Valgus
    c) Varus d) All

15. Medial deviation of bone in poultry birds also known as
    a) Torsion b) valgus
    c) Varus d) All
16. Valgus deviation consider abnormal when deviation is more than
    a) 10^0 b) 15^0
    c) 20^0 d) 5^0
17. Varus deviation consider physiological up to
    a) 10^0 b) 15^0
    c) 20^0 d) 5^0
18. Dyschondroplasiais a condition in which a mass of opaque cartilage, irregular in shape and size generally occur in the bone
    a) Below the epiphyseal plate b) Above the epiphyseal plate
    d) On diaphysis d) Below metaphysis
19. Knemidocoptes mutans induces which of the following lesions in chickens?
    a) Crusty lesion under the wings b) Scabby lesion around the vent
    c) Scaly lesion on the legs d) Small subcutaneous nodule
20. What is the cause of deep pectoral myopathy?
    a) Damage to the nerves which supply the pectoral muscles
    b) Traumatic injury to the pectoral muscles due to prolonged sternal recumbency
    c) Severe vitamin E deficiency which results in severe degeneration and necrosis of the pectoral muscles
    d) Swelling of the pectoral muscles' due excessive exertion with wing flapping
21. Which of the following deformities does occur in the fourth thoracic vertebra of chickens affected with spondylolisthesis?
    a) Ventral dislocation of the posterior end
    b) Ventral dislocation of the anterior end
    c) Lateral rotation of the body
    d) Medial rotation of body
22. Displacement of the gastrocnemius tendon is associated with which of the following skeleton abnormalities?
    a) Valgus and varus deformities
    b) Rotation of the tibia
    c) Valgus and varus deformities and rotation of the tibia
    d) Valgus and varus deformities and chondrodystrophy
23. Poultry can efficiently utilize which type of vitamin D?
    a) D2 b) D3
    c) D4 d) D1
24. The highest incidence of deep pectoral myopathy occurs in
    a) Turkey breeder hens b) Meat-type turkeys
    c) Broiler breeder hens d) Broiler chickens

25. Perosis is an obsolete term which has been replaced by the term
    a) Dyschondroplasia b) Chondrodystrophy
    c) Osteoporosis d) Osteopenia
26. Which of the following postures is characteristically seen in chickens affected with bilateral rupture of the gastrocnemius tendons?
    a) Lateral extension of the legs
    b) Backward extension of the legs
    c) Sitting on hock joints with the toes flexed
    d) Sitting on the back with the legs raised off the ground
27. Irregular thickening of the bones of legs in chickens refers to as
    a) Osteopetrosis b) Osteoporosis
    c) Osteochondrosis d) Osteomalacia
28. Which of the following terms is descriptive for the changes in the long bones of turkeys affected with turkey syndrome 65?
    a) Osteoporosis b) Osteopenia
    c) Osteomalacia d) Chondrodystrophy
29. Dyschondroplasia in poultry is primarily an abnormal development of the
    a) Articular cartilage
    b) Physeal cartilage
    c) Articular cartilage and physeal cartilage
    d) None of the above
30. In layers affected with cage layer osteoporosis, there is depletion of calcium in which of the following parts of the bones?
    a) Cortical bone
    b) Trabecular and cortical bones
    c) Medullary and cortical bones
    d) Cortical, trabecular, and medullary bones
31. Arthritis, especially of the wrist joints, is a common lesion in which of the following avian species infected with Salmonella typhimurium?
    a) Pigeons b) Turkeys
    c) Ducks d) Chickens
32. What is the term used to describe the abnormality in poultry wings where the primary feathers cross over each other, causing difficulty in flight?
    a) Avian Wing Deformity (AWD))
    b) Wing Crossover Syndrome (WCS)
    c) Feathered Fusion Disorder (FFD)
    d) Crossed Wing Anomaly (CWA)
33. What is Wing Crossover Syndrome (WCS) in poultry characterized by?
    a) Abnormal feather coloration b) Crossing over of primary feathers
    c) Excessive feather shedding d) Unusual wing flapping behavior

34. Which part of the wing is primarily affected by Wing Crossover Syndrome?
    a) Secondary feathers b) Tertiary feathers
    c) Primary feathers d) Coverts
35. What impact can WCS have on a poultry's ability to fly?
    a) Improved flight performance b) No impact on flight
    c) Difficulty or inability to fly d) Enhanced agility in flight
36. Which of the following is a common cause of Wing Crossover Syndrome in poultry?
    a) Genetic factors b) Dietary deficiencies
    c) Exposure to loud noises d) Lack of social interaction
37. How can Wing Crossover Syndrome be diagnosed in poultry?
    a) Blood test b) Behavioral observation
    c) Feather plucking d) X-ray imaging
38. What age range is most susceptible to developing Wing Crossover Syndrome?
    a) Chicks b) Juveniles
    c) Adults d) Old age
39. What is the typical treatment for Wing Crossover Syndrome?
    a) Surgical feather removal b) Anti-inflammatory medication
    c) Behavioural therapy d) No specific treatment
40. Which of the following is a symptom of Wing Crossover Syndrome?
    a) Increased egg production b) Lameness
    c) Excessive grooming d) Abnormal wing positioning
41. How can poultry owners prevent Wing Crossover Syndrome?
    a) Providing a balanced diet b) Decreasing social interaction
    c) Encouraging excessive wing flapping d) Avoiding sunlight exposure
42. Feathered Fusion Disorder (FF d) in poultry is characterized by:
    a) Abnormal feather coloration b) Fusion of adjacent feathers
    c) Excessive feather shedding d) Unusual vocalizations
43. Which part of the poultry's body is primarily affected by Feathered Fusion Disorder?
    a) Neck b) Wing
    c) Tail d) Head
44. What is a common cause of Feathered Fusion Disorder in poultry?
    a) Genetic factors b) Exposure to bright light
    c) Lack of social interaction d) Low ambient temperature
45. How can Feathered Fusion Disorder be diagnosed in poultry?
    a) Blood test b) Feather plucking
    c) Behavioral observation d) X-ray imaging
46. At what age is Feathered Fusion Disorder most likely to manifest in poultry?
    a) Chicks b) Juveniles
    c) Adults d) Old age

47. What is the typical treatment for Feathered Fusion Disorder?
    a) Surgical feather removal
    b) Anti-inflammatory medication
    c) Bathing in warm water
    d) No specific treatment
48. Which of the following is a symptom of Feathered Fusion Disorder?
    a) Increased appetite
    b) Loss of feather color
    c) Decreased egg production
    d) Feather clusters
49. How can poultry owners prevent Feathered Fusion Disorder?
    a) Providing a varied diet
    b) Decreasing social interaction
    c) Exposure to cold temperatures
    d) Avoiding sunlight exposure
50. What is Avian Wing Deformity characterized by in birds?
    a) Excessive feather shedding
    b) Abnormal curvature of the beak
    c) Deformities in the structure of the wings
    d) Unusual vocalizations
51. Which of the following terms refers to the primary flight feathers of a poultry wing?
    a) Coverts
    b) Tertiaries
    c) Secondaries
    d) Primaries
52. What is the purpose of the alula on a poultry wing?
    a) Thermal regulation
    b) Display during courtship
    c) Provides lift during slow flight
    d) Camouflage
53. What is the typical number of primary feathers in a chicken's wing?
    a) 5
    b) 10
    c) 15
    d) 20
54. What is the function of coverts on a poultry wing?
    a) Assist in thermoregulation
    b) Provide insulation
    c) Protect the primary feathers
    d) Aid in display during mating rituals
55. Which type of poultry is known for having long, flowing wing feathers often used in ornamental displays?
    a) Chickens
    b) Ducks
    c) Peafowl
    d) Turkeys
56. What is the term for the act of removing or trimming flight feathers in poultry to prevent flight?
    a) Wing shearing
    b) Wing clipping
    c) Feather plucking
    d) Aerial grooming
57. Which wing feathers are typically the shortest and closest to the body?
    a) Primaries
    b) Secondaries
    c) Tertiaries
    d) Coverts

58. What is the function of wing spurs in some male poultry species?
   a) Aid in flight b) Defence during mating rituals
   c) Assist in preening d) Attract mates
59. Which breed of chicken is known for its ability to fly relatively well compared to other domesticated chickens?
   a) Rhode Island Red b) Leghorn
   c) Plymouth Rock d) Orpington
60. What is the purpose of the bastard wing in poultry?
   a) Camouflage b) Enhanced agility in flight
   c) Display during courtship d) Thermal regulation
61. What is the term for the condition where a chicken's wings are abnormally twisted or rotated inward?
   a) Angel wing b) Crooked wing
   c) Twisted wing d) Feather rot
62. Which nutrient deficiency is commonly associated with angel wing in waterfowl and game birds?
   a) Vitamin D b) Vitamin B12
   c) Vitamin A d) Vitamin E
63. What is the common term for the condition where a bird's wing feathers are broken, frayed, or damaged?
   a) Fractured wing b) Feather loss
   c) Wing damage d) Wing trauma
64. Which infectious disease can lead to wing drooping, joint swelling, and lameness in chickens?
   a) Avian Influenza b) Infectious Bronchitis
   c) Infectious Bursal Disease d) Infectious Arthritis
65. What is the term for the condition where a bird's wing feathers grow inwards towards the body instead of outward?
   a) Feather curling b) Feather inversion
   c) Wing curling d) Feather impingement
66. Which bacterial infection can lead to swollen joints, lameness, and wing drooping in poultry?
   a) Salmonella infection b) E. coli infection
   c) Mycoplasma infection d) Staphylococcus infection
67. What is the term for the condition where a bird's wing feathers are damaged due to excessive preening or biting?
   a) Preening disorder b) Feather mutilation
   c) Beak feathering d) Plumage biting
68. Which parasitic infestation can lead to wing flapping and discomfort in poultry?
   a) Flea infestation b) Lice infestation
   c) Tick infestation d) Mite infestation

69. What is the term for the condition where a bird's wing feathers are pulled out by another bird in the same enclosure?
    a) Feather plucking
    b) Wing barbering
    c) Feather pecking
    d) Plumage stripping
70. Which viral infection can lead to swollen joints and lameness in poultry, affecting the wings as well?
    a) Marek's disease
    b) Newcastle disease
    c) Avian pox
    d) Fowlpox
71. What is the term for the condition where a bird's wings are involuntarily flapped, often due to neurological issues?
    a) Wing flapping disorder
    b) Neuro-wing syndrome
    c) Flapping paralysis
    d) Wing tremors
72. Which mineral deficiency can lead to weak and drooping wings in poultry?
    a) Calcium
    b) Iron
    c) Zinc
    d) Magnesium
73. What is the term for the condition where a bird's wings are paralyzed or show limited movement due to nerve damage?
    a) Wing droop
    b) Wing nerve disorder
    c) Brachial paralysis
    d) Neuro-wing palsy
74. Which fungal infection can cause lesions and swelling in the wing joints of poultry?
    a) Aspergillosis
    b) Candidiasis
    c) Ringworm
    d) Histoplasmosis
75. What is the common term for the condition where a bird has one wing shorter than the other, making it difficult to fly?
    a) Uneven wing syndrome
    b) Asymmetric wing development
    c) Single-winged disorder
    d) Short-winged condition
76. Which bacterial infection can lead to joint swelling, lameness, and wing drooping in poultry?
    a) Escherichia coli (E. coli)
    b) Salmonella enteritidis
    c) Clostridium perfringens
    d) Pasteurella multocida
77. What is the term for the condition where a bird's wing feathers are excessively pulled out by self-preening?
    a) Self-feathering
    b) Self-plucking
    c) Wing preening disorder
    d) Auto-barbering
78. Which protozoal infection can lead to joint inflammation and lameness in poultry, affecting the wings?
    a) Coccidiosis
    b) Toxoplasmosis
    c) Cryptosporidiosis
    d) Histomoniasis
79. What is the term for the condition where a bird has difficulty extending or flexing its wing joints?
    a) Wing contracture
    b) Joint stiffness syndrome
    c) Brachial limitation
    d) Wing articulation disorder

80. Which external injury can cause wing fractures or dislocations in poultry?
 a) Frostbite b) Sunburn
 c) Traumatic injury d) Electrical shock

81. What is the term for the condition where a bird's wings are affected by inflammation of the air sacs?
 a) Air sacculitis b) Wing pneumonitis
 c) Pulmonary inflammation d) Avian bronchitis

82. Which mite infestation can lead to feather loss and irritation in the wings of poultry?
 a) Red mites b) Northern fowl mites
 c) Scaly leg mites d) Feather mites

83. What is the term for the condition where a bird has difficulty folding or unfolding its wings due to stiffness?
 a) Wing folding disorder b) Feather rigidity syndrome
 c) Brachial rigidity d) Wing lock

84. Which nutritional deficiency can lead to weakened wing muscles and poor feather development in poultry?
 a) Vitamin K deficiency b) Vitamin C deficiency
 c) Protein deficiency d) Thiamine deficiency

85. What is the term for the condition where a bird's wings have an abnormal curvature or twist due to developmental issues?
 a) Wing torsion b) Feather curling syndrome
 c) Twisted wing disorder d) Curved wing anomaly

86. What is the term for the condition where a bird's wings have excessive feather loss without apparent injury?
 a) Feather shedding syndrome b) Wing alopecia
 c) Pterylomania d) Wing denudation

87. Which bacterial infection can cause abscesses in the wings of poultry, leading to swelling and discomfort?
 a) Avian tuberculosis b) Mycoplasma gallisepticum
 c) Erysipelas d) Clostridium botulinum

88. What is the term for the condition where a bird's wings exhibit excessive flapping and restlessness due to discomfort?
 a) Wing hyperactivity b) Wing agitation syndrome
 c) Flap-induced distress d) Wing restlessness disorder

89. Which viral infection can cause wing hemorrhages and clotting disorders in poultry?
 a) Avian pox b) Newcastle disease
 c) Infectious bronchitis d) Avian influenza

90. What is the term for the condition where a bird's wings show signs of edema and swelling due to fluid retention?
 a) Wing hydrops b) Edematous wing syndrome
 c) Fluid-wing disorder d) Wing effusion

91. Which fungal infection can lead to nodules and granulomas in the wings of poultry?
   a) Aspergillosis b) Cryptococcosis
   c) Histoplasmosis d) Candidiasis
92. What is the term for the condition where a bird's wings exhibit a peculiar odor due to bacterial infection?
   a) Wing rot b) Odoriferous wing syndrome
   c) Bacterial wing malodour d) Wing putrefaction
93. Which viral infection can lead to wing lesions and necrosis in poultry?
   a) Fowlpox b) Marek's disease
   c) Avian leukosis d) Infectious laryngotracheitis
94. What is the term for the condition where a bird's wings exhibit abnormal growth or development, leading to deformities?
   a) Wing dysplasia b) Wing malformation
   c) Avian wing dystrophy d) Dysmorphic wing syndrome
95. Which parasitic infestation can cause severe irritation and inflammation in the wings of poultry?
   a) Sticktight fleas b) Northern fowl mites
   c) Lice infestation d) Scaly leg mites
96. What is the term for the condition where a bird's wings show signs of erythema and heat due to inflammation?
   a) Wing fever b) Hot wing syndrome
   c) Inflamed wing disorder d) Erythematous wing condition
97. Which bacterial infection can cause cellulitis and abscesses in the wings of poultry?
   a) Clostridium perfringens b) Escherichia coli (E. coli)
   c) Mycoplasma gallisepticum d) Pasteurella multocida
98. What is the term for the condition where a bird's wings show signs of cyanosis and lack of oxygenation due to respiratory issues?
   a) Wing hypoxia b) Cyanotic wing syndrome
   c) Respiratory wing disorder d) Hypoxic wing condition
99. Which fungal infection can cause skin lesions and ulcers in the wings of poultry?
   a) Candidiasis b) Aspergillosis
   c) Fusarium infection d) Trichophyton infection
100. What is the term for the condition where a bird's wings show signs of necrosis and tissue death due to bacterial infection?
   a) Necrotic wing syndrome b) Gangrenous wing disorder
   c) Wing tissue necrosis d) Avian wing putrefaction
101. What is a feather cyst?
   a) A growth caused by overgrown feathers
   b) A type of skin infection in birds
   c) A lump or mass formed when a growing feather curls within the follicle
   d) A genetic disorder affecting feathers

102. Which birds are most commonly affected by feather cysts?
   a) Parrots and canaries
   b) Blue and gold macaws and certain breeds of canaries
   c) Falcons and eagles
   d) Pigeons and doves

103. What can feather cysts look like?
   a) Circular bumps
   b) Star-shaped masses
   c) Oval or elongated swellings
   d) Smooth, flat patches

104. What is a possible cause of feather cysts in some canaries?
   a) Trauma to the wings
   b) Genetic predisposition
   c) Viral infections
   d) Lack of proper nutrition

105. How can feather cysts be treated?
   a) Topical ointments
   b) Antibiotic medications
   c) Surgical removal of the involved feather follicles
   d) Natural remedies

106. Why may surgery not be practical for canaries with multiple feather cysts?
   a) High risk of infection
   b) Genetic complications
   c) Feather regrowth issues
   d) Multiple cysts make surgery impractical

107. What is feather plucking in birds?
   a) A grooming behavior
   b) A mating ritual
   c) A disease caused by parasites
   d) A range of behaviors from mild overpreening to self-mutilation

108. Why is good communication with a veterinarian important for addressing feather plucking in birds?
   a) Veterinarians can provide feathers for replacement
   b) Veterinarians can offer psychological counseling to birds
   c) To improve the health of the bird and reduce or eliminate plucking behavior
   d) Veterinarians can teach owners how to groom their birds

109. What is a common contributing factor to feather plucking according to the information provided?
   a) Genetic predisposition
   b) Heavy metal poisoning
   c) Nutritional deficiencies
   d) Lack of social interaction

110. What is a feather cyst?
   a) A growth caused by overgrown feathers
   b) A lump or mass formed when a growing feather curls within the follicle
   c) A type of skin infection in birds
   d) A genetic disorder affecting feathers

111. In poultry birds, maximum callus formation in the radius was achieved in

a) Two to three weeks
b) Three-four weeks
b) Four-five weeks
d) Five-six weeks

112. Avian bones heal .... in comparison to mammalian bones

a) slower
b) Faster
b) Equally
d) May be faster or slower

113. Which of the following is a common type of tumor that may affect the wings of poultry birds?

a) Ovarian tumor
b) Lipoma
c) Avian influenza tumor
d) Marek's disease tumor

114. What is a common fungal infection affecting the wings of poultry birds?

a) Aspergillosis
b) Candidiasis
c) Histoplasmosis
d) Cryptococcosis.

115. Which part of the wing is commonly affected by fungal infections?

a) Primary feathers
b) Secondary feathers
c) Coverts
d) Alula

116. Which antifungal agent is commonly used for the treatment of fungal infections in poultry?

a) Penicillin
b) Tetracycline
c) Amphotericin B
d) Ivermectin

117. What is the common method of transmission of fungal infections in poultry flocks?

a) Direct contact
b) Airborne spores
c) Ingestion of contaminated feed
d) Biting insects

118. Which of the following is a symptom of an advanced stage of wing fungal infections?

a) Increased preening behaviour
b) Swollen joints
c) Improved feather quality
d) Vocalization changes

119. What is a common viral infection affecting the wings of poultry birds?

a) Aspergillosis
b) Avian Influenza
c) Marek's Disease
d) Fowl Pox

120. What is the primary mode of transmission for most viral infections affecting poultry wings?

a) Direct contact
b) Airborne droplets
c) Ingestion of contaminated feed
d) Biting insects

121. Which viral infection can lead to the formation of wart-like lesions on the comb, wattles, and wings of poultry?

a) Infectious bronchitis
b) Fowl pox
c) Avian influenza
d) Newcastle disease

122. What is a common clinical sign of viral infections in poultry wings?

a) Feather loss
b) Lameness
c) Beak deformities
d) Wing drooping

123. Which of the following viruses can cause respiratory signs in addition to affecting the wings of poultry?
   a) Infectious laryngotracheitis
   b) Infectious bursal disease
   c) Avian leukosis virus
   d) Infectious bronchitis virus
124. Which viral infection is characterized by nervous signs such as twisting of the neck and paralysis?
   a) Marek's disease
   b) Avian influenza
   c) Newcastle disease
   d) Fowl pox
125. Which virus is associated with the "blue wing disease" in poultry?
   a) Avian adenovirus
   b) Avian encephalomyelitis virus
   c) Avian paramyxovirus
   d) Avian reovirus
126. Which viral infection is known for causing a drop in egg production in addition to affecting the wings?
   a) Fowl cholera
   b) Avian infectious bronchitis
   c) Avian leucosis
   d) Infectious bursal disease
127. Which of the following viruses is known to cause feather picking and cannibalism in poultry?
   a) Avian adenovirus
   b) Marek's disease virus
   c) Avian leukosis virus
   d) Infectious laryngotracheitis virus
128. Which viral infection can result in swollen sinuses, facial edema, and respiratory distress in addition to wing manifestations?
   a) Avian influenza
   b) Newcastle disease
   c) Fowl pox
   d) Avian encephalomyelitis
129. Which viral infection is characterized by the presence of tumors in various organs, including the wings?
   a) Avian leucosis
   b) Infectious bronchitis
   c) Avian reovirus
   d) Infectious laryngotracheitis
130. What is a common method for diagnosing viral infections in poultry wings?
   a) Feather plucking
   b) Blood smear examination
   c) Polymerase chain reaction (PCR)
   d) Increased temperature
131. Which virus can cause conjunctivitis in addition to wing lesions in poultry?
   a) Fowl pox
   b) Infectious bronchitis
   c) Avian adenovirus
   d) Avian paramyxovirus
132. What is a common route of entry for viruses causing wing infections in poultry?
   a) Skin contact
   b) Ingestion
   c) Respiratory route
   d) Conjunctival route
133. Which viral infection is associated with haemorrhages on the comb and wattles, along with wing manifestations?
   a) Avian influenza
   b) Marek's disease
   c) Infectious bursal disease
   d) Infectious laryngotracheitis

134. Which viral infectiton is characterized by yellowish nodules on the skin and mucous membranes, including the wings?
   a) Infectious laryngotracheitis
   b) Newcastle disease
   c) Avian adenovirus
   d) Fowl pox

Answer Key

1	c	2	b	3	d	4	a	5	b	6	b	7	b
8	d	9	c	10	c	11	c	12	c	13	d	14	b
15	c	16	c	17	a	18	a	19	c	20	d	21	b
22	d	23	b	24	b	25	b	26	c	27	a	28	d
29	b	30	d	31	a	32	c	33	b	34	c	35	c
36	a	37	b	38	b	39	d	40	d	41	a	42	b
43	b	44	a	45	c	46	c	47	d	48	d	49	a
50	c	51	c	52	b	53	b	54	c	55	c	56	b
57	d	58	b	59	b	60	c	61	a	62	a	63	c
64	d	65	b	66	c	67	b	68	d	69	c	70	a
71	a	72	a	73	c	74	c	75	a	76	a	77	b
78	a	79	a	80	c	81	a	82	b	83	d	84	c
85	a	86	b	87	c	88	a	89	b	90	a	91	a
92	b	93	a	94	a	95	a	96	b	97	a	98	b
99	c	100	a	101	b	102	b	103	c	104	b	105	c
106	d	107	d	108	c	109	c	110	b	111		112	
113	d	114	a	115	a	116	c	117	b	118	b	119	c
120	b	121	b	122	d	123	b	124	a	125	c	126	b
127	b	128	b	129	a	130	c	131	a	132	c	133	a
134	d												

26

Disorders of Reproductive System

Felix Uchenna Samuel[1] and Ibrahim Mohammed Abdul[2]

[1]*Animal Science Program, Alabama Cooperative Extension*
Alabama A&M University, Normal
[2]*National Animal Production Research Institute, Ahmadu Bello University, Nigeria*

Introduction

The reproductive system is fundamental to poultry production, playing a crucial role in both the quantity and quality of eggs laid. Its importance goes beyond mere biology, impacting the profitability and long-term sustainability of poultry operations (Abbasi *et al.*, 2024). Central to this is the egg, the ultimate product of avian reproduction. The reproductive system coordinates complex processes to ensure eggs meet high standards. Any disruption to this delicate balance can have far-reaching effects on the economic and environmental aspects of poultry farming. Disorders affecting the avian reproductive system pose significant challenges to the poultry industry. Whether they are minor disturbances or major disruptions, these disorders can undermine the foundation of successful production. They can lead to reduced egg production and compromised egg quality, affecting productivity, efficiency, and ultimately, profitability. In today's poultry management landscape, where efficiency is paramount, the impact of reproductive disorders cannot be overstated. Beyond economic concerns, these disorders also affect sustainability and environmental responsibility. A healthy reproductive system is not only crucial for financial success but also for upholding ethical and responsible poultry practices. As such, ensuring the reproductive health of poultry is of utmost importance. It requires dedicated effort, attention to detail, and a comprehensive approach. By strengthening the reproductive system against various threats, poultry producers can secure not only the current success of their operations but also a legacy of responsible stewardship for future generations (Habibi *et al.*, 2024).

Causes of Reproductive Disorders:

Reproductive disorders in poultry can arise from a multitude of factors, including infectious agents, nutritional deficiencies, environmental stressors, genetic predisposition, and management practices. Understanding these underlying causes is essential for effective prevention and management (Verma *et al.*, 2024). Here are some common causes of reproductive disorders in poultry:

Infectious Diseases: Bacterial, viral, fungal, and parasitic infections can target the reproductive organs of poultry, leading to inflammation, organ damage, and functional impairment. Common pathogens implicated in reproductive disorders include Escherichia coli, Mycoplasma spp., Avian Leukosis Virus, Infectious Bronchitis Virus, and Avian Influenza Virus.

Nutritional Deficiencies: Inadequate intake of essential nutrients, such as vitamins, minerals, and proteins, can disrupt reproductive function in poultry. Calcium deficiency, in particular, can lead to soft-shelled eggs, egg binding, and decreased hatchability.

Environmental Stressors: Adverse environmental conditions, such as extreme temperatures, poor ventilation, high stocking densities, and inadequate lighting, can induce stress in poultry, disrupting hormonal balance and reproductive cycles.

Genetic Factors: Genetic abnormalities or predispositions can increase the susceptibility of poultry to reproductive disorders. Breeding for specific traits, such as high egg production or rapid growth, may inadvertently introduce genetic defects that compromise reproductive health.

Management Practices: Inappropriate management practices, such as improper handling of breeding stock, inadequate sanitation, and insufficient biosecurity measures, can facilitate the transmission of pathogens and predispose poultry to reproductive disorders.

Common Reproductive Disorders in Poultry:

The reproductive disorders of poultry are outlined below (Thomas *et al.*, 2024)

Egg Binding (Dystocia):

Egg binding, also known as dystocia, is a condition where a hen is unable to expel an egg from the oviduct. This can occur due to various reasons, including oversized eggs, oviductal abnormalities, calcium deficiency, and hormonal imbalances. When a hen experiences egg binding, it may exhibit symptoms such as abdominal distension, lethargy, reluctance to move, and vocalization during egg laying. The inability to pass the egg can lead to discomfort and even life-threatening complications if left untreated.

Oversized eggs, often produced by young or immature hens, can become lodged in the oviduct, particularly if the hen's pelvic canal is not adequately developed. Oviductal abnormalities, such as strictures or adhesions, can impede the passage of eggs through the reproductive tract. Calcium deficiency can weaken the muscles of the oviduct, making it difficult for the hen to expel the egg. Hormonal imbalances, such as inadequate levels of progesterone or oxytocin, can affect the contraction of the oviduct muscles, further exacerbating the problem.

Treatment for egg binding typically involves providing supportive care to the affected hen. This may include gently massaging the abdomen to stimulate egg movement, providing warm baths to relax the muscles, and administering calcium supplements to strengthen uterine contractions. In severe cases, manual egg removal or surgical intervention may be necessary to alleviate the obstruction and prevent complications.

Salpingitis:

Salpingitis is a common reproductive disorder in poultry characterized by inflammation of the oviduct. This condition is often caused by bacterial infections, such as Escherichia coli or Mycoplasma spp., which can ascend the reproductive tract and colonize the oviduct. Salpingitis can result in a range of clinical signs, including reduced egg production, poor egg quality, internal egg laying, and peritonitis.

Bacterial infections are typically introduced into the reproductive tract through contaminated feed, water, or bedding. Once established, these bacteria can proliferate within the oviduct, leading to inflammation, tissue damage, and the formation of pus-filled lesions. In severe cases, the oviduct may become obstructed, preventing the passage of eggs and leading to internal egg laying. Additionally, bacterial toxins released into the abdominal cavity can trigger peritonitis, causing inflammation and infection of the peritoneum.

Treatment for salpingitis involves administering appropriate antibiotics to target the underlying bacterial infection. Supportive care, including fluid therapy and analgesics, may also be necessary to alleviate symptoms and support the hen's overall health. In some cases, surgical intervention may be required to remove severely damaged portions of the oviduct and prevent further complications.

Egg Peritonitis:

Egg peritonitis is a serious condition that occurs when a ruptured egg spills its contents into the abdominal cavity, leading to inflammation, infection, and septicemia. This condition is often secondary to underlying reproductive disorders, such as salpingitis or egg binding, which weaken the integrity of the oviduct and increase the risk of egg rupture.

When an egg ruptures within the oviduct or abdominal cavity, its contents, including egg yolk, egg white, and shell fragments, can trigger a severe inflammatory response. This inflammatory cascade can lead to the formation of adhesions, abscesses, and fibrinous exudates within the abdominal cavity, resulting in peritonitis. Clinical signs of egg peritonitis may include lethargy, abdominal distension, respiratory distress, and a palpable mass in the abdomen.

Treatment for egg peritonitis is challenging and often involves aggressive medical management to control infection and inflammation. This may include administering broad-spectrum antibiotics, anti-inflammatory medications, and supportive care to stabilize the hen and alleviate symptoms. In severe cases, surgical drainage of abdominal fluid or removal of the affected reproductive organs may be necessary to prevent further complications.

Ovarian Cysts:

Ovarian cysts are fluid-filled sacs that develop on the surface of the ovary, disrupting normal follicular development and ovulation. These cysts can vary in size and may be single or multiple. Ovarian cysts can interfere with the release of mature follicles from the ovary, leading to reduced fertility, irregular egg production, and hormonal imbalances.

The exact cause of ovarian cysts in poultry is not fully understood, but hormonal imbalances, genetic predisposition, and environmental factors may play a role in their development. Hormonal disruptions, such as elevated levels of estrogen or luteinizing hormone, can stimulate the formation of cystic follicles and inhibit ovulation. Genetic factors may also influence the susceptibility of hens to ovarian cysts, with certain breeds or lines being more predisposed to this condition.

Treatment for ovarian cysts typically involves hormonal therapy to regulate ovarian function and induce ovulation. Gonadotropin-releasing hormone (GnRH) agonists or human chorionic gonadotropin (hCG) injections may be used to stimulate follicular growth and trigger ovulation. In some cases, surgical removal of the cystic ovaries may be necessary to restore normal reproductive function.

Testicular Abnormalities:

Testicular abnormalities can affect the reproductive health and fertility of roosters, leading to impaired sperm production and reduced fertility. Common testicular disorders in poultry include orchitis, epididymitis, prostatitis, and testicular tumors. These conditions can result from bacterial infections, hormonal imbalances, genetic factors, or environmental stressors.

Orchitis refers to inflammation of the testes, often caused by bacterial infections such as Escherichia coli or Mycoplasma spp. Epididymitis is inflammation of the epididymis, the tube that stores and transports sperm from the testes. Prostatitis is inflammation of the prostate gland, which produces seminal fluid. Testicular tumors may be benign or malignant and can interfere with normal spermatogenesis.

Clinical signs of testicular abnormalities may include swollen or painful testes, abnormal sperm morphology, reduced sperm motility, and infertility. Diagnosis typically involves a combination of physical examination, ultrasound imaging, and laboratory tests to identify the underlying cause.

Treatment for testicular abnormalities depends on the specific disorder and its severity. Antibiotic therapy may be used to treat bacterial infections, while hormonal therapy may be employed to regulate reproductive hormone levels. In some cases, surgical removal of the affected testicle or tumor may be necessary to alleviate symptoms and restore fertility.

Infertility:

Infertility is a multifactorial condition characterized by the inability to achieve successful reproduction despite regular mating or insemination. Various factors can contribute to infertility in poultry, including age, genetics, nutrition, health status, and environmental conditions. Reduced fertility rates can manifest as poor hatchability, low egg fertility, or high embryonic mortality.

Advanced age can negatively impact fertility in both hens and roosters, leading to decreased reproductive performance and increased embryonic mortality. Genetic factors, such as inbreeding depression or genetic defects, can also affect fertility rates and hatchability percentages. Nutritional deficiencies, particularly deficiencies in essential nutrients such as calcium, vitamin D3, and selenium, can impair reproductive function and egg quality.

Environmental stressors, such as extreme temperatures, poor ventilation, high stocking densities, and inadequate lighting, can induce stress in poultry, disrupting hormonal balance and reproductive cycles. Infectious diseases, such as Newcastle disease, Infectious Bronchitis, or Avian Influenza, can also affect reproductive health and fertility.

Diagnosing and treating infertility in poultry requires a systematic approach, including thorough health assessments, reproductive evaluations, and diagnostic tests. Treatment options may include optimizing nutrition, reducing environmental stressors, implementing vaccination programs, and selecting breeding stock with desirable reproductive traits.

Prevention Strategies:

Preventing reproductive disorders in poultry requires a multifaceted approach encompassing nutrition management, environmental control, biosecurity measures, genetic selection, and health monitoring. Key prevention strategies include:

Nutritional Management: Providing a balanced diet formulated to meet the specific nutritional requirements of breeding poultry, including adequate levels of calcium, phosphorus, protein, vitamins, and minerals.

Environmental Control: Maintaining optimal housing conditions, including temperature, humidity, ventilation, lighting, and stocking density, to minimize stress and promote reproductive health.

Biosecurity Measures: Implementing strict biosecurity protocols to prevent the introduction and spread of infectious agents, including quarantine procedures, disinfection protocols, and pest control measures.

Genetic Selection: Selecting breeding stock with desirable traits, including reproductive fitness, disease resistance, and genetic diversity, to improve overall flock health and productivity.

Health Monitoring: Conducting routine health assessments, including physical examinations, laboratory tests, and flock performance evaluations, to detect early signs of disease or reproductive dysfunction.

Treatment Options:

Treatment of reproductive disorders in poultry varies depending on the specific disorder, its severity, and underlying causes. Treatment options may include:

Supportive Care: Providing supportive therapy, such as fluid therapy, analgesics, and nutritional support, to alleviate symptoms, maintain hydration, and support overall health.

Antibiotic Therapy: Administering appropriate antibiotics to treat bacterial infections associated with reproductive disorders, such as salpingitis or oviductal infections.

Hormonal Therapy: Using hormone therapy to induce ovulation, regulate reproductive cycles, or address hormonal imbalances that may affect fertility.

Surgical Intervention: Performing surgical procedures, such as oviductal surgery, egg removal, cystectomy, or castration, to alleviate obstruction, correct abnormalities, or remove diseased tissue.

Nutritional Supplements: Supplementing the diet with calcium, vitamin D3, or other essential nutrients to address nutritional deficiencies and support reproductive health.

Conclusion

Reproductive disorders pose significant challenges to poultry producers worldwide, impacting both commercial and backyard poultry operations. Understanding the common reproductive disorders in poultry, their causes, symptoms, diagnostic approaches, prevention strategies, and treatment options is essential for effective management and control. Through proactive management practices, including proper nutrition, environmental control, health monitoring, and genetic selection, producers can minimize the incidence of reproductive disorders and optimize flock health and productivity. Collaboration with veterinary professionals, extension specialists, and industry experts is crucial for developing comprehensive disease management programs tailored to the specific needs of each poultry operation. By implementing sound management practices and employing evidence-based interventions, poultry producers can mitigate the risks associated with reproductive disorders and ensure the long-term sustainability of their operations.

References

Abbasi, I.A, Shamim, A, Shad, M. K., Ashari, H., & Yusuf, I. (2024). Circular economy-based integrated farming system for indigenous chicken: Fostering food security and sustainability. Journal of Cleaner Production, 436, 140368.

Habibi, H., Rahmatnejad, E., Tohidifar, S. S., Afshar, A, Kameli,A, Jafari, M., & Mohammadi, M. (2024). Improving performance, reproduction, and immunity in laying Japanese quail with algal derivatives. Poultry Science, 103(2), 103295.

Thomas, K. S., Vasanthakumar, T., Mehala, C, Nithiaselvi, R., & Maheshwari, S. (2024). A retrospective study on the diseases and conditions causing mortality in a poultry farm.

Verma, S., Malik, Y. S., Singh, G., Dhar, P., & Singla, A.K. (2024). Comprehensive Knowledge of Non-infectious Diseases of Livestock Including Pets, Birds, and Wildlife. In Core Competencies of a Veterinary Graduate (pp. 67-76). Singapore: Springer Nature Singapore.

Multple Choice Questions and Answers

1. What are some common causes of reproductive disorders in poultry?
   a) Genetic abnormalities only
   b) Environmental stressors and management practices only
   c) Nutritional deficiencies and infectious diseases only
   d) Infectious diseases, nutritional deficiencies, environmental stressors, genetic predisposition, and management practices
2. Which of the following infectious agents can target the reproductive organs of poultry?
   a) Salmonella spp. b) Aspergillus spp.
   c) Escherichia coli d) Candida albicans
3. What deficiency can lead to soft-shelled eggs and egg binding in poultry?
   a) Iron b) Calcium
   c) Vitamin C d) Potassium
4. How do adverse environmental conditions affect poultry reproduction?
   a) They promote hormonal balance
   b) They enhance reproductive cycles
   c) They induce stress and disrupt hormonal balance
   d) They have no impact on reproduction
5. What can increase the susceptibility of poultry to reproductive disorders?
   a) Proper management practices b) Genetic diversity
   c) Nutritional supplements d) Genetic abnormalities
6. What is the primary symptom of egg binding in poultry?
   a) Increased egg production
   b) Vocalization during egg laying
   c) Laying eggs with hard shells
   d) Lethargy and abdominal distension
7. What may cause oversized eggs to become lodged in the oviduct?
   a) Weak oviduct muscles b) Hormonal imbalances
   c) Adequately developed pelvic canal d) Excessive calcium levels
8. Which bacterial infections are common causes of salpingitis in poultry?
   a) Salmonella spp. b) Mycoplasma spp.
   c) Streptococcus spp. d) Clostridium spp.

9. What condition can result from egg peritonitis in poultry?
   a) Reduced egg production
   b) Internal egg laying
   c) Increased hatchability
   d) Elevated egg fertility
10. What is a potential consequence of ruptured eggs in the abdominal cavity?
   a) Decreased inflammation
   b) Increased egg production
   c) Formation of abscesses
   d) Improved reproductive health
11. How are ovarian cysts characterized in poultry?
   a) Solid masses on the surface of the ovary
   b) Fluid-filled sacs on the surface of the ovary
   c) Abnormal enlargement of the oviduct
   d) Calcified structures within the oviduct
12. What is a potential consequence of ovarian cysts in poultry?
   a) Increased fertility
   b) Hormonal balance
   c) Reduced egg production
   d) Improved hatchability
13. Which of the following hormones can stimulate the formation of ovarian cysts?
   a) Testosterone
   b) Luteinizing hormone
   c) Progesterone
   d) Prolactin
14. What can lead to testicular abnormalities in roosters?
   a) Excessive vitamin intake
   b) Genetic factors
   c) Proper hormonal balance
   d) Adequate environmental conditions
15. What is orchitis in roosters?
   a) Inflammation of the oviduct
   b) Inflammation of the testes
   c) Inflammation of the epididymis
   d) Inflammation of the prostate gland
16. Which diagnostic method is typically used to identify testicular abnormalities in poultry?
   a) Blood test
   b) Ultrasound imaging
   c) Feather analysis
   d) Vocalization assessment
17. What are some clinical signs of testicular abnormalities in roosters?
   a) Increased sperm motility
   b) Reduced fertility
   c) Normal testicular size
   d) Improved egg production
18. What is a multifactorial condition characterized by the inability to achieve successful reproduction in poultry?
   a) Egg binding
   b) Salpingitis
   c) Infertility
   d) Ovarian cysts
19. How can advanced age affect fertility in poultry?
   a) It improves reproductive performance
   b) It decreases embryonic mortality
   c) It has no impact on fertility
   d) It decreases reproductive performance and increases embryonic mortality

20. What nutritional deficiencies can impair reproductive function and egg quality in poultry?
    a) Excess calcium
    b) Vitamin B12 deficiency
    c) Selenium deficiency
    d) Iron overdose
21. What environmental stressors can disrupt hormonal balance and reproductive cycles in poultry?
    a) Adequate lighting
    b) Proper ventilation
    c) Extreme temperatures
    d) Low stocking densities
22. Which infectious diseases can affect reproductive health and fertility in poultry?
    a) Newcastle disease
    b) Avian Leukosis Virus
    c) Infectious Bronchitis
    d) All of the above
23. What is the primary cause of egg binding in poultry?
    a) Excessive egg production
    b) Hormonal imbalances
    c) Oviductal abnormalities
    d) Calcium deficiency
24. What are some symptoms of egg binding in hens?
    a) Increased activity
    b) Abdominal distension
    c) Improved egg laying
    d) Vocalization during egg laying
25. Which of the following is NOT a common cause of egg binding in poultry?
    a) Oversized eggs
    b) Genetic factors
    c) Adequate calcium levels
    d) Hormonal imbalances
26. What treatment approach is typically used for egg binding in poultry?
    a) Administering antibiotics
    b) Providing warm baths
    c) Increasing egg production
    d) Reducing calcium intake
27. What is the primary cause of salpingitis in poultry?
    a) Bacterial infections
    b) Viral infections
    c) Nutritional deficiencies
    d) Genetic abnormalities
28. How do bacterial infections typically enter the reproductive tract of poultry?
    a) Through airborne transmission
    b) Through contaminated feed or water
    c) Through genetic inheritance
    d) Through hormonal imbalances
29. Which of the following is a symptom of salpingitis in poultry?
    a) Increased egg production
    b) Improved egg quality
    c) Internal egg laying
    d) Decreased peritonitis
30. What treatment is commonly used for salpingitis in poultry?
    a) Surgical removal of eggs
    b) Antibiotic therapy
    c) Increasing calcium intake
    d) Hormonal therapy
31. What is the primary cause of egg peritonitis in poultry?
    a) Genetic abnormalities
    b) Bacterial infections
    c) Hormonal imbalances
    d) Nutritional deficiencies

32. How does egg peritonitis develop in poultry?
    a) Due to viral infections
    b) Through hormonal imbalances
    c) As a result of egg rupture into the abdominal cavity
    d) Genetic abnormalities
33. What are some clinical signs of egg peritonitis in poultry?
    a) Increased egg production b) Respiratory distress
    c) Improved overall health d) Normal abdominal size
34. What is the primary treatment approach for egg peritonitis in poultry?
    a) Surgical drainage b) Hormonal therapy
    c) Antibiotic therapy d) Nutritional supplements
35. What are ovarian cysts in poultry?
    a) Fluid-filled sacs on the surface of the oviduct
    b) Abnormal growths on the testes
    c) Fluid-filled sacs on the surface of the ovary
    d) Hormonal imbalances in hens
36. What can ovarian cysts interfere with in poultry?
    a) Digestive function
    b) Normal follicular development and ovulation
    c) Respiratory function
    d) Egg production
37. What is a potential cause of ovarian cysts in poultry?
    a) Genetic abnormalities b) Nutritional deficiencies
    c) Hormonal imbalances d) Bacterial infections
38. How are ovarian cysts typically treated in poultry?
    a) Surgical removal b) Hormonal therapy
    c) Antibiotic therapy d) Nutritional supplements
39. What are common testicular disorders in poultry?
    a) Egg binding b) Ovarian cysts
    c) Orchitis and epididymitis d) Salpingitis
40. Which condition refers to inflammation of the testes?
    a) Prostatitis b) Orchitis
    c) Epididymitis d) Testicular tumors
41. What is the tube that stores and transports sperm from the testes called?
    a) Uterus b) Oviduct
    c) Epididymis d) Prostate gland
42. What is the function of the prostate gland in poultry?
    a) Produces seminal fluid b) Stores and transports sperm
    c) Regulates hormonal balance d) Stimulates egg production

43. What may be a consequence of testicular tumors in poultry?
   a) Reduced egg production
   b) Internal egg laying
   c) Abnormal sperm morphology
   d) Increased hatchability
44. What are the clinical signs of testicular abnormalities in roosters?
   a) Lethargy and respiratory distress
   b) Swollen or painful testes
   c) Abdominal distension and peritonitis
   d) Abnormal egg production
45. How are testicular abnormalities typically diagnosed in poultry?
   a) Ultrasound imaging
   b) Blood tests
   c) Fecal examination
   d) Egg quality assessment
46. What treatment may be necessary for testicular abnormalities in severe cases?
   a) Hormonal therapy
   b) Antibiotic therapy
   c) Surgical removal
   d) Nutritional supplements
47. What is infertility in poultry characterized by?
   a) Decreased reproductive performance
   b) Increased hatchability
   c) Improved egg quality
   d) Normal embryonic mortality
48. How can advanced age affect fertility in poultry?
   a) Increases egg production
   b) Decreases reproductive performance
   c) Improves hatchability
   d) Reduces embryonic mortality
49. What role do genetics play in poultry infertility?
   a) Improves fertility rates
   b) Decreases egg production
   c) Can affect fertility rates and hatchability percentages
   d) Reduces embryonic mortality
50. What environmental factor can disrupt hormonal balance in poultry?
   a) Adequate lighting
   b) Optimal ventilation
   c) Extreme temperatures
   d) High stocking densities
51. Which infectious diseases can affect reproductive health in poultry?
   a) Fungal infections
   b) Viral infections
   c) Parasitic infections
   d) All of the above
52. What nutrient deficiency can lead to soft-shelled eggs in poultry?
   a) Vitamin A deficiency
   b) Protein deficiency
   c) Calcium deficiency
   d) Vitamin D deficiency

53. Which environmental condition can induce stress in poultry?
  a) Adequate lighting
  b) Proper ventilation
  c) Extreme temperatures
  d) Low stocking densities
54. What genetic factor may predispose poultry to reproductive disorders?
  a) Genetic diversity
  b) Rapid growth
  c) High egg production
  d) Genetic abnormalities
55. Which management practice can contribute to the transmission of pathogens in poultry?
  a) Proper biosecurity measures
  b) Adequate sanitation
  c) Appropriate handling of breeding stock
  d) Insufficient biosecurity measures
56. What is another term for egg binding in poultry?
  a) Oviductal inflammation
  b) Dystocia
  c) Peritonitis
  d) Egg peritonitis
57. What symptom may indicate egg binding in a hen?
  a) Increased egg production
  b) Abdominal distension
  c) Normal vocalization during egg laying
  d) Improved appetite
58 What is a possible consequence of severe egg binding if left untreated?
  a) Increased egg production
  b) Normal reproductive function
  c) Life-threatening complications
  d) Improved hatchability
59. How is egg binding typically treated in poultry?
  a) Surgical removal of the egg
  b) Providing warm baths
  c) Administering calcium supplements
  d) All of the above
60. What is salpingitis characterized by?
  a) Inflammation of the oviduct
  b) Inflammation of the ovary
  c) Inflammation of the testes
  d) Inflammation of the prostate gland
61. Which bacterial infections can cause salpingitis in poultry?
  a) Salmonella spp.
  b) Escherichia coli
  c) Staphylococcus aureus
  d) Bacillus cereus
62. How do bacterial infections typically enter the reproductive tract in poultry?
  a) Through airborne transmission
  b) Through contaminated feed, water, or bedding
  c) Through direct contact with wild birds
  d) Through ingestion of infected prey

63. What can bacterial toxins released into the abdominal cavity lead to in cases of salpingitis?
   a) Decreased egg production
   b) Reduced egg quality
   c) Peritonitis
   d) Ovarian cysts
64. What is a potential consequence of severe salpingitis?
   a) Internal egg laying
   b) Increased hatchability
   c) Improved reproductive performance
   d) Normal egg production
65. How is salpingitis typically treated in poultry?
   a) Surgical removal of the oviduct
   b) Administration of appropriate antibiotics
   c) Providing warm baths
   d) All of the above
66. What is egg peritonitis caused by?
   a) Rupture of the egg within the oviduct
   b) Bacterial infections of the ovary
   c) Rupture of the egg into the abdominal cavity
   d) Inflammation of the uterine wall
67. What symptoms may indicate egg peritonitis in poultry?
   a) Increased egg production
   b) Lethargy
   c) Normal respiratory rate
   d) Improved appetite
68. What can trigger a severe inflammatory response in cases of egg peritonitis?
   a) Rupture of the egg into the oviduct
   b) Presence of benign ovarian cysts
   c) Rupture of the egg into the abdominal cavity
   d) Inflammation of the uterine wall
69. What is a possible complication of untreated egg peritonitis?
   a) Improved hatchability
   b) Respiratory distress
   c) Increased egg production
   d) Normal reproductive function
70. How is egg peritonitis typically managed in poultry?
   a) Surgical drainage of abdominal fluid
   b) Administration of broad-spectrum antibiotics
   c) Providing warm baths
   d) All of the above

Answer Key

1	d	2	c	3	b	4	c	5	d	6	d	7	c
8	b	9	b	10	c	11	b	12	c	13	b	14	b
15	b	16	b	17	b	18	c	19	d	20	c	21	c
22	d	23	d	24	b	25	c	26	b	27	a	28	b

29	c	30	b	31	b	32	c	33	b	34	c	35	c
36	b	37	c	38	b	39	c	40	b	41	c	42	a
43	c	44	b	45	a	46	c	47	a	48	b	49	c
50	c	51	d	52	c	53	c	54	d	55	d	56	b
57	b	58	c	59	c	60	a	61	b	62	b	63	c
64	a	65	b	66	c	67	b	68	c	69	b	70	d

27

Pain Management

Richa Chourasia

Department. of Veterinary Surgery & Radiology, CVAS, Jodhpur

Introduction

Pain management in poultry is an important aspect of animal welfare and overall production efficiency in the poultry industry. Poultry birds, such as chickens and turkeys, can experience pain due to various reasons including routine management procedures, injuries, and diseases. Managing pain in poultry is crucial not only for ethical reasons but also because pain can lead to decreased productivity and increased susceptibility to diseases. For the better management First step is identification of pain in birds which can only be possible with the thorough knowledge of their behaviour. Second step is the selection of appropriate analgesics and their dosing's as there are various species of birds. Commonly used analgesics for birds includes, NSAID's, opioids etc.

1. **Routine Management Procedures:** Many routine procedures in the poultry industry, such as beak trimming, toe clipping, and wing clipping, can cause pain and distress to birds if not done properly. Beak trimming, for example, is often performed to reduce feather pecking and cannibalism in crowded conditions but can cause acute pain if not done correctly. Proper techniques and pain management strategies must be employed during such procedures to minimize pain and distress in birds.
2. **Injuries and Diseases:** Poultry birds can suffer from various injuries and diseases that cause pain. Leg injuries, such as fractures and sprains, are common in poultry due to overcrowding or improper flooring. Diseases like necrotic enteritis and infectious bursal disease can also cause pain and discomfort in birds. Prompt diagnosis and treatment of injuries and diseases are essential for effective pain management in poultry.
3. **Nutritional Management:** Proper nutrition plays a crucial role in maintaining the health and well-being of poultry birds. Nutritional deficiencies or imbalances can lead to conditions such as skeletal deformities and metabolic disorders, which can cause pain and discomfort in birds. Formulating balanced diets with adequate levels of vitamins, minerals, and other nutrients is essential for preventing nutritional-related pain in poultry.
4. **Environmental Management:** The poultry housing environment significantly impacts the welfare of birds and their susceptibility to pain. Overcrowding, poor ventilation, and inadequate litter management can increase stress levels and predispose birds to injuries and diseases, exacerbating pain. Providing adequate

space, proper ventilation, and clean litter can help reduce stress and promote overall well-being in poultry.

5. **Pain Relief Measures:** While pain management in poultry is still an evolving field, there are some pain relief measures that can be implemented. For example, local anaesthesia or analgesics can be used during routine management procedures to alleviate pain. Additionally, providing environmental enrichments, such as perches and dust baths, can help distract birds from pain and promote natural behaviours.
6. **Genetic Selection:** Selective breeding for traits related to robustness and resilience can also indirectly contribute to pain management in poultry. By breeding birds with traits that make them less prone to injuries and diseases, such as stronger bones and immune systems, the incidence of painful conditions can be reduced.

In conclusion, pain management in poultry is essential for ensuring the welfare and productivity of birds in the poultry industry.

1. An ideal pain scale considers patient characteristics like
   a) Species & Breed
   b) External environment and Rearing condition
   c) Age and sex
   d) All
2. Academy of Animal Pain Management was formed in
   a) 2000 b) 2001
   c) 2002 d) 2003
3. IASP stands for
   a) International Association for the Study of Pain
   b) Indian Association for the Study of Pain
   c) International Association for the Specific Pain
   d) International Association for the Species specific Pain
4. Avianpulmonary system component responsible for the exchange of gases
   a) Bronchi b) Parabronchial lungs
   c) Pneumatic bones d) Air sac
5. The pain manifest in poultry as
   a) Anorexia b) Head shaking
   c) Biting d) None
6. Dose of Methadone in poultry is
   a) 6 mg/ kg IM or IV b) 4 mg/ kg IM or IV
   c) 8 mg/kg IM or IV d) 10 mg/kg IM or IV
7. Dose of Mophine in poultry is
   a) 6 mg/ kg SC b) 4 mg/ kg SC
   c) 8 mg/kg SC d) 2 mg/kg SC
8. Dose of Buprenorphine in poultry is
   a) 0.1 mg/ kg IM b) 1 mg/ kg IM
   c) 2 mg/kg IM d) 0.01 mg/kg IM

9. Drugs that can be used as local anaesthesia, nerve blocks & spinal anesthesia in birds
   a) Lidocaine b) Bupivacaine
   c) Both d) None
10. Analgesic agents worked by blocking/ interfering with conduction of action potential
   a) Local Anaesthetics b) NSAID's
   c) Opioids d) Steroids
11. Maximum dose of Lignocaine given to the Birds
   a) 5 to 6 mg/ kg b) 10 to 15 mg/ kg
   c) 2 to 3 mg/ kg d) 25 to 30 mg/kg
12. What is the recommended dosage range of Butorphanol for analgesia?
   a) 0.25–0.5 mg/kg IM q6h b) 0.5–3.0 mg/kg IM q4–6h
   c) 10 mg/kg PO q12h d) 0.6 mg/kg IM q6h
13. What is the dosage range of Buprenorphine for analgesia?
   a) 0.2–0.5 mg/kg PO or IM q24h b) 0.5–3.0 mg/kg IM q4–6h
   c) 0.25–0.5 mg/kg IM q6h d) 15–30 mg/kg q6h
14. What is the recommended dosage of Gabapentin for analgesia?
   a) 0.6 mg/kg IM q6h b) 0.5–3.0 mg/kg IM q4–6h
   c) 10 mg/kg PO q12h d) 5–11 mg/kg PO q12h
15. What is the dosage range of HydromorphoneHCl for analgesia?
   a) 0.6 mg/kg IM q6h b) 10 mg/kg PO q12h
   c) 5–11 mg/kg PO q12h d) 0.25–0.5 mg/kg IM q6h
16. Which of the following is the recommended dosage of Meloxicam for analgesia?
   a) 0.2–0.5 mg/kg PO or IM q24h b) 0.5–3.0 mg/kg IM q4–6h
   c) 15–30 mg/kg q6h d) 0.6 mg/kg IM q6h
17. What is the recommended dosage of Tramadol HCl for raptors for analgesia?
   a) 0.6 mg/kg IM q6h b) 5–11 mg/kg PO q12h
   c) 0.25–0.5 mg/kg IM q6h d) 0.5–3.0 mg/kg IM q4–6h
18. What is the dosage range of Tramadol HCl for psittacines for analgesia?
   a) 0.5–3.0 mg/kg IM q4–6h b) 15–30 mg/kg q6h
   c) 10 mg/kg PO q12h d) 0.6 mg/kg IM q6h
19. Which of the following challenges are associated with the adequate use of analgesics in backyard poultry?
   a) Lack of availability of analgesics for chickens
   b) Difficulty in recognizing and assessing pain in chickens
   c) Limited options for analgesics, primarily restricted to opiates
   d) All

20. Which homeopathic remedy can be used for chickens experiencing bruising, injury, and shock?
    a) Aconite
    b) Traumeel
    c) CBD oil
    d) Arnica Montana
21. How is Arnica Montana administered to chickens for pain management?
    a) Orally
    b) Topically
    c) Intramuscular
    d) All of the above
22. What is the recommended dosage of Arnica Montana pellets for chickens?
    a) One or two 30x pellets
    b) Five pellets per day
    c) One pellet per gallon of water
    d) One pellet per week
23. Which natural remedy is commonly used for inflammation, muscle, and joint pain in poultry?
    a) CBD (Cannabidiol) oil
    b) Aconite
    c) Traumeel
    d) Arnica Montana
24. Which of the following is NOT a form in which CBD products for animals are available?
    a) Edibles
    b) Topical creams
    c) Injectable solution
    d) Oils
25. What is Traumeel primarily used for in poultry?
    a) Shock
    b) Bruising
    c) Inflammation, muscle, and joint pain
    d) None of the above
26. What is the primary reason for performing beak trimming in layer flocks?
    a) To increase egg production
    b) To prevent feather pecking and cannibalism
    c) To improve feed conversion ratio
    d) To reduce aggression among chickens
27. Which method has replaced the traditional use of a hot blade for beak trimming?
    a) Laser treatment
    b) Infra-red (IR) beak treatment
    c) Cryotherapy
    d) Chemical cauterization
28. How long does it take for the beak tip to be lost after Infra-red (IR) beak treatment?
    a) 1 week
    b) 4 weeks
    c) 2 weeks
    d) 6 weeks
29. At what age is beak trimming likely to be acutely painful according to the study?
    a) 10 days
    b) 15 days
    c) One day
    d) Six weeks
30. What behavioural effects were observed immediately after beak trimming in young birds?
    a) Increased feed intake
    b) Decreased activity
    c) Aggressive behavior
    d) Nesting behaviour

31. In older birds, what is the composition of the beak tip after trimming?
    a) Scar tissue
    b) Neuroma
    c) Healthy tissue
    d) Bone

32. What evidence suggests the presence of chronic pain following beak trimming in older birds?
    a) Reduced food intake
    b) Neuroma formation at the end of the nerve stump
    c) Increased beak activity six weeks after trimming
    d) Absence of scar tissue formation

33. Why is beak trimming used in the egg industry?
    a) To improve egg quality
    b) To increase egg production
    c) To enhance chicken comfort
    d) To prevent feather pecking and cannibalism

34. How do birds typically react during feather removal?
    a) They become agitated and show wing flapping and vocalization
    b) They become lethargic and show decreased heart rate
    c) They show increased feeding behaviour
    d) They exhibit no noticeable behavioural changes

35. What physiological responses were observed during feather removal?
    a) Decrease in blood pressure and EEG arousal
    b) Increase in blood pressure and EEG arousal
    c) Decrease in heart rate and blood pressure
    d) Increase in heart rate and EEG arousal

36. What characteristic EEG pattern was observed during the period of immobility following feather removal?
    a) Low amplitude high frequency activity
    b) Low amplitude low frequency activity
    c) High amplitude high frequency activity
    d) High amplitude slow wave activity

37. What term is used to describe the immobility seen following feather removal, similar to an anti-predator strategy?
    a) Learned helplessness
    b) Stress-induced analgesia
    c) Tonic immobility
    d) Flight response

38. What is the potential purpose of the immobility seen following feather removal?
    a) To increase pain sensation
    b) To facilitate feather regrowth
    c) To prevent further damage from struggling
    d) To signal distress to other chickens

39. Why might the immobility seen following feather removal be counterproductive in production systems?
   a) It increases egg production
   b) It decreases stress levels in chickens
   c) It makes hens more susceptible to predation
   d) It prevents further feather pecking
40. What does shackling of commercial poultry involve?
   a) Restraining the wings of the bird
   b) Inserting each leg into parallel metal slots and holding the bird inverted for stunning & slaughter
   c) Placing the bird in a cage for transportation
   d) Administering medication to the bird
41. Why is shackling considered likely to be a very painful procedure?
   a) It causes psychological distress to the bird
   b) It results in feather loss
   c) It is a suprathreshold stimulus for cutaneous nociceptors in the leg
   d) It leads to increased egg production
42. What types of nociceptors were found in the scaly skin of the adult chicken leg?
   a) A-delta fibres mechanothermalnociceptors
   b) C-fibre polymodalnociceptors
   c) A-delta fibres responding only to thermal stimulation
   d) None, as chickens lack nociceptors in their legs
43. What is the potential consequence of footpad dermatitis in broiler chickens?
   a) Increased egg production
   b) Enhanced mobility
   c) Severe lesions to the feet
   d) Improved feather quality
44. How does footpad dermatitis impact the pain experience of chickens?
   a) It has no effect on pain perception
   b) It leads to increased egg production
   c) It causes pain, especially in severe lesions
   d) It reduces stress levels in chickens
45. What environmental factor could potentially cause pain to poultry?
   a) High levels of carbon dioxide
   b) Low humidity
   c) Clean air
   d) Controlled temperature
46. What conclusion can be drawn regarding ammonia pollution in poultry houses and its effect on nasal pain?
   a) Ammonia pollution is likely to cause severe nasal pain
   b) Ammonia pollution is unlikely to cause nasal pain based on available nociceptive thresholds
   c) Ammonia pollution has no effect on poultry health
   d) Ammonia pollution only affects the respiratory system of poultry

47. What is a major problem in the poultry industry related to skeletal disorders?
    a) Feather pecking
    b) Beak abnormalities
    c) Bone breakage and lameness
    d) Decreased egg production
48. In laying hens, what is the major problem associated with skeletal disorders?
    a) Angular and torsional deformities
    b) Osteoarthosis and lameness
    c) Bone breakage usually resulting from osteoporosis
    d) Gout and metabolic disorders
49. What is the prevalence figure for keel bone fracture in laying hens?
    a) Up to 20%
    b) Up to 30%
    c) Up to 40%
    d) Up to 50%
50. What is a major problem in broiler chickens related to skeletal disorders?
    a) Feather loss
    b) Beak abnormalities
    c) Decreased egg production
    d) Rapid growth rate leading to pathologies in the growth plate
51. What can be inferred about broken bones in birds based on physiological similarities with humans?
    a) They are not painful
    b) They are likely to be very painful
    c) They cause discomfort but not pain
    d) They are only painful in laying hens
52. What is a possible cause of lameness in broiler chickens?
    a) Viral infections only
    b) Bacterial infections only
    c) Both infectious and non-infectious causes
    d) Metabolic disorders only
53. According to research, what was found to be a possible cause of lameness in broiler chickens?
    a) Increased activity
    a) Inflammatory joint disease
    b) Decreased bone density
    c) Genetic abnormalities
54. What evidence supports the conclusion that inflammatory joint disease in broiler chickens is likely painful?
    a) Changes in gait only
    b) Blood in the synovia and behavioural responses
    c) Synovial fluid analysis only
    d) Histopathological examinations
55. What conclusion can be drawn about the walking ability of modern broilers?
    a) They walk efficiently due to their rapid growth rate
    b) They walk similarly to lightweight laying strains of birds
    c) They experience pain due to altered gait patterns
    d) They walk differently from lightweight laying strains due to morphological changes

56. What is the primary peripheral process involved in the physiology of pain?
    a) Transmission of impulses to the spinal cord
    b) Activation of pain receptors
    c) Modulation of impulses in the brain
    d) Withdrawal response activation
57. Which of the following statements regarding nociceptive pain is true?
    a) It is usually prolonged and diffuse.
    b) It does not involve tissue damage or inflammation.
    c) It typically activates a withdrawal response.
    d) It is considered pathological in nature.
58. Peripheral sensitization occurs due to:
    a) Decreased response to painful stimuli.
    b) Activation of "silent" nociceptors.
    c) Decreased sensitivity of peripheral receptors.
    d) Reduced excitability of spinal cord neurons.
59. What is central sensitization?
    a) Decrease in excitability of spinal cord neurons
    b) Recruitment of neurons not involved in pain perception
    c) Activation of pain receptors in the brain
    d) Reduction in pain perception in the central nervous system
60. How does early administration of analgesics affect spinal excitability?
    a) It increases spinal excitability.
    b) It has no effect on spinal excitability.
    c) It dampens spinal excitability.
    d) It activates silent nociceptors.
61. What is the benefit of providing analgesia before a painful event?
    a) It reduces the need for postoperative analgesics.
    b) It decreases the total drug requirement.
    c) It prolongs the postoperative recovery period
    d) It has no effect on postoperative discomfort.
62. What are the advantages of receiving butorphanol before and after orthopaedic surgery in birds?
    a) They required higher doses of butorphanol.
    b) They experienced prolonged postoperative recovery.
    c) They returned to normal behaviours sooner.
    d) They had increased spinal excitability.
63. How do local anaesthetics produce regional anaesthesia?
    a) By activating opioid receptors
    b) By blocking sodium channels in nerve axons
    c) By inhibiting cyclooxygenase enzymes
    d) By increasing serotonin synthesis

64. What is the primary mechanism of action of lidocaine and bupivacaine?
   a) Inhibition of prostaglandin synthesis
   b) Activation of opioid receptors
   c) Blockade of sodium channels
   d) Enhancement of GABAergic transmission
65. Which of the following methods is commonly used for local anaesthetic administration in birds?
   a) Intravenous infusion b) Intramuscular injection
   c) Regional infiltration or line block d) Oral administration
66. Why are local anaesthetic dosage recommendations lower for birds compared to mammals?
   a) Birds have higher tissue sensitivity to local anaesthetics.
   b) Birds have slower systemic uptake of drugs.
   c) Birds have fewer pain receptors.
   d) Birds have more rapid systemic uptake of drugs.
67. Which adverse effect can occur if local anaesthetics are accidentally injected intravenously?
   a) Hypotension b) Respiratory depression
   c) Gastric ulceration d) Fine tremors and ataxia
68. What is the primary mechanism of action of opioids?
   a) Inhibition of sodium channels
   b) Activation of GABA receptors
   c) Reversible binding to specific receptors
   d) Inhibition of cyclooxygenase enzymes
69. Which opioid receptor type primarily mediates pain relief?
   a) Mu b) Delta
   c) Kappa d) Sigma
70. What is the current recommendation for opioid analgesia in parrots?
   a) Buprenorphine b) Fentanyl
   c) Morphine d) Butorphanol
71. How are NSAIDs believed to exert their analgesic effects?
   a) By activating opioid receptors
   b) By blocking sodium channels
   c) By inhibiting cyclooxygenase enzymes
   d) By enhancing GABAergic transmission
72. Which NSAID is commonly used for chronic pain management in birds?
   a) Ketamine b) Acetaminophen
   c) Carprofen d) Diazepam

73. What is the primary mechanism of action of NSAIDs?
    a) Activation of opioid receptors
    b) Inhibition of cyclooxygenase enzymes
    c) Blockade of sodium channel
    d) Enhancement of GABAergic transmission
74. Which of the following NSAIDs is NOT recommended for use in birds due to significant toxic effects?
    a) Meloxicam b) Diclofenac
    c) Carprofen d) Piroxicam
75. Why is diclofenac not recommended for use in birds?
    a) It causes muscle necrosis at the injection site.
    b) It interferes with uric acid transport.
    c) It causes gastrointestinal ulceration.
    d) It increases serum uric acid concentrations
76. What is the advantage of using meloxicam in birds compared to other NSAIDs?
    a) It has a longer duration of analgesic effect.
    b) It has a higher oral bioavailability.
    c) It is less likely to cause renal toxicity.
    d) It has a shorter half-life.
77. Which parameter should be monitored before NSAID administration in birds?
    a) Plasma uric acid levels b) Serum phosphorous levels
    c) Hepatic enzyme concentrations d) All
78. What is the recommended route of administration for NSAIDs in birds to avoid myositis and muscle necrosis?
    a) Intravenous b) Subcutaneous
    c) Intramuscular d) Oral
79. Which NSAID has been shown to be effective for up to 6 hours in Parrots with chronic arthritis?
    a) Ketoprofen b) Piroxicam
    c) Carprofen d) Meloxicam
80. What adverse effect has been associated with high doses of piroxicam in chickens with ascites syndrome?
    a) Gastrointestinal ulceration b) Muscle necrosis
    c) Glomerular congestion d) Tubular necrosis
81. What is the first-line therapy for chronic pain disorders in birds?
    a) Opioids b) NSAIDs
    c) Tramadol d) Butorphanol
82. How should NSAID dosage be adjusted over time in birds with chronic pain?
    a) Increased gradually b) Decreased gradually
    c) Maintained at a constant level d) Stopped completely after a certain period

83. Which of the following behaviours may indicate pain in birds?
   a) Increased activity
   b) Improved feather quality
   c) Decreased weight-bearing
   d) Vocalizing more than usual
84. What type of analgesic drugs are commonly used in avian patients?
   a) Antidepressants
   b) Corticosteroids
   c) Opioids
   d) Antihistamines
85. Which statement accurately reflects the challenges in researching avian pain?
   a) Birds have similar responses to pain across species
   b) Pain behaviours are consistent within each bird species
   c) Avian pharmacokinetics and responses to drugs vary widely
   d) Pain scales for birds are well-established and widely used
86. What is recommended in the absence of specific pain scales for avian patients?
   a) Administer pain relief based on clinical judgment
   b) Delay treatment until pain behaviours are observed
   c) Rely solely on owner's assessment of pain
   d) Use only NSAIDs for pain management
87. What is the primary goal of developing species-specific pain scales for birds?
   a) To justify the use of analgesia in veterinary practice
   b) To measure the effectiveness of therapy
   c) To ensure consistent pain assessment and management
   d) To reduce the cost of pain treatment
88. What is the primary reason for the increasing trend of backyard poultry keeping?
   a) Cultural traditions
   b) Emotional value
   c) Economic benefits
   d) Pest control
89. Which of the following is NOT mentioned as a motive for keeping chickens according to the survey in the USA?
   a) Food for home use
   b) Gardening partners - fertilization
   c) Income generation
   d) Pets
90. Why do small animal veterinarians hesitate to become actively involved with backyard chicken care?
   a) Lack of interest from poultry owners
   b) Inadequate training in avian medicine
   c) Strict regulations on chicken keeping
   d) High cost of treatment
91. What is identified as a significant challenge in providing analgesia to backyard poultry?
   a) Lack of available analgesic drugs
   b) Variation in food safety regulations
   c) Difficulty in restraining the chickens
   d) Owners' reluctance to medicate their poultry

92. Which of the following analgesics is recommended for severe pain, including surgery and trauma, in birds?
    a) Meloxicam b) Butorphanol
    c) Tramadol d) Carprofen
93. What is the primary adverse effect associated with the use of opioids in birds?
    a) Gastrointestinal upset b) Renal pathology
    c) Hepatic lipidosis d) Cardiovascular depression
94. What is recommended regarding the dosage of tramadol for backyard poultry?
    a) Start with a high dose and adjust based on response
    b) Administer a fixed dose irrespective of the bird's weight
    c) Start with a lower dose and titrate to effect
    d) Avoid using tramadol due to its potential adverse effects
95. Which NSAID is considered the most commonly prescribed analgesic in backyard poultry?
    a) Carprofen b) Ketoprofen
    c) Ibuprofen d) Meloxicam
96. How euthanasia is typically performed in backyard poultry?
    a) Intravenous injection of a sedative
    b) Administration of oral medication
    c) Inhalation of anaesthetic gases
    d) Intramuscular injection of a barbiturate
97. What is the recommended dosage of carprofen for poultry?
    a) 1-2 mg/kg IM, IV SID b) 3-5 mg/kg IM, IV SID
    c) 5-10 mg/kg IM, IV SID d) 10-15 mg/kg IM, IV SID
98. Which of the following physiological parameters would commonly be associated with acute pain in birds?
    a) Tachycardia b) Overgrooming
    c) Loss of muscle mass d) Hypotension
99. Which of the following changes in temperament or personality could indicate pain in a bird?
    a) Hypertension b) Sleep deprivation
    c) Constipation d) Tachypnoea
100. Which opioid pain receptor is predominant in the forebrain of avian species?
    a) μ-receptors b) α2-receptors
    c) K-receptors d) δ-receptors
101. Which of the following opioids is an agonist at K-receptors?
    a) Buprenorphine b) Methadone
    c) Morphine d) Butorphanol
102. Which of the following is a purpose of sedation in birds?
    a) Increase vocalization b) Heighten stress response
    c) Facilitate immobilization d) Enhance manual restraint

103. What is the most commonly used drug for sedation of pet birds?
a) Midazolam b) Butorphanol
c) Flumazenil d) Ketamine

104. Which route of administration is considered a non-invasive alternative to intramuscular (IM) administration for sedating birds?
a) Intravenous (IV) b) Intranasal
c) Subcutaneous (SC) d) Intraperitoneal (IP)

105. What can be administered to reverse the effects of midazolam if needed?
a) Ketamine b) Atipamezole
c) Flumazenil d) Butorphanol

106. Which of the following is recommended as part of the pre-anaesthetic evaluation for birds undergoing long anaesthesia?
a) Blood glucose measurement only
b) Complete blood count and biochemistry panel
c) Physical examination only
d) History and radiography

107. What is the fasting period recommended for most raptor species before anaesthesia?
a) 12 hours b) 24 hours
c) 6 hours d) 2 hours

108. Which drug is preferred over diazepam for premedication in birds due to its minimal adverse effects and ability to decrease the minimum alveolar concentration (MAC) of inhalants?
a) Atropine b) Glycopyrrolate
c) Midazolam d) Butorphanol

109. Which inhalation agent is considered the anaesthetic agent of choice in avian clinical practice?
a) Halothane b) Desflurane
c) Isoflurane d) Nitrous oxide

110. Which opioid drug is routinely used in parrots for peri-operative analgesia and MAC reduction during anaesthesia?
a) Fentanyl b) Hydromorphone
c) Butorphanol d) Methadone

111. What is considered the most important aspect of avian anaesthesia due to the rapid rate at which birds may decompensate?
a) Pre-anaesthetic assessment b) Fluid therapy
c) Monitoring d) Drug administration

112. Which monitoring technique is recommended for assessing cardiovascular parameters during avian anaesthesia?
a) Electrocardiogram (ECG) b) Pulse oximetry
c) Oesophageal stethoscope d) Capnography

113. What loss of reflexes indicates that a bird is in a medium (surgical) plane of anaesthesia?
    a) Palpebral and corneal reflexes
    b) Withdrawal reflexes
    c) Corneal reflexes only
    d) Palpebral reflexes only
114. How is respiratory rate and character typically monitored during avian anaesthesia?
    a) Auscultation
    b) Observation of sternal motion
    c) Pulse oximetry
    d) End-tidal carbon dioxide (PETCO2) measurement
115. What temperature range is considered normal for avian core body temperature?
    a) 35-37°C
    b) 37-39°C
    c) 38-40°C
    d) 39-41°C
116. What is the primary goal of pre-emptive analgesia?
    a) To completely eliminate pain sensation
    b) To reduce the overall potential for pain and inflammation
    c) To induce sedation before a painful event
    d) To increase the likelihood of adverse effects
117. How does pre-emptive analgesia work in reducing pain sensation?
    a) By blocking sensory noxious stimuli from transmission to the central nervous system
    b) By directly targeting the central nervous system receptors
    c) By increasing the sensitivity of pain receptors
    d) By reducing the production of endogenous opioids
118. What is the main advantage of multimodal or balanced analgesia?
    a) It reduces the need for anaesthesia during painful procedures
    b) It increases the likelihood of adverse effects
    c) It enhances the analgesic efficacy and reduces adverse effects
    d) It eliminates the need for pre-emptive analgesia
119. Which of the following is NOT a type of drug commonly used for pre-emptive analgesia in birds?
    a) Opioid drugs
    b) Non-steroidal anti-inflammatory drugs (NSAIDs)
    c) Antibiotics
    d) Local anaesthetics
120. What is the purpose of combining different analgesics with different pharmacologic profiles and mechanisms?
    a) To increase the likelihood of adverse effects
    b) To reduce the overall potential for pain and inflammation
    c) To simplify the administration of analgesic drugs
    d) To eliminate the need for pre-emptive analgesia1

121. Why is recognition and appropriate treatment of pain in birds challenging for practitioners?
   a) Birds do not experience pain due to their physiology
   b) There is a lack of published information on analgesic efficacy in birds
   c) Birds do not possess neurologic components to respond to painful stimuli
   d) Birds show overt pain-associated behaviour that is easily recognizable
122. What are the primary reason birds do not indicate pain in an obvious manner?
   a) They lack the neurologic components to respond to pain
   b) They are prey species and are less likely to display overt pain-associated behaviour
   c) They do not experience pain due to their physiology
   d) They have a higher threshold for pain sensation compared to mammals
123. Which of the following is NOT mentioned as a method of nonpharmacologic analgesia for birds?
   a) Support or bandaging of the traumatized area
   b) Provision of appropriate bedding and perches
   c) Administration of opioids and NSAIDs
124. What is the purpose of pre-emptive analgesia in birds?
   a) To induce prolonged changes in CNS activity
   b) To decrease the intensity of pain experienced after tissue damage
   c) To reduce the need for postoperative analgesia
   d) To inhibit central sensitization caused by nociceptive stimulation
125. Which class of drugs is often used for pre-emptive analgesia in birds?
   a) Corticosteroids b) NSAIDs
   c) Alpha2-agonists d) Local anaesthetics
126. How do corticosteroids reduce pain associated with tissue damage?
   a) By directly blocking pain receptors in the CNS
   b) By increasing fibroblast proliferation
   c) By suppressing inflammatory responses to tissue damage
   d) By activating macrophage response to migration inhibition factor
127. Which of the following statements about betamethasone is NOT true?
   a) It reduces pain associated with degenerative hip disorders in adult male turkeys
   b) It decreases inflammation associated with sodium urate–induced synovitis in chickens
   c) It is administered at a dosage of 0.04 mg/kg in birds
   d) It decreases pain-related behaviours in birds
128. How do corticosteroids affect responses to opioids?
   a) They enhance the antinociceptive properties of agonists
   b) They reverse the analgesic effects of opioids
   c) They have no effect on responses to opioids
   d) They reduce the antinociceptive properties of agonists

129. Why should caution be used when considering administration of corticosteroids to birds?
   a) Because they may enhance the analgesic effects of opioids
   b) Because they may reverse stress-induced analgesia
   c) Because they have no effect on stress-induced analgesia
   d) Because they may directly stimulate pain receptors in birds
130. In what situations are NSAIDs preferable over corticosteroids?
   a) When dealing with chronic pain
   b) When the bird is experiencing high levels of stress
   c) When tissue damage is severe
   d) When immunosuppression is desired
131. Which of the following is NOT a typical effect of alpha2-agonists?
   a) Sedation
   b) Anxiolytics
   c) Hypertension
   d) Analgesia
132. Why alpha2-agonists are not usually administered to birds in the postoperative period?
   a) Due to their ineffectiveness as analgesics
   b) Because they can cause muscle tremors and respiratory depression
   c) Because they are only effective when combined with other drugs
   d) Due to their high cost
133. How does atipamezole affect unwanted side effects of alpha2-agonists?
   a) It enhances the side effects
   b) It has no effect on the side effects
   c) It reverses the side effects
   d) It prolongs the duration of the side effects
134. What is the role of ketamine in analgesia when combined with alpha2-agonists?
   a) It enhances the sedative effects
   b) It reverses the analgesic effects
   c) It prevents sensitization of nociceptive pathways in the CNS
   d) It increases the risk of postoperative complications
135. Which type of pain is ketamine NOT effective in controlling?
   a) \Sharp, superficial pain
   b) Visceral, dull pain
   c) Orthopaedic pain
   d) Laparotomy pain
136. How do local anaesthetics such as lidocaine and bupivacaine function?
   a) By enhancing nociceptive impulses
   b) By blocking sodium ion channels
   c) By increasing CNS changes
   d) By activating nociceptive pathways

137. What effect does local anaesthesia before tissue trauma have on postoperative pain?
   a) It increases postoperative pain
   b) It prevents nociceptor sensitization
   c) It enhances CNS changes
   d) It decreases the duration of action of local anaesthetics

138. What is the effect of topical bupivacaine on chickens after amputation?
   a) It reduces feed intake
   b) It increases postoperative pain
   c) It maintains pretrimming feed intake levels
   d) It has no effect on feed intake

139. Why are birds potentially more sensitive to local anaesthetics compared to mammals?
   a) Because they require higher doses for effect
   b) Because their blood-brain barrier is less structured
   c) Because they have fewer nociceptive pathways
   d) Because they have higher tolerance levels

140. What is a potential sign of toxicity associated with the administration of higher doses of bupivacaine in chickens?
   a) Increased activity levels
   b) Increased feeding behaviour
   c) Recumbency with outstretched legs
   d) Increased pecking behaviour

141. What is recommended regarding the dosage of lidocaine in birds to prevent adverse effects?
   a) It should not exceed 2 mg/kg
   b) It should not exceed 3 mg/kg
   c) It should not exceed 4 mg/kg
   d) It should not exceed 5 mg/kg

142. What is the primary mechanism of action of analgesics in birds?
   a) Stimulation of ascending spinal pathways
   b) Activation of endogenous descending pain modulation pathways
   c) Inhibition of COX-2 enzyme activity
   d) Activation of COX-1 enzyme activity

143. Why is timely administration of analgesics important in birds?
   a) To induce loss of consciousness
   b) To minimize the risk of hyperalgesia
   c) To prevent nociceptive sensitization
   d) To avoid adverse effects on homeostasis and healing

144. Which of the following is NOT a recommended nonpharmacologic method of analgesia for birds?
   a) Bandaging the traumatized area
   b) Modifying the environment with appropriate choices of perches and bedding
   c) Administering anxiolytics and tranquillizers
   d) Providing a dry, warm, quiet, nonstressful environment

145. What is the term used to describe pain perception in birds?
a) Hyperalgesia
b) Nociception
c) Analgesia
d) Sensitization

146. Which analgesic acts by preventing onward transmission of sensory nociceptive stimuli?
a) Ketamine
b) Buprenorphine
c) Butorphanol
d) NSAIDs

147. What is the primary concern regarding the use of inhaled anaesthetics in birds?
a) Risk of hyperalgesia during recovery
b) Risk of respiratory depression during anaesthesia
c) Risk of cardiac instability during recovery
d) Risk of thromboembolism during anaesthesia

148. Which class of analgesics is known to produce analgesia in birds but with variable and conflicting results?
a) Steroidal anti-inflammatories
b) α2-adrenergic agonists
c) NSAIDs
d) Opioids

149. What role do prostaglandins play in avian pain modulation?
a) They act as central nervous system depressants.
b) They lower the activation threshold for pain stimuli.
c) They decrease the synthesis of COX enzymes.
d) They modulate pain responses through spinal cord mechanisms.

150. Which analgesic is known to function by blocking ion channels, thereby preventing the generation and conduction of pain impulses?
a) Ketamine
b) Lidocaine
c) Meloxicam
d) Flunixin

151. What is the primary purpose of pre-emptive analgesia in birds?
a) To reduce overall pain experienced by the bird
b) To block sensory nociceptive stimuli from onward transmission
c) To induce loss of consciousness before the onset of pain
d) To prevent prolonged changes in CNS function after tissue injury

152. Which of the following veins are mentioned as easily accessible for injection of euthanasia solution in chickens?
a) Right jugular, ulnar, and femoral veins
b) Left jugular, radial, and femoral veins
c) Right jugular, ulnar, and tibiotarsal veins
d) Left jugular, ulnar, and tibiotarsal veins

153. Why is inhalational anaesthesia often used prior to euthanasia in chickens?
a) To induce agitation
b) To decrease the cost of euthanasia
c) To induce unconsciousness
d) To hasten the euthanasia process

154. Which combination of injectable anaesthesia is recommended for chickens prior to euthanasia?

a) Ketamine 5 mg/kg and xylazine 0.5 mg/kg

b) Ketamine 10 mg/kg and xylazine 1 mg/kg

c) Propofol 5 mg/kg and dexmedetomidine 0.5 μg/kg

d) Propofol 10 mg/kg and dexmedetomidine 1 μg/kg

155. What is the recommended dose range of pentobarbital for intravenous injection in chickens?

a) 50 to 100 mg/kg
b) 100 to 200 mg/kg
c) 200 to 400 mg/kg
d) 300 to 600 mg/kg

156. How is death confirmed after euthanasia in chickens?

a) By checking for pupil dilation

b) By assessing respiratory rate

c) By determining final cessation of heartbeat

d) By observing muscle twitching

157. What is the recommended alternative to burial for euthanized backyard poultry?

a) Donation to research facilities
b) Incineration or cremation
c) Composting
d) Disposal in landfill sites

158. Owners taking home their chicken following euthanasia should be advised of the risks, especially regarding:

a) Exposure to sunlight
b) Risk of infection transmission
c) Risk of necropsy
d) None of the above

159. Which of the following statements regarding backyard poultry euthanasia is NOT true?

a) Withdrawal times must be considered, especially if their meat and eggs are used for human consumption.

b) Burial of euthanized backyard poultry is always recommended.

c) The presence of pentobarbital or other anaesthetics in the carcass could represent a risk to other animals.

d) Propagation of infectious diseases such as avian influenza must be considered.

160. What medical condition frequently necessitates the use of analgesics in backyard poultry presented as patients in small animal practices?

a) Feather pecking
b) Egg binding
c) Molting
d) Beak trimming

Answer Key

1	d	2	c	3	a	4	b	5	a	6	a	7	d
8	a	9	c	10	a	11	c	12	b	13	c	14	c
15	a	16	a	17	b	18	b	19	d	20	d	21	a
22	a	23	c	24	d	25	c	26	b	27	b	28	c
29	c	30	b	31	a	32	a	33	d	34	a	35	d
36	d	37	c	38	c	39	d	40	b	41	c	42	a
43	c	44	c	45	a	46	b	47	c	48	c	49	c
50	d	51	b	52	c	53	b	54	b	55	d	56	a
57	c	58	b	59	b	60	c	61	b	62	c	63	b
64	c	65	c	66	a	67	d	68	c	69	a	70	d
71	c	72	c	73	b	74	b	75	b	76	c	77	d
78	d	79	c	80	a	81	b	82	b	83	d	84	c
85	c	86	a	87	c	88	b	89	c	90	b	91	b
92	b	93	d	94	c	95	d	96	d	97	c	98	a
99	d	100	a	101	d	102	c	103	a	104	b	105	c
106	b	107	b	108	c	109	c	110	c	111	c	112	a
113	b	114	b	115	c	116	b	117	a	118	c	119	c
120	b	121	b	122	b	123	c	124	d	125	d	126	c
127	c	128	d	129	b	130	b	131	c	132	b	133	c
134	c	135	b	136	b	137	b	138	c	139	b	140	c
141	c	142	b	143	d	144	c	145	b	146	a	147	a
148	d	149	b	150	b	151	d	152	c	153	c	154	b
155	d	156	c	157	b	158	b	159	b	160	b		

28

Disorders of the Integumentary System

Bhavanam Sudhakara Reddy, Sirigireddy Sivajothi, Malaka Malavika Reddy and Gongati Abhinethri

College of Veterinary Science - Proddatur, Sri Venkateswara Veterinary University Andhra Pradesh, India

The skin of the birds provides a physical barrier between the birds its environment, protecting the birds from bacteria and physical injury. The health of the bird can be compromised, and the value of the end-product can dramatically decrease. Bird's skin differs from that of mammals by its thinness, by the presence of feathers instead of hair, and by the absence of sebaceous glands (sweat glands), although the overall histological structure is similar. Bird's skin is composed of an epidermis separated from a dermis by a basal membranes to protect the body from infection. The integumentary system consists of the skin, the feathers and the appendages (claws and beak). The skin covers the majority of the body and contains glands in the outer ear canal and the preen gland at the base of the tail, that the bird uses to preen its feathers. The integumentary system is very important in providing protection to the bird from a number of potentially dangerous situations. The functions provided by the integumentary system include: A barrier between the external environment and the internal systems and organs thus provides support and protection from infection by microorganisms and from physical injury. Excellent thermal insulation to help regulate body temperature in a variable environment. Numerous nerve endings for the senses to enable the bird to be aware of potentially harmful situations. Pigments for display and protection from the elements. The compounds capable of conversion into vitamin D when exposed to sunlight. Avian skin is relatively thin with the epidermis consisting of only 2-10 cell layers. There are no sweat glands; instead heat is lost via the respiratory tract and by radiation from featherless areas. The brood patch is a featherless area that can occur in both sexes and is either seasonal or permanent depending on species. The feet have shield-like plates of keratin named scutes. The foot has various digital pads to aid grip. The uropygial gland or preen gland is bilobed gland that secrets lipoid sebaceous material that is spread by the beak over the plumage during preening. The gland lies dorsally near the tip of the tail. Feathers function not only to facilitate flight but also insulate, waterproof and protect the bird. Feathers are keratinized epidermis derived from follicles in the dermis. New feathers developing in the dermal papilla force the shedding of old feathers above it. The shedding and replacement of feathers occurs at least once a year usually after breeding but can occur more frequent or purposeful moulting. Dermatologic disease is sporadic poultry, and most commonly involves trauma and ectoparasites. Other infectious skin diseases can occur, but are less frequently encountered in poultry flocks. Skin quality is affected by a number of husbandry factors, including diet and sanitation.

Dermatitis: In broilers it is caused by a combination of moisture and chemical irritants like ammonia in the litter material during natural decomposition. These conditions affect areas of the skin greatly exposed, like the feet, hocks and breast.

Footpad dermatitis: It is also called paw burns, ammonia burns and pododermatitis.

Dermatitis with cellulitis: Dermal carcinomatosis, skin tares, scabby hip, and breast blisters are the most frequent ones. However, the permanent increasing dermatitis with cellulitis as well as the frequency rank following dermal carcinomatosis are of utmost importance.

Contact dermatitis: It is a common finding in commercial poultry kept for meat production that has both economic and welfare implications. The disease commonly affects the epidermis of the foot pad, hock joint and skin covering the breast muscles that are in contact with the litter or other floor materials.

Staphylococcal infection of poultry: This infection is commonly associated with infection of skin, bones, joints, and navel. There is a potential risk for human food poisoning.

Gangrenous dermatitis (GD): It is characterized with nercotization of different skin areas and a severe cellulitis of the subcutaneous tissue. The sudden and quick increase in death rates is often the first signal for the incidence of GD. The affected birds die after less than 24 hours with mortality rate from 1% to 60%. The lesions are dark red to blue green macerated skin areas, usually featherless, beginning generally from wings and the adjacent areas.

Blue wing disease: It is consequent to chicken infectious anaemia infection. It is an acute disease in chickens that causes high mortality in 2-3 week-old chickens. The major pathological lesions are haemorrhages in skin and muscles especially on the wings, and gangrenous dermatitis and depletion of lymphocytes in lymphoid tissues; the thymuses being most severely damaged)

Ulcerative dermatitis: Ulcerative dermatitis of brown cage-free layers. It results in high mortality. The birds get an ulcer right in the middle of their back, and we're not sure how it starts.

Skin Tumors: Marek's Disease (MD) affects chicken breeds for meat production and those for egg production, even though these two types of productions may not be equally affected in some countries due to breeding practices. It is also called as skin leucosis or cutaneous leucosis/ cutaneous MD.

Skin leucosis: Noted in broiler chicken on postmortem examination as enlargement of feather follicles and associated lymphoid infiltrations. Enlarged feather follicles may be noted in broilers after defeathering during processing and are a cause for condemnation.

Footpad dermatitis: It is a type of skin inflammation that causes necrotic lesions on the plantar surface of the footpads in commercial poultry, with significant animal welfare, and economic implications.

Cutaneous fowl pox: Avian pox is a highly contagious viral disease caused by avipox viruses Fowl pox *virus causes crusty and nodular lesions primarily on the un*-feathered portions of the bird. Occasionally, poxvirus can cause lesions in the mouth and trachea, causing death due to suffocation (wet form). If the bird recovers, immunity is generally lifelong.

Favus dermatophytic fungus: Favus is a chronic skin condition that afflicts poultry and mammals, including humans. It is normally caused by the dermatophytic fungus *Trichophyton megninii*. The fungi *Microsporum gypseum*, *Mycosporum gallinae* and *Trichophyton simii* have also been identified with some cases of favus. The first symptoms include the development of lesions on non-feathered skin, such as the lower leg, comb and wattle. Some loss of feathers and skin scales may occur although there are normally no significant signs.

Parasites: External parasites such as ticks, mites and lice are common in poultry. Scaly leg mites (*cnemidokoptes mutans*), Sticktight fleas (*Echidnophaga gallinacea*), *Dermanyssus gallinae*, the red mite, is probably the most common parasitic problem encountered by poultry keepers. It is easily spread by wild birds.

Write correct alphabet of the answer in the given bracket

1. Acquired loss of feathers on head in birds

   a) Molting b) Shedding

   c) Baldness d) Sloughing

2. Baldness is commonly seen in

   a) Canaries b) Parrots

   c)Ostrich d) Peacock

3. Etiology of baldness in birds

   a) Hormonal imbalance b) Genetic effect

   c) Diseased follicles d) All

4. Patchy feather loss in a bird indicative of

   a) Vitamin A deficiency b) Ringworm

   c) A and B d) None

5. Loss of head feathers at once

   a) Abnormal molt b) Shedding

   c) Ecdysis d) Sloughing

6. In birds, feather changes due to over supplementation with

   a) Vitamin A b) Zinc

   c) Vitamin C d) Copper

7. Changes in the temporary feather coloration in birds can be noticed in molting period

   a) Supplementation with vitamins

   b) Administration of antibiotics

   c) Administration of inflammatory medicines

   d) None

8. Brown hypertrophy can be noticed in Budgies

   a) Scaly lesions b) Nodules

   c) Tail like appearance d) Horn like appearance

9. Growth of multiple feather from one follicle

   a) Hyper follicles b) Poly follicles

   c) Both A and B d) None

10. Itchy poly folliculitis has seen in which birds
    a) Love birds
    b) Budgies
    c) A and B
    d) None
11. In birds poly folliculitis has seen in which areas
    a) Tail
    b) Dorsal neck
    c) Abdomen
    d) A and B
12. In birds, poly folliculitis is caused by
    a) Bacteria
    b) Fungi
    c) Prions
    d) Virus
13. Poor feather condition, conjunctivitis and diarrhea noticed in birds with
    a) Chlamydia infection
    b) Salmonellosis
    c) Giardia infection
    d) All the above
14. In birds brittle frayed feathers and itchy skin, discoloration of feathers can be seen in deficiency of
    a) Calcium
    b) Zinc, Manganese
    c) Selenium
    d) All
15. Poor feather condition long molts and flaky beaks or results of dietary deficiency of which amino acid
    a) Methionine
    b) Tryptophan
    c) Lysine
    d) All the above
16. High levels of methionine can be found in
    a) Sesame seeds
    b) Pumpkin seeds
    c) Sunflower seeds
    d) All
17. Duration of clinical improvement after dietary changes in birds with flaky beak
    a) 9-12 months
    b) 10 days
    c) 12 weeks
    d) 14 weeks
18. Name of fungus can cause dermatological signs in birds
    a) Epidermophyton
    b) Mycosis
    c) Trichophyton
    d) All the above
19. Red, dozing and ulcerative skin is termed as.
    a) Ulcerative dermatitis
    b) Decubitus sores
    c) Sores
    d) All the above
20. In birds ulcerative dermatitis can be associated with
    a) Intestinal parasites
    b) Wound
    c) Diabetes
    d) All
21. Dry itchy scaly skin is due to — in birds
    a) Diabetes
    b) Giardia
    c) A and B
    d) None
22. In which condition birds will do plucking and self mutilation
    a) Ca deficiency
    b) Vitamin deficiency
    c) Food allergy
    d) All the above

23. Blackened feathers are due to deficiency of
    a) Vitamin D b) Vitamin C
    c) Zinc d) Copper
24. Clubbed down condition in chicks due to deficiency of
    a) Niacin b) Riboflavin
    c) Cynocobalamin d) All the above
25. Strange feathering in birds
    a) Niacin b) Folic acid
    c) A and B d) Riboflavin
26. Loss of pigmentation in birds due to deficiency of
    a) Methionine b) Lysine
    c) Cobalt d) All the above
27. Decreased red pigmentation in birds due to deficiency of
    a) Copper b) Iron
    c) Zinc d) A and B
28. Inflammation of skin can be result of dietary lacking of
    a) Niacin b) Biotin
    c) Pantothenic acid d) All
29. Irritation or inflammation of foot pad in birds due to deficiency of
    a) Biotin b) Niacin
    c) Pantothenic acid d) All the above
30. In birds keratinization impaired by deficiency of
    a) Vitamin A b) Vitamin B complex
    c) Zinc d) Vitamin D
31. In birds depletion of muscles caused due to deficiency of
    a) Vitamin E b) Thymine
    c) Vitamin C d) A and B
32. Ginger hairs on neck region of newly hatched chicks due to
    a) Deficiency of copper b) Deficiency of molybdenum
    c) Deficiency of zinc d) Deficiency of sodium chloride
33. Another name for clubbed down condition in chicks
    a) Round syndrome b) Ascites syndrome
    c) Defective down syndrome d) Both A and B
34. Spoon shaped feathers are due to
    a) Copper deficiency b) Molybdenum deficiency
    c) Manganese deficiency d) Zinc deficiency
35. Which toxins can cause feather abnormalities in birds
    a) Epsilon toxin b) Tetanus toxins
    c) Mycotoxins (T2 toxins) d) All the above

36. Which toxicity delays feathering in broilers
    a) T2 toxins   b) Epsilon toxins
    c) Ochratoxin   d) All the above
37. Depigmentation and shorter shaft of wing feather are due to deficiency of
    a) Vitamin A   b) Selenium
    c) Vitamin C   d) A and B
38. Frayed feathers can be noticed in birds due to deficiency of
    a) Copper   b) Zinc
    c) Molybdenum   d) All the above
39. In which toxicity sparse covering of feathers and sticking out of feathers from the body is observed in birds
    a) Na Cl toxicity   b) Mycotoxins
    c) Ochratoxins   d) All the above
40. Which causes increased injurious pecking in laying hens
    a) Na Cl toxicity   b) Over feeding of Ca
    c) Both A and B   d) Crude protein <13%
41. What is the best roughage to decrease injurious pecking behavior
    a) Maize silage   b) Barley silage
    c) Carrot   d) All
42. Which amino acids reduces the incidence of feather pecking in birds
    a) Methionine   b) Lysine
    c) Tryptophan   d) All the above
43. What is most common and challenging syndrome in birds
    a) Clubbed feet   b) Cannibalism
    c) Feather plucking   d) All the above
44. Which viral disease can cause psittacine disease and feather disease
    a) Sarco virus   b) Orbi virus
    c) Morbilli virus   d) All the above
45. The most common mites in birds
    a) Demodex   b) Cnemidocoptes
    c) Clover mite   d) Psoroptes
46. Etiology for scaly face of parrots
    a) Demodex   b) Psoroptes
    c) Clover mite   d) Cnemidocoptes
47. Etiology of tassel foot of passerines
    a) Sarcoptes   b) Psoroptes
    c) Demodex   d) Cnemidocoptes
48. In birds feather cysts are considered as
    a) SCC   b) Sertoli cell tumour
    c) Mast cell tumour   d) Basal cell tumors

49. Psittacine beak and feather disease transmitted by
    a) Inhalation b) Ingestion(d)
    c) Vertical d) All
50. Avian polyoma virus can cause
    a) Budgerigar fledgling disease b) Mange
    c) Clubbed feet d) Tassal feet
51. Pox virus in birds transmitted by
    a) Direct contact b) Biting insects
    c) Inhalation d) All
52. In birds wet box can cause development of signs in
    a) Feet b) Oral cavity and trachea
    c) Abdomen d) All
53. Cutaneous pox can cause development of
    a) Nodules b) Papules
    c) Vesicles d) All
54. Cutaneous form of pox in birds can be demonstrated by
    a) Intracytoplasmic eosinophilic bodies b) Negri bodies
    c) Within the RBC d) All
55. Cutaneous form of pox is self limiting, when it requires antibiotic therapy
    a) First day b) CHF
    c) Diarrhoea d) Secondary bacterial infection
56. Benign epithelial tumors in birds caused by
    a) Circo virus b) Papilloma virus
    c) Orbi virus d) All
57. Location of papilloma virus lesions in birds
    a) Cloaca b) Oral cavity
    c) Skin d) All
58. Mite infestation in birds most commonly seen in
    a) Abdomen b) Feather areas
    c) Featherless areas d) All
59. Mite infestation in birds can cause
    a) Hyperplasia b) Hyperkeratosis
    c) Aplasia d) A and B
60. Red mites in poultry
    a) Demodex b) Sarcoptes
    c) Notoedres d) Dermanyssus
61. Which mite is visible at night in birds
    a) Notoedres b) Dermanyssus
    c) Demodex d) Sarcoptes

62. Blood sucking mites in birds
   a) Notoedres b) Dermanyssus
   c) Demodex d) Sarcoptes
63. Protozoa responsible for feather plucking behavior in birds
   a) Giardia b) Theileria
   c) Coccidia d) Babesia
64. In giardiosis feather plucking behavior is due to
   a) Hypersensitivity b) Malabsorption
   c) Nutritional deficiency d) All
65. Most commonly isolated bacteria from skin infection in birds
   a) Staphylococcus b) Mycobacterium
   c) Aromonas d) All
66. Candida has been associated with deficiency of ……. in birds
   a) Vitamin B b) Vitamin A
   c) Vitamin E d) Vitamin D
67. Reported fungi can cause dermatological lesions in birds
   a) Microsporum b) Trichophyton
   c) Cryptococcus d) All
68. Ulcerative dermatitis in love birds caused by
   a) Poor nutrition b) Giardia
   c) Agapornis pox virus d) All
69. Reduced protein levels result in poor feather condition on
   a) Fret marks b) Pug marks
   c) Dermatitis d) All
70. Essential amino acid necessary for feather quality
   a) Lysin b) Methionine
   c) Cysteine d) All
71. Hypovitaminosis A can effects the —in birds
   a) Moulting b) Hyperkeratosis
   c) Glandular metaplasia d) All
72. Hypothyroidism in birds leads to
   a) Retardation of feather growth b) Over weight
   c) Increased of feather growth d) All
73. Confirmatory test for hypothyroidism in birds
   a) Ultrasonography b) TSH
   c) ECG d) All
74. Clinical signs for hypothyroidism in birds
   a) Obesity b) Lipaemia
   c) Abnormal feathers d) All

75. Hyperthyroidism in birds can cause
   a) Polyurea & Polydypsia b) Regurgitation & Tachycardia
   c) Weight loss d) All
76. Follicular cyst are commonly noticed in
   a) Wing b) Along the back
   c) A and B d) None
77. Squamous cell carcinomas are considered as —in birds
   a) Mast cells b) Benign
   c) Malignant tumors d) All
78. Squamous cell carcinomas can be managed by
   a) Medical therapy b) Cryosurgery
   c) A and B d) Quarantine
79. Benign proliferation of lipocytes in birds called as
   a) Lipomas b) SCC
   c) Melanoma d) None
80. Lipomas in birds commonly noticed in
   a) Abdominal skin b) Sternum
   c) A and B d) Feathers
81. Predisposing factors for development of lipomas in birds
   a) Obesity b) Advanced age
   c) A and B d) Gender
82. In birds locally invasive benign masses are known as
   a) Xanthomas b) SCC
   c) Mast cells d) All
83. In which skin disorders in birds multinucleated giant cells and cholesterol crystals are noticed
   a) SCC b) Mast cells
   c) A and B d) Xanthomas
84. Crusty pruritic skin lesions that do not respond to therapy
   a) SCC b) Xanthomas
   c) Epithelio lymphosarcoma d) All
85. Bumble foot can be
   a) Pododermatitis b) Metatarsal pad
   c) Digital pad d) All
86. In parrots, bumble foot can be caused by
   a) Poor perches b) Obesity
   c) Hypovitaminosis A d) All
87. In birds chronic pyoderma will be associated with
   a) MRSA b) Streptococci
   c) E coli d) All

88. Effective antimicrobials for skin lesions in birds
a) Chlorhexidine b) Povidone iodine
c) A and B d) DNS
89. Drugs used to prevent antibiotic resistant bacteria
a) Mupiromycin b) Cephalexin
c) Povidne iodine d) Gentamicin
90. Drug effective against gram positive and negative and fungi in birds
a) Povidone iodine b) Gentamicin
c) Silver sulpha diazene d) All
91. Supplements used for treating the dermatological disorder in birds
a) Cholesterol b) Omega-3 fatty acids
c) Triglycerides d) All
92. In birds papova virus can cause— disease
a) Over weight b) Dermatitis
c) Fledgling d) All
93. General symptoms of skin infection in birds
a) Itching b) Redness
c) Swelling d) All
94. Bumble foot in birds caused by
a) Staphylococcus b) Streptococcus
c) E coli d) All
95. Another name for bumble foot disease
a) Tassal foot b) Pododermatitis
c) Foot ball d) None
96. Location of yeast infection in birds
a) Neck b) Head
c) Around beak d) Wing
97. Facial dermatitis in birds caused by which fungi
a) Cryptococcus b) Demodex
c) Trichophyton d) All
98. Most common diagnostic methods in avian skin diseases
a) Skin scrapings b) Culture
c) Biopsy d) All
99. Congenital beak abnormalities are encountered due to
a) Improper transport b) Improper nutrition
c) Improper incubation d) All
100. Best example for congenital beak abnormalities
a) Scissor beak b) Mandibular prognathism
c) A and B d) Mange

101. Hepatopathy in birds can be linked to
   a) Beak and nail deformities   b) Scaling
   c) Dermatitis   d) Feather loss
102. In which condition contour tail and flight feathers grow continuously
   a) Folliculitis   b) Scaling
   c) Feather duster   d) All
103. Feathers fail to emerge from their sheaths
   a) Hereditary condition   b) Recessive genetic effect
   c) Improper ventilation   d) A and B
104. In which disease honey comb encrustations on featherless part of the skin is noticed
   a) Mite infestation   b) Mange
   c) Tick infestation   d) Lice infestation
105. Drug of choice for mite infestation in birds
   a) Amprolium   b) Albendazole
   c) Ivermectin   d) All
106. External preparations for management of lice infestation in birds
   a) Amprolium   b) Pyrethrum spray
   c) Ivermectin   d) All
107. Dry flaky skin, granulomas and raised ulcers in birds due to
   a) Mycobacterium   b) Gentamicin
   c) Pox   d) All
108. Candida species are most commonly seen as lesions at
   a) Head   b) Commissures
   c) Beak   d) All
109. Favus in poultry caused by
   a) Microsporum   b) Trichophyton
   c) A and B   d) Demodex
110. Treatmemt of dermatomycosis by
   a) Gentamicin   b) Itraconazole
   c) Tylosin   d) All
111. Granulomatous lesions on the face, beak and sinuses in birds
   a) Streptococci   b) Cryptococcus
   c) Coccidia   d) All
112. Parasitic fungal infection in birds
   a) Malassezia   b) Trichophyton
   c) Coccidia   d) Demodex
113. Avian pox virus transmitted by
   a) Mosquitoes   b) Pecking
   c) Fighting   d) All

114. Agalinis pox virus can cause — lesions at
   a) Face   b) Nasal cavity
   c) Axillae   d) All
115. Amazon pox virus causes cutaneous lesions at
   a) Eyes   b) Beak
   c) Nares   d) All
116. Budgerigar pox is confined as
   a) Apathogenic   b) Pathogenic
   c) Low virulent   d) All
117. In birds haemorrhages within the pulp cavity is caused by
   a) Pox virus   b) Circo virus
   c) MD   d) All
118. Detection of virus in the feathers by
   a) HA test   b) HI test
   c) DNA probs   d) all
119. Polyoma virus can cause
   a) Subcutaneous edema   b) Subcutaneous haemorrhages
   c) Subcutaneous nodules   d) A and B
120. Dystrophic primary flight feathers caused by
   a) Mange   b) Psittacine circo virus
   c) Sarcoptes   d) All
121. Cannabilsm is also known as
   a) Feather pecking   b) Loss of hair
   c) Loss of weight   d) All
122. Metal causing feather mutilation in birds
   a) Lead   b) Zinc
   c) Iron   d) A and B
123. Which rickettsial disease can cause feather mutilation in birds
   a) Streptococci   b) Anaplasma
   c) Chlamydia   d) All
124. Mal nutrition role as self mutilation
   a) Hepatic lipidosis   b) Ketosis
   c) Obesity   d) All
125. Self mutilation prevent by providing
   a) Bones   b) Calcium
   c) Minerals   d) All
126. Nesting behavior in pet birds results in
   a) Pecking   b) Torticollis
   c) Seasonal feather self mutilation   d) All

127. Drug to prevent nesting behavior
   a) Gnrh b) LH
   c) TSH d) ACTH
128. Self mutilation prevented by application of
   a) Elizabethan collar b) Neck braces
   c) A and B d) None
129. In birds pruritus prevented by
   a) Aloe vera & Ammonium solution b) Povidone iodine
   c) Gentamicin d) All
130. Psychotropic drugs used to treat
   a) Cannibalism b) Nesting behavior
   c) Self mutilation d) All
131. Self mutilation treated with
   a) Diazepam b) Phenobarbitol
   c) Haloperidol d) All
132. Uropygial gland tumors in birds
   a) SCC b) Mast cell tumour
   c) Adeno carcinoma d) All
133. Common neoplasms affecting the dermis
   a) Mast cell tumour b) Adenoma
   c) Basal cell tumour d) Fibrosarcoma
134. Hemangioma are like —in birds
   a) Melanomas b) Adenoma
   c) A and B d) Sarcoma
135. Brown cere hypertrophy
   a) Hyperplasia of corniefied layers of cere b) Hyperplasia of tail skin
   c) Hypoplasia d) All
136. Subcutaneous air in birds due to
   a) Ruptured air sac b) Pleural injury
   c) Trauma d) All
137. Involved air sac in airsac rupture
   a) Cranial thoracic airsac b) Cervical airsac
   c) Cervicocephalic airsac d) None
138. Gland can swollen at the tail head in birds
   a) Uropygial gland b) Adrenal gland
   c) Thyroid gland d) Pineal gland
139. Medications with .... based should be avoided in birds
   a) Water based b) Powders
   c) A and B d) Oil based

140. Common feather mutilations
   a) Picking b) Plucking
   c) Chewing d) All
141. Feather cysts are ……. in nature
   a) Acquired b) Neonatal
   c) Congenital d) Genetic
142. Types of feathers in fowls
   a) Contour b) Plumules
   c) Filoplumes, Bristles d) All
143. Characteristics pin point tunnels in the skin due to
   a) Knemidocoptes spp mite b) Sarcoptes
   c) Notoedres d) Demodex
144. Follicular swelling, hyperkeratosis and crust formation in birds is due to
   a) Malassezia b) Streptococci
   c) A and B d) Dermatomycosis
145. Which is considered as under-reported syndrome related to feather destructive behavior
   a) Malassezia dermatitis b) Dermatomycosis
   c) Mange d) All
146. Localized perioccular inflammation and minimal feather loss due to
   a) Orbi virus b) Circovirus infection
   c) Morbili virus d) Adeno virus
147. Quaker mutilation syndrome is due to
   a) Viral b) Obesity
   c) Hepatic lipidosis, Lipoma d) All
148. Nodular lesions that may have a white chalky, glossy appearance due to
   a) Calcinosis b) Gout
   c) Pox d) All
149. Gangrenous dermatitis in poultry commonly noticed in
   a) Turkey b) Domestic birds
   c) Layers d) Commercial broiler production
150. Necrotization of skin areas in birds with cellulitis is due to
   a) Pyoderma b) Gangrenous dermatitis
   c) Ulcerative dermatitis d) All

Answer Key

1	c	2	a	3	d	4	c	5	a	6	a	7	b
8	d	9	b	10	c	11	d	12	d	13	a	14	d
15	a	16	d	17	a	18	c	19	a	20	d	21	c
22	c	23	a	24	a	25	c	26	b	27	d	28	d
29	a	30	a	31	d	32	b	33	c	34	d	35	c
36	c	37	d	38	b	39	b	40	d	41	d	42	c
43	c	44	a	45	b	46	d	47	d	48	d	49	d
50	a	51	d	52	b	53	d	54	a	55	d	56	b
57	d	58	c	59	d	60	d	61	b	62	b	63	a
64	d	65	d	66	b	67	d	68	d	69	a	70	d
71	d	72	a	73	b	74	d	75	d	76	c	77	c
78	b	79	a	80	c	81	c	82	a	83	d	84	c
85	d	86	d	87	a	88	c	89	a	90	c	91	b
92	c	93	d	94	d	95	a	96	c	97	a	98	d
99	c	100	c	101	a	102	c	103	d	104	a	105	c
106	b	107	a	108	b	109	c	110	b	111	b	112	a
113	d	114	d	115	d	116	a	117	b	118	b	119	d
120	b	121	d	122	d	123	c	124	a	125	d	126	c
127	a	128	c	129	a	130	d	131	d	132	a	133	d
134	a	135	a	136	d	137	c	138	a	139	d	140	d
141	d	142	d	143	a	144	d	145	a	146	b	147	d
148	a	149	d	150	b								

29

Disorders of Eye and Ear

M.P.S. Tomar[1], Rahul Singh Arya[2], Abhishek Gupta[3] and Chetna Mahajan[4]

[1]*Sri Venkateswara Veterinary University, Tirupati*

[2]*Central Agricultural University, Aizawl*

[3]*Rajasthan University of Veterinary & Animal Sciences, Bikaner*

[4]*Guru Angad Dev Veterinary & Animal Sciences University, Ludhiana*

Introduction

Eye

Avian ocular apparatus includes eyeball, optic nerve, and accessary structures e.g., eyelids, lacrimal glands, and muscles etc. The eyeball is composed of three tunics namely the fibrous (cornea and sclera), vascular (choroid, iris, ciliary body) and nervous tunic (retina). The histological structures of all these tunics are similar to mammals except the Bowman's membrane (the basal lamina of corneal epithelium) is not distinct. Similar to the mammals, they also have three refractive media viz., aqueous humour, lens, and vitreous humour. The cornea does not refract light.

There are some important diseases and disease conditions of eye in poultry birds. The common aetiology of eye diseases in poultry birds has a wide range and includes heredity, nutritional deficiency, infections (microbial and parasitic) and managemental failure. Some of them are not seen often in the modern intensive rearing systems like the deficiency diseases while others are seen associated only with the intensive system housing of birds like the ammonia burns. The infectious diseases of only eyes, are not encountered in poultry birds. The diseases like the colibacillosis, pasteurellosis and Marek's disease can affect eyes along with other body systems. Understanding of eye diseases of poultry birds requires basic knowledge of ophthalmic anatomy, concepts and terminology of eye associated pathological changes. The affected birds generally show ocular lesions and loss of condition due to starvation as they are unable to search for feed and water. Some conditions are reversible while others may be irreversible according to the extent of damage. Nutritional and managemental diseases in most cases are relatively easy to diagnose and manage, while infectious and hereditary diseases may require deeper investigation. Some diseases like endophthalmitis, eye notch syndrome and ophthalmopathy have been recorded but their causes could not be found out.

Ear

The avian ear is composed of external ear, middle ear, and inner ear. The external appendages of ear i.e., pinnae and its cartilages are absent in birds, and the external auditory meatus leads to the canal and is closed by tympanic membrane (ear drum) which separate the external ear from middle ear. The middle ear is irregular cavity and has columella (the cartilaginous rod similar to ear ossicles of mammals) and the paired auditive tubes (connection between the middle ear and pharynx). The inner ear is composed of bony and membranous labyrinths and divided in to vestibular and cochlear segments. The vestibular segment comprises of the central cavity and three semi-circular ducts while the cochlea is slightly curved tube with blind end i.e., the *lagena.* The vestibules and cochlea are filled with endolymph and the basilar membrane possess the hair cells. The vestibule is related to balance while the cochlea is related to hearing.

The pathology of ear may involve any part of ear. The external ear infections (Otitis externa) are generally bacterial or fungal in origin. The most common microbes related to it are *Pseudomonas aeuroginosa*, *Klebsiella spp.*, *Enterobacter spp.*, and *Kocuria kristinae*. The middle ear infections (Otitis media) are generally due to chronic bacterial infections and the isolated bacteria are *Enterococcus faecalis*, *Escherichia coli*, *Pasteurella multocida*, and *Pseudomonas aeuroginosa.* The most challenging problem with the middle ear infection is the involvement of opportunist bacteria, therefore, prior antibiotic sensitivity gives better results. The inner ear infections exhibit mostly the nervous signs and are mostly related to viral infections which makes them difficult to treat.

1. The bony scleral ring present in the eye of birds

   a) Os phrenis b) Ossa opticus
   c) Os penis d) Os cordis

2. The transparent fibrous layer present in front of lens is

   a) Choroid b) Ciliary body
   c) Cornea d) Sclera

3. The lining epithelium of cornea is

   a) Simple squamous b) Simple cuboidal
   c) Stratified cuboidal d) Stratified squamous

4. An internal layer of hyaline cartilage is present in .... layer of avian eye.

   a) Sclera b) Cornea
   c) Retina d) Lens

5. The posterior limiting membrane of cornea is called

   a) Descemet's membrane b) Bowman's membrane
   c) Nictitating membrane d) Iris

6. A highly vascular-pigmented membranous organ arising from the retina is called

   a) Pecten b) Iris
   c) Ciliary body d) Choroid

7. The third eyelid of bird is

   a) Well-developed but non-functional b) Ill developed but functional
   c) Vestigial d) Well-developed and functional

8. Which statement is correct
   a) Gland of third eyelids is absent in birds
   b) Gland of third eyelid is smaller than the lacrimal gland
   c) Gland of third eyelid is larger than the lacrimal gland
   d) Gland of third eyelid is similar to the lacrimal gland
9. About the avian ears, which is the correct statement
   a) The external appendages are absent
   b) It has well-developed ear pinnae
   c) The ears are absent in birds
   d) Tympanic membrane is absent in birds
10. The auditive tube is connection between
   a) External ear and middle ear
   b) Middle ear and pharynx
   c) Middle ear and internal ear
   d) External ear and pharynx
11. Which statement is correct
   a) Both auditive tubes join before opening in pharynx.
   b) Both auditive tubes are blind diverticula in birds.
   c) Both auditive tubes have separate openings in pharynx.
   d) Auditive tubes are absent in birds.
12. The only ear ossicle (cartilaginous) present in birds
   a) Malleus
   b) Incus
   c) Columella
   d) Stapes
13. The avian cochlea
   a) Forms 2.5 coils
   b) Forms slight curve
   c) Forms 1.5 coils
   d) Straight in orientation
14. The blind end of the cochlear duct carries
   a) Maculae
   b) Saccule
   c) Lagena
   d) Organ of Corti
15. The lagena
   a) Responds for lower notes to leave higher frequency for basilar membrane.
   b) Responds for higher notes to leave lower frequency for basilar membrane.
   c) Responds for lower notes to leave higher frequency for tectorial membrane.
   d) Responds for higher notes to leave lower frequency for tectorial membrane.
16. The inflammation of eyelids is called as ....
   a) Conjunctivitis
   b) Blepharitis
   c) Scleritis
   d) Keratitis
17. The inflammation of white part of eye is called as ....
   a) Conjunctivitis
   b) Blepharitis
   c) Scleritis
   d) Keratitis

18. The inflammation of cornea is called as ....
    a) Conjunctivitis
    b) Blepharitis
    c) Scleritis
    d) Keratitis
19. The inflammation of conjunctiva is called as ....
    a) Conjunctivitis
    b) Blepharitis
    c) Scleritis
    d) Keratitis
20. The inflammation of eye is called as ....
    a) Conjunctivitis
    b) Blepharitis
    c) Scleritis
    d) Ophthalmitis
21. The inflammation of tear glands of eyes is called as ....
    a) Conjunctivitis
    b) Blepharitis
    c) Dacryoadenitis
    d) Ophthalmitis
22. The inflammation of iris of eye is called as ....
    a) Iritis
    b) Blepharitis
    c) Scleritis
    d) Ophthalmitis
23. The inflammation of iris, ciliary body and choroid of the eye is called as ....
    a) Conjunctivitis
    b) Uveitis
    c) Scleritis
    d) Ophthalmitis
24. Inflammation of retina is called as ....
    a) Conjunctivitis
    b) Uveitis
    c) Retinitis
    d) Ophthalmitis
25. The opacity of the eye lens is called as ....
    a) Conjunctivitis
    b) Cataract
    c) Scleritis
    d) Ophthalmitis
26. The congenital fusion of the eyes is called as ....
    a) Cyclopia
    b) Anophthalmia
    c) Buphthalmos
    d) Triple eye
27. The congenital failure of formation of the eyes is called as ....
    a) Cyclopia
    b) Anophthalmia
    c) Buphthalmos
    d) Triple eye
28. The congenital failure of complete development leading to formation of small rudimentary eyes is called as ....
    a) Triple eye
    b) Anophthalmia
    c) Microphthalmia
    d) Cyclopia
29. The thin and bulging cornea are called as ....
    a) Corneal bulging
    b) Cataract
    c) Corneal atrophy
    d) Corneal ectasia

30. Triple eyes, optic nerve hypoplasia, cataracts, retinal dysplasia and corneal oedema seen in poultry birds are of .... origin
    a) Infectious b) Managemental
    c) Congenital d) All
31. The deficiency of vit A in chicken leads to ....
    a) Excessive lacrimation b) Eyelids stuck together
    c) Caseous deposits on eyes d) All
32. The deficiency of vit B complex in chicken leads to ....
    a) Trachoma b) Encrustations around eyelids
    c) Caseous deposits on eyes d) All
33. Ammonia burns in chicken is characterized by ....
    a) Ophthalmitis b) Blepharitis
    c) Keratoconjunctivitis d) Uveitis
34. The corneal opacity develop in birds suffering from ammonia burns due to ....
    a) Oedema b) Ulceration
    c) Inflammatory cell infiltration d) All
35. A chicken farm revealed strong putrid ammoniacal odour with off feed emaciated birds showing signs of photophobia, excess lacrimation, rubbing of head and eyelids against wings, grey cloudy or ulcerated cornea, variable conjunctival congestion and respiratory distress, the disease is ....
    a) Vit A deficiency b) CRD
    c) RD d) Ammonia burns
36. Microscopic lesions of the ammonia burns in the eye are: necrosis of the epithelium of the cornea, ulceration, and infiltration into the epithelium and substantia propria by the ....
    a) Heterophils b) Lymphocytes
    c) Fibroblasts d) Macrophages
37. Cataract in chicken can be caused by ....
    a) Avian encephalomyelitis virus b) Vit-E deficiency
    c) Heredity d) All
38. Histopathological lesions of degeneration of lens fibres, epithelial hyperplasia, formation of bladder cells and liquefaction in advance stages, are characteristic of .....
    a) Conjunctivitis b) Cataract
    c) Scleritis d) Ophthalmitis
39. Gray eyes with misshapen iris in chicken are caused by ....
    a) Marek's disease b) Vit A deficiency
    c) Congenital microphthalmia d) Ophthalmitis
40. Gray eyes in Marek's disease infected chicken develops due to ....
    a) Keratitis b) Cataract
    c) Infiltration of MDV infected cells in iris d) All

41. The congenital enlargement of the eyes is called as ....
    a) Cyclops b) Anophthalmia
    c) Buphthalmos d) Ophthalmitis
42. The congenital retinal dysplasia is inherited .... gene
    a) Autosomal recessive b) Autosomal dominant
    c) Sex chromosomal d) Mitochondrial
43. Chorioretinitis is the inflammation of type of posterior uveitis affecting ....
    a) Lens only b) Retina only
    c) Choroid and retina both d) Lens and retina both
44. Turkey blindness syndrome seen in turkey's raised on artificial light is characterized by ....
    a) Chorioretinitis and Buphthalmos b) Cyclops
    c) Anophthalmia d) Cataract
45. Ossifying cartilage in posterior chamber of eye in turkey are seen in disease ....
    a) Xerophthalmia b) Marek's disease
    c) Cataract d) Turkey blindness syndrome
46. Blepharoconjunctivitis characterized by excess lacrimation, later white frothy foam at the anterior canthus followed by accumulation of caseous exudate, the eyelids are swollen, encrusted & closed, presence of corneal ulcerations and later panophthalmitis, are seen in ocular infection of ....
    a) *Pasteurella multocida* b) Marek's disease
    c) *Mycoplasma* d) *E. coli*
47. Eye notch syndrome of caged layers of unknown aetiology is microscopically ....
    a) Blepharoconjunctivitis b) Panophthalmitis
    c) Retinitis d) Uveitis
48. Inflammation of complete Eye ball is called as ....
    a) Blepharoconjunctivitis b) Panophthalmitis
    c) Keratoconjunctivitis d) Uveoretinitis
49. Turkey blindness syndrome is causes by ....
    a) Vit A deficiency b) *E coli*
    c) Ammonia d) Rearing on artificial light
50. An eye disease of broiler chicken of unknown aetiology characterized grossly by pupillary opacity, cataract, detachment & thickening of retina, shrinking of vitreous humour and microscopically by presence of granulation tissue throughout the eye with atrophy of optic nerves is ....
    a) Blepharoconjunctivitis b) Panophthalmitis
    c) Endophthalmitis d) Uveitis

51. Eye worm found in poultry is-
    a) *Oxyspirura mansoni* b) *Thelazia rhodesii*
    c) *Gangylonema pulchurum* d) None
52. Which of the following is responsible for the blindness in poultry
    a) *Ceratophyllus gallinae* b) *Echidnophaga gallinacean*
    c) *Tunga penetrans* d) *Goniocotes gallinae*
53. What is the common name for the parasitic infection caused by *Thelazia spp.* in poultry eyes?
    a) Avian coccidiosis b) Avian leukosis
    c) Avian conjunctivitis d) Avian eyeworm disease
54. Which of the following is a preventative measure against parasitic eye diseases in poultry?
    a) Vaccination b) Antibiotic treatment
    c) Providing vitamin supplements d) Environmental sanitation
55. Which of the following parasites commonly affects the external ear canal of poultry, leading to irritation and discomfort?
    a) *Ascaridia galli* b) *Syngamus trachea*
    c) *Oxyspirura mansoni* d) *Ornithonyssus sylviarum*
56. Which nematode parasite is responsible for causing conjunctivitis and corneal lesions in poultry?
    a) *Toxoplasma gondii* b) *Thelazia spp.*
    c) *Histomonas meleagridis* d) *Haemoproteus spp.*
57. Which of the following measures is effective in preventing parasitic eye and ear disorders in poultry?
    a) Providing antihistamine supplements
    b) Isolating infected birds
    c) Using insecticide-treated bedding
    d) Administering deworming medication orally
58. Parasites infesting the conjunctival sac, causing irritation, lacrimation, and in severe cases, corneal ulcers
    a) *Oxyspirura mansoni* b) *Thelezia gulosa*
    c) Both of these d) None of these
59. Single-celled parasites that can cause ocular lesions in poultry leading to conjunctivitis, corneal opacity, and in some cases, granulomatous inflammation in the eye tissues
    a) *Ascaridia galli* b) *Syngamus trachea*
    c) *Oxyspirura mansoni* d) *Encephalitozoon hellem*
60. Kerato-conjunctivitis is associated with which of the following infection in poultry
    a) Microsporidiosis b) Coccidiosis
    c) Ascariosis d) All of these

61. The retina may show detachment in
    a) Marek's disease
    b) Vit A deficiency
    c) Congenital microphthalmia
    d) Ophthalmitis
62. Which vitamin deficiency can lead to eye problems such as swelling and cloudiness in poultry?
    a) Vitamin D
    b) Vitamin E
    c) Vitamin A
    d) Vitamin B12
63. What mineral deficiency is associated with eye disorders like blindness and cataracts in poultry?
    a) Calcium
    b) Iron
    c) Zinc
    d) Magnesium
64. Which vitamin deficiency can cause dryness and irritation of the eyes in poultry?
    a) Vitamin K
    b) Vitamin C
    c) Vitamin A
    d) Vitamin B6
65. Lack of which mineral can result in eye abnormalities and impaired vision in poultry?
    a) Phosphorus
    b) Selenium
    c) Potassium
    d) Sodium
66. What vitamin deficiency can lead to decreased tear production and eye inflammation in poultry?
    a) Vitamin A
    b) Vitamin D
    c) Vitamin B12
    d) Vitamin E
67. Which vitamin deficiency can lead to ear problems such as head tilt and balance issues in poultry?
    a) Vitamin C
    b) Vitamin D
    c) Vitamin B12
    d) Vitamin E
68. What mineral deficiency is associated with inner ear disorders and hearing loss in poultry?
    a) Calcium
    b) Iron
    c) Zinc
    d) Magnesium
69. Which vitamin deficiency can cause inflammation and infection of the ear canal in poultry?
    a) Vitamin K
    b) Vitamin A
    c) Vitamin B6
    d) Vitamin E
70. Lack of which mineral can result in ear abnormalities and impaired hearing in poultry?
    a) Phosphorus
    b) Selenium
    c) Potassium
    d) Sodium
71. What vitamin deficiency can lead to decreased ear function and balance problems in poultry?
    a) Vitamin A
    b) Vitamin D
    c) Vitamin B12
    d) Vitamin E

72. In poultry suffering from Vitamin A deficiency, which of the following biochemical processes is most likely affected in the eye?
   a) Increased synthesis of rhodopsin
   b) Decreased synthesis of retinol-binding protein
   c) Increased synthesis of tear film components
   d) Decreased synthesis of visual pigments
73. Which biochemical pathway is primarily involved in the pathogenesis of zinc deficiency-related ear diseases in poultry?
   a) Glycolysis b) Krebs cycle
   c) DNA replication d) Protein synthesis
74. In Vitamin E deficiency-related ear disorders in poultry, which of the following biochemical roles of Vitamin E is compromised?
   a) Antioxidant protection of cell membranes
   b) Coenzyme function in electron transport chain
   c) Regulation of calcium homeostasis
   d) Synthesis of haem in haemoglobin
75. Which biochemical marker is often elevated in poultry with ear infections caused by bacterial pathogens?
   a) C-reactive protein (CRP) b) Alanine aminotransferase (ALT)
   c) Creatinine kinase (CK) d) Lipase
76. In avian species, which biochemical mechanism is critical for maintaining the balance of ions and fluids in the inner ear, contributing to proper auditory function?
   a) Activation of Na+/K+-ATPase pump
   b) Inhibition of calcium channels
   c) Increase in GABAergic neurotransmission
   d) Suppression of glutamate receptors

Answer Key

1	b	2	c	3	d	4	a	5	a	6	a	7	d
8	c	9	a	10	b	11	a	12	c	13	b	14	c
15	a	16	b	17	c	18	d	19	a	20	d	21	c
22	a	23	b	24	c	25	b	26	a	27	b	28	c
29	d	30	c	31	d	32	b	33	c	34	d	35	d
36	a	37	d	38	b	39	a	40	c	41	c	42	a
43	c	44	a	45	d	46	a	47	a	48	b	49	d
50	c	51	a	52	b	53	c	54	d	55	d	56	b
57	d	58	c	59	d	60	a	61	a	62	c	63	c
64	c	65	b	66	d	67	a	68	c	69	b	70	b
71	a	72	d	73	d	74	a	75	a	76	a		

30

Disorder of Hemolyphatic and Immune System

Ganesh K. Sawale[1] *and G.P. Bharkad*[2]

[1]*Department of Veterinary Pathology, Mumbai Veterinary College, Parel, Mumbai*

[2]*Department of Veterinary Parasitology, College of Veterinary & Animal Sciences Udgir, Maharashtra*

Introduction

Disorders of the hemopoietic system in poultry can significantly impact the health and productivity of these birds. The hemopoietic system is responsible for the production of blood cells, including red blood cells, white blood cells, and platelets. Disorders within this system can lead to various health issues, including anemia, immunodeficiency, and impaired blood clotting. Some of the common disorders of hemopoietic system include:

1. **Anemia**: Anemia is a condition characterized by a decrease in the number of red blood cells or hemoglobin in the blood. In poultry, anemia can be caused by various factors, including nutritional deficiencies (such as iron deficiency), infectious diseases (such as avian malaria or chicken infectious anemia), and parasitic infestations (such as blood-sucking parasites like *leucocytozooncaulleryi*, ticks, lice and mites).
2. **Avian Leukosis**:Avian leucosis is a viral disease caused by avian leukosis virus (ALV). It primarily affects young birds, causing tumors in various organs, including the spleen, liver, and bursa of Fabricius. Avian leukosis can lead to immunosuppression, anemia, and increased susceptibility to secondary infections. The avian leucosis diseases include lymphoid leucosis (affecting lymphoid cells), myeloid leucosis (affecting myeloid cells), osteoptrosis, etc. and can result in immunodeficiency, increased susceptibility to infections, and other systemic symptoms. It also affects blood-forming tissues, including the bone marrow and lymphatic system, leading to an overproduction of abnormal white blood cells.
3. **Thrombocytopenia**: Thrombocytopenia is a condition characterized by a low platelet count, which can impair blood clotting. It can be caused by viral infections (such as avian leukosis virus), toxic substances, immune-mediated destruction of platelets, or certain medications.
4. **Hemorrhagic disorders**: Disorders affecting blood clotting can lead to hemorrhage or excessive bleeding. These disorders may be inherited (such as hemophilijn a) or acquired (such as vitamin K deficiency or exposure to certain toxins).

5. **Nutritional deficiencies**: Deficiencies in essential nutrients like iron, vitamin B12, and folic acid can impair the production of blood cells, leading to various hematopoietic disorders.

Lymphatic system disorders are rare in poultry.

The immune system is essential for defending the body against pathogens, including bacteria, viruses, fungi, and parasites. Disorders of the immune system in poultry can result from various factors, including infectious agents, nutritional deficiencies, genetic predispositions, and environmental stressors. The common disorders of immune system includes:

1. **Immunosuppression/ immunodeficiency disorders**: Immunosuppression is defined as "A state of temporary or permanent dysfunction of the immune response resulting from insults to the immune system and leading to increased susceptibility to disease with suboptimal innate and cell-mediated responses (Schat and Skinner, 2014).Immunodeficiency disorders in poultry can result in compromised immune function, leading to increased susceptibility to infections. These disorders can be congenital or acquired and may affect innate immunity, cellular immunity, or humoral immunity. Examples include congenital immunodeficiency syndromes and acquired immunodeficiency due to viral infections like Marek's disease or infectious bursal disease (Schat and Skinner, 2014).
2. **Infectious Diseases**: Various infectious agents can directly affect the immune system of poultry, leading to immunosuppression or dysregulation. For example, viruses like avian influenza virus, Newcastle disease virus, infectious bursal disease virus, Marek's disease virus, chicken anaemia virus, and avian leukosis virus can directly infect immune cells or impair immune function, leading to increased susceptibility to secondary infections.
3. **Autoimmune Disorders**: Autoimmune disorders occur when the immune system mistakenly targets and attacks the body's own tissues. While autoimmune disorders are less common in poultry compared to mammals, they can still occur and lead to various health issues, including organ damage and systemic inflammation (Erf, 2022).
4. **Stress-induced immunosuppression**: Environmental stressors such as high stocking densities, poor ventilation, temperature extremes, and transportation can induce stress in poultry, leading to immunosuppression. Stress hormones like corticosterone can modulate immune function, making birds more susceptible to infections.
5. **Nutritional Immunodeficiency**: Nutritional deficiencies, particularly of essential nutrients like vitamins (e.g., vitamin A, vitamin D, vitamin E), minerals (e.g., zinc, selenium), and amino acids, can compromise immune function in poultry. Proper nutrition is essential for maintaining optimal immune health and disease resistance.
6. **Allergic Reactions**: While less common in poultry, allergic reactions can occur, leading to hypersensitivity responses and inflammation. Allergens may include certain feed ingredients, environmental contaminants, or microbial antigens.
7. **Vaccination Failure**: Improper vaccination protocols, vaccine handling, or inadequate immune responses to vaccines can result in vaccination failure, leaving birds susceptible to preventable diseases.

Diagnosis of hemolyphatic and immune system disorders in poultry typically involves a combination of clinical examination, laboratory testing (including serological assays, histopathology, and molecular diagnostics), and assessment of management practices. Treatment and management strategies depend on the specific disorder and may include vaccination, antimicrobial therapy, nutritional supplementation, environmental management, and stress reduction. Prevention strategies focus on implementing biosecurity measures, maintaining optimal nutrition and management practices, vaccination programs, and minimizing stressors to support immune health and overall flock welfare.

1. The primary lymphoid organs of birds includes
   a) Thymus b) Spleen
   c) Caecal tonsil d) All of these
2. The primary lymphoid organs of birds includes
   a) Thymus b) Bursa of fabricious
   c) Spleen d) Only a and b
3. The lymphoid system of poultry includes all except
   a) Thymus b) Bursa of fabricious
   c) Lymph node d) Caecal tonsil
4. The secondary lymphoid organs of birds includes all except
   a) Harderian gland b) Bursa of fabricious
   c) Spleen d) Caecal tonsil
5. The infectious agent which multiply in lymphoid organs and causes of immuno-suppression includes the all except
   a) Marek;s disease b) Infectious bursal disease
   c) Rickets d) Chicken infectious anaemia
6. The infectious agent which multiply in lymphoid organs and causes of immuno-suppression includes the all except
   a) Lymphoid leucosis b) Reo viruses
   c) Reticuloendotheliosis d) Ascites
7. The most striking feature of mycotoxicosis in poultry is
   a) Increase body weight of chicken
   b) Decrease fatty liver syndrome incidences
   c) Immunosuppression
   d) All of these
8. The non-infectious causes of immunosuppression includes the following except
   a) Stress b) Lead toxicity
   c) Corticosteroid therapy d) High protein diet
9. In poultry, the humoral mediated immunity is mediated by
   a) B cell b) T cell
   c) Both a and b d) None of these

10. In poultry, the cell mediated immunity is mediated by
    a) B cell b) T cell
    c) Both a and b d) None of these
11. The following statement(s) is/are true with regards to involution of Thymus and Bursa of fabricious in birds
    a) At the onset of sexual maturity b) At the age of 4 month of age
    c) Both a and b are true d) All are the statements are false
12. In adult birds, role of immunity is played by
    a) Thymus b) Bursa of Fabricious
    c) Bone marrow d) All of these
13. The T (lymphocytes) cellmature and differentiate in
    a) Thymus b) Bursa of Fabricious
    c) Spleen d) Caecal tonsil
14. The B (lymphocytes) cell mature and differentiate in
    a) Thymus b) Bursa of Fabricious
    c) Spleen d) Caecal tonsil
15. In humoral immunity, the predominant antibody generated in primary immune response i.e immediately after infection is
    a) IgG b) IgM
    c) IgA d) IgY
16. In humoral immunity, the predominant antibody generated in secondary immune response
    a) IgG b) IgM
    c) IgA d) IgY
17. The most common antibody found in natural secretions is
    a) IgG b) IgM
    c) IgA d) IgY
18. The antibody maternally transferred to chick via yolk is
    a) IgG b) IgM
    c) IgA d) IgY
19. The highest concentration of antibody maternally transferred to chick was found on
    a) Day of hatch b) Day two of age of chick
    c) Day five of ageof chick d) Day 10 of ageof chick
20. In birds, the antibodies are produced by
    a) B cell b) T cell
    c) Spleen d) Antigen presenting cell

21. The following statements are true for cell mediated immunity (CMI) of chicken except
    a) CMI play major role in destruction of virus infected cells
    b) CMI playsa role in destruction of*Mycobacterium avium*
    c) CMI plays a role in destruction of intracellular fungi
    d) CMI plays a role in antibody mediated killing of bacteria
22. The aflatoxin depresses immunity by following mechanism except
    a) Depresses complement activity
    b) Decreases phagocytic activity
    c) Inhibition of thymic associated lymphocytes
    d) By increases in protein synthesis
23. The following statements are true for viral causes of immunosuppression in wild birds except
    a) The psittacine beak and feather disease virus
    b) Circovirus
    c) Avian coronavirus
    d) Avian polyomavirus
24. The psittacine beak and feather disease virus (PBFDV) is a immunosuppressive disease of parrots caused by
    a) Avian reovirus *b)* Circovirus
    c) Avian rota virus d) Herpes virus
25. The target organs for psittacine beak and feather disease virus includes all except
    a) Bursa *b)* Thymus
    c) Epidermis d) Lung
26. The diagnosis of psittacine beak and feather disease virus includes
    a) Intranuclear inclusion body in macrophages and lymphocytes
    b) Intracytoplasmic inclusion body in macrophages and lymphocytes
    c) Eosinophilicintranuclear inclusion bodies in epithelial cells
    d) All of these
27. The avian polyoma virus diseases is a immunosuppressive disease seen in
    a) Parrot *b)* Finch
    c) Budgerigar d) All of these
28. Cryptosporidiosis in chicken is a protozoan parasite with target organ(s) includes
    a) Intestinal mucosa *b)* Bursa of Fabricious
    c) Tracheal mucosa d) All of these
29. The following statement(s) is/ are true for Cryptosporidiosis in chicken
    a) It is immunosuppressive protozoan disease of chicken
    b) It is protozoan disease of chicken seen after immunosuppression
    c) Its target organ is liver
    d) It may also affect cardiovascular system

30. Cryptosporidiosis in chicken is a protozoan parasite commonly occurs in concurrent with
    a) Chicken infectious anaemia
    b) Infectious bursal disease
    c) The psittacine beak and feather disease in parrots
    d) All of these
31. The neoplastic (tumour) disease of Bursa of Fabricious is seen due to
    a) Lymphoid leucosis
    b) Mareks disease virus
    c) Reticuluendothelial virus
    d) All of these
32. The Pacheco's disease is an immunosuppressive disease commonly seen in
    a) Hawks
    b) Falcons
    c) Parrots
    d) All of these
33. The Pacheco's disease is an immunosuppressive disease of parrots caused by
    a) Avian reovirus
    b) Circovirus
    c) Herpes virus
    d) Retrovirus
34. The following statement(s) is/ are true for diagnosis of Pacheco's disease in parrot
    a) Intranucleareosinophilic inclusion bodies in Histocytes
    b) Lymphoid tumours in bursa of Fabricious
    c) Lymphoproliferation in skin epithelium
    d) None of these
35. The Lymphoid leucosis is immunosuppressive and neoplastic disease of chicken caused by
    a) Avian reovirus
    b) Circovirus
    c) Herpes virus
    d) Retrovirus
36. Methyl green pyronin staining is used for diagnosis of
    a) Marek's disease
    b) Erythroid leucosis
    c) Lymphoid leucosis
    d) Myeloid leucosis
37. Uniform population of lymphocytes on cytology of poultry tumor is seen in
    a) Marek's disease
    b) Erythroid leucosis
    c) Myeloid leucosis
    d) Lymphoid leucosis
    e) None of these
38. Gumboro disease is immunosuppressive disease of chicken caused by a
    a) Double stranded RNA virus
    b) Single stranded RNA virus
    c) Double stranded DNA virus
    d) Single stranded DNA virus
39. The RIF is a test is used for the diagnosis of one of the immunospressive disease
    a) Marek's disease
    b) Avian Leukosis Complex
    c) New Castle disease
    d) All of the above
40. The Marek's Disease virus matures and reaches fully infectious stage in
    a) Skin epithelium
    b) Spleen
    c) Gastrointestinal tract
    d) Brain

41. The target cell for Marek's disease virus is
    a) T-lymphocytes b) B-lymphocytes
    c) Plasma cell d) Macrophages
42. The target cell for Lymphoid leucosis virus is
    a) T-lymphocytes b) B-lymphocytes
    c) Plasma cell d) Macrophages
43. The Marek's disease is immunosuppressive disease of chicken caused by
    a) Avian reovirus b) Circovirus
    c) Herpes virus d) Retrovirus
44. Marek's disease is an immunosuppressive disease of chicken clinically characterized by
    a) Neural form in grower birds b) Visceral form in adult birds
    c) Both a and b d) None of these
45. Neural form of Marek's disease is most commonly seen in birds of age group
    a) 4-10 wks b) 10-20 wks
    c) 20-30 wks d) 30-40 wks
46. Cytological examination of sample collected from tumour masses ofMarek's disease affected bird show
    a) Uniform population of lymphocytes
    b) Pleomorphic population of lymphocytes
    c) Only lymphoblast
    d) None of these
47. Infectious bursal disease is an immunosuppressive disease of chicken caused by
    a) Corona virus b) Avibirna virus
    c) Avian rota virus d) Avian paramyxovirus
48. Infectious bursal disease is an immunosuppressive disease of chicken commonly called as
    a) Ranikhet disease b) Gumboro disease
    c) Hjarre's disease d) All of these
49. The main target organ for Gumboro disease in chicken is
    a) Liver b) Kidney
    c) Bursa of Fabricious d) None of these
50. The primary target organs for Gumboro disease in chicken is
    a) Spleen b) Liver
    c) Bone marrow d) Bursa of Fabricious
51. The important diagnostic gross lesions of Gumboro disease in chicken include
    a) Enteritis
    b) Enlargement of liver
    c) Enlarged and haemorrhagic Bursa of Fabricious
    d) Enlarged thymus

52. The chicken infectious anaemia is immunosuppressive disease of chicken caused by
    a) Avian gyrovirus b) Avian rota virus
    c) Herpes virus d) Retrovirus
53. The primary target organforchicken infectious anaemia is
    a) Bone marrow b) Thymus
    c) Heart d) Only a and b
54. Theclinical signs of chicken infectious anaemia are primarily seen in
    a) Grower age (6-12 weeks) b) Mid lay age
    c) Old age (>50 weeks) d) All of these
55. Clinically, chicken infectious anaemia is characterized by
    a) Anaemia b) Leucopenia
    c) Thrombocytopenia d) All of these
56. Chicken infectious anaemia, a immunosuppressive disease of chicken is caused by
    a) Single stranded RNA virus b) Single stranded DNA virus
    c) Double stranded RNA virus d) Double stranded DNA virus
57. In India, chicken infectious anaemia, an immunosuppressive disease is major issue in
    a) Broiler type birds b) Layer type birds
    c) Broiler parent birds d) None of these
58. In USA, chicken infectious anaemia, an immunosuppressive disease is major issue in
    a) Broiler type birds b) Layer type birds
    c) Layer parent birds d) None of these
59. The mechanism of immunosuppression in stress in birds is due to release of
    a) Alkaline phosphatase b) Corticosterone
    c) Histamine d) All of these
60. The mechanism of immunosuppression in aflatoxin toxicity in birds is due to
    a) Binding of epoxide to DNA b) Cytotoxicity to lymphoid cells
    c) Release of corticosterone d) Both a and b
61. The bioactivation of aflatoxinB_1in liver is due to
    a) Aflatoxin-aldehyde reductase b) Glutathione-S-transferases
    c) Cytochrome P450 d) None of these
62. The immunosuppression in Infectious bursal disease id mediated through
    a) Cytochrome P450 b) Production of iNOS by $CD4^+$
    c) Production of Nitric oxide d) Only b and c
63. The necrosis and apoptosis in lymphoid cellsis major cause of immunosuppression in
    a) Infectious bursal disease virus infection
    b) Chicken infectious anaemia virus infection
    c) Marek's disease virus infection
    d) All of these

64. The common causes of anaemia in poultry includes the following except
   a) *Plasmodium* parasites b) *Leucocytozooncaulleryi*
   c) Vitamin A deficiency d) Chicken anaemia virus
65. The main target cells for *Plasmodium* parasites in birds is
   a) White blood cell b) Red blood cell
   c) Platelets d) None of these
66. The Avian malaria in chicken is transmitted by
   a) Mosquitoes b) Ticks
   c) Mites d) All of these
67. The Leucocytozoonosis in chicken is transmitted by
   a) *Leucocytozooncaulleryi* b) *Cryptocporidiumbaileyi*
   c) *Plasmodium spp.* d) All of these
68. The main target cells for *Leucocytozooncaulleryi*in birds is
   a) Epithelial cell b) Red blood cell
   c) Histiocytes d) None of these
69. The protozoan diseases of birds associated with anaemia includes all except
   a) Coccidiosis b) Haemproteus infection
   c) Leucocytozoonosis d) Histomoniasis
70. The Haemproteus infection associated with anaemia is mainly seen in
   a) Pigeon b) Turkey
   c) Quails d) All of these
71. The main target cell for Haemproteus parasite (gamotes) in birds is
   a) White blood cell b) Red blood cells
   c) Platelets d) All of these
72. One of the important clinical sign of Haemproteus in birds is
   a) Diarrhoea b) Anaemia
   c) Torticolis d) All of these
73. The Haemproteusinfection in pigeon is caused by
   a) *Leucocytozooncaulleryi* b) *Cryptocporidiumbaileyi*
   c) *Plasmodium vivax* d) *Haemoproteuscolumbae*
74. The natural host for *Haemoproteuscolumbae*is
   a) Birds b) Pigeon
   c) Peacock d) All of these
75. The *Haemoproteuscolumbae*in poultry is transmitted by
   a) Tick b) Mites
   c) Louse flies d) Mosquitoes

76. The immune mediated disorders of poultry reported worldwide include following except
    a) Idiopathic pulmonary arterial hypertension
    b) Ovarian autoimmune disease
    c) Epididymallithiasis in roosters
    d) Salmonellosis
77. One of the best chicken model to study spontaneous Hashimoto thyroiditis is
    a) White leghorn b) Obese-strain chicken
    c) Rhode Island Red d) Smyth-Line chicken
78. One of the best chicken model to study autoimmune vitiligois
    a) White leghorn b) Obese-strain chicken
    c) Rhode Island Red d) Smyth-Line chicken
79. In autoimmune Vitiligo, the antibodyare produced against
    a) Melanin pigment b) Melanocyte
    c) Both of these d) None of these
80. The most common cause of thrombocytopenia in chicken is
    a) *Escherchia coli* b) Chicken infectious anaemia virus
    c) Avian reo virus d) Vitamin A deficiency
81. One of the disease associated with thrombocytopenia in chicken is
    a) Avian leucosis virus b) *Salmonella galinarum*
    c) Avian nephritis virus d) Vitamin B_{12} deficiency
82. The causes of stress induced immunosuppression includes
    a) High stocking density b) High temperature
    c) Transportaion d) All of these
83. The nutritional causes of anaemia in birds includes all except
    a) Iron deficiency b) Copper deficiency
    c) Vitamin B_{12} deficiency d) Vitamin A deficiency
84. The haemorrhagic disorders in birds seen in
    a) Vitamin K deficiency b) Infectious bursal disease virus
    c) Chicken anaemia virus d) All of these
85. The vaccination failure in poultry is associated with
    a) Infectious bursal disease virus b) Marek's disease virus
    c) Chicken anaemia virus d) All of these
86. The vaccination failure in poultry is associated with
    a) Mycotoxin toxicity b) Salmonellosis
    c) Vitamin K deficiency d) None of these

References

Schat KA, Skinner MA. Avian Immunosuppressive Diseases and Immunoevasion.Avian Immunology. 2014:275–97. doi: 10.1016/B978-0-12-396965-1.00016-9. Epub 2013 Jul 12. PMCID: PMC7150009.

Erf GF. Autoimmune diseases of poultry.In:Avian Immunology 2022 Jan 1 (pp. 437-455). Academic Press.

Answer Key

1	a	2	d	3	c	4	b	5	c	6	d	7	c
8	d	9	a	10	b	11	c	12	c	13	a	14	b
15	b	16	a	17	c	18	a	19	b	20	a	21	d
22	d	23	c	24	b	25	d	26	d	27	d	28	d
29	b	30	d	31	d	32	d	33	c	34	a	35	d
36	c	37	d	38	a	39	b	40	a	41	a	42	b
43	c	44	c	45	a	46	b	47	b	48	b	49	c
50	d	51	c	52	a	53	d	54	a	55	d	56	b
57	b	58	a	59	b	60	d	61	c	62	d	63	d
64	c	65	b	66	a	67	a	68	b	69	d	70	d
71	b	72	b	73	d	74	b	75	c	76	d	77	b
78	d	79	b	80	b	81	a	82	d	83	d	84	d
85	d	86	a										

31

Production and Metabolic Disorders

Bhavanam Sudhakara Reddy*, Sirigireddy Sivajothi, Rangappagari Tejeswar Reddy & Dadireddy Narmada Raghavi

College of Veterinary Science - Proddatur, Sri Venkateswara Veterinary University Andhra Pradesh, India

Metabolic disorders are classed as illness associated with a failure in one of the body hormone or enzyme systems, storage disease related to lack of metabolism of secretory products because of the lack of production of a specific enzyme, or the failure or reduced activity of some metabolic function. There are numerous genetic, metabolic disorders in poultry but these are rare in commercial poultry. In poultry it is usual to include under the heading of metabolic disorders those conditions associated with increased metabolism, rapid growth rate or high egg production that result in the failure of a body system because of the increased work-load on that organ or system. Metabolic disorders that result from an increase production of, or deficiency of or failure in the production, synthesis, or transport of an enzyme, hormone or secretary mechanism. Metabolic disorders that result from high nutrient intake, rapid growth, high metabolic rate, pulmonary or systemic hypertension, and high egg production or a rapid increase in egg production. Other conditions that could be classed as metabolic disorders related to: (a) management defects; (b) nutritional deficiency or excess; (c) infectious agents; (d) toxins.

In poultry two defects of amino acid metabolisms, tyrosinase-positive albinism and protein binding riboflavin uria; one defect of lipid metabolism, hyperlipidaemia, two defects in connective tissue, muscle and bone, inherited muscular dystrophy, two defects in transport, ADH-responsive (kidney) nephrogenic diabetes and uric acid. Increased metabolism, rapid growth or high egg production that results in the failure of a body system because of the increased work-load on an organ or system. These make up the largest group of poultry diseases classified as metabolic disorders and cause more economic loss than infectious agents. Poultry metabolic diseases occur primarily in two body systems: (1) cardiovascular ailments, which in broiler chickens and turkeys are responsible for a major portion of the flock mortality; (2) musculoskeletal disorders, which account for less mortality, but in broilers and turkeys slow down growth (thereby reducing profit), and cause lameness, which remains a major welfare concern. In addition, conditions such as osteoporosis and hypocalcaemia in table-egg chickens reduce egg production and can kill.

Fatty liver and kidney syndrome which is a biotin deficiency-related metabolic disease in broiler and layers chicks of 2–3 weeks of age. When the bird is subject to a mild stress through high or low temperatures, a lighting failure or short term fasting, liver glycogen reserves become rapidly depleted and a progressive hypoglycemia develops that ultimately proves fatal. Affected chicks are hyperlipaemic showing increase in the free fatty acid and triglyceride levels in the plasma and there is a 2- to 5-fold increase in the lipid content of the liver and kidneys. Ascites is caused by an increased production or decreased removal of peritoneal lymph results in accumulation of serous fluid in body cavity leading to carcass condemnation or death. The etiology of ascites may be associated with the typical lesions, like obstruction of lymph drainage, decreased plasma oncotic pressure, increased vascular permeability and increased hydrostatic pressure in the vascular system. The most frequent cause of ascites in birds is increased portal pressure, secondary to right ventricular failure (RVF) or liver damage. Genetic selection of broilers for fast growth rate or body weight gain predisposes them for ascites compared with slow-growing strains, because a fast growth rate increases the demand for oxygen and hence the workload on the heart predispose broiler for the development of pulmonary hypertension syndrome. Presence of major antioxidant compounds such as vitamin E, selenium, vitamin A, vitamin C, and glutathione in the circulation or at the level of the respiratory membrane plays vital role in protecting damage at cellular levels, prevent the induction of hypoxia and thus reduce the incidence of ascites. Sudden death syndrome is normally occurs in healthy, fast-growing, commercial broilers. In fast growing broilers have a large proportion of muscles compared to visceral organs which are not proportionally developed leading to inadequate supply of oxygen to muscles, which leads to hypoxic condition. Lack of aerobic metabolism in hypoxic condition result in production of more lactate leads to systemic acidosis, change in blood pH, cardiovascular disturbance leads cardiac failure" which increases the incidence of sudden death syndrome. More feed intake and continuous lighting for long period of time in broiler house results in higher mortality due to sudden death syndrome compared to intermittent lighting. The incidence of non-infectious leg problems such as chondrodystrophy, valgus-varus deformities, spondylolisthesis are probably related to rapid growth of broiler chickens. The production of strong tissue, remodeling and alignment of bone requires more time than rapid growth allows. The use of management methods to reduce metabolic diseases by decreasing feed consumption, without increasing mineral concentration in the pre-starter diet, affect the healthy bone development and predisposes the broilers for different leg problems. It can be reduced by slowing early growth and by extended daily rest (dark) periods. Vitamin D plays important role in proliferating chondrocytes, deficiency of this leads to Tibial dyschondroplasia and ratio of Ca and P in the diet also plays vital role and influence the incidence and severity of tibial dyschondroplasia in broiler chicken. Birds excrete nitrogenous wastes as urates bound in colloidal form with mucus in their urine. Renal dysfunction decreases the clearance of uric acid from the blood, which results in hyperuricemia with precipitation of insoluble products within the kidney itself or other organs, leading to urate deposition or urolithiasis. Visceral urate deposition occurs after rapidly progressing renal failure or as a terminal event with acute decompensation of chronic renal disease. Deposits develop most commonly on the pericardium, peritoneum, and liver capsule and rarely on synovial surfaces of joints and tendons. Predisposing factors for visceral urate deposition and urolithiasis in poultry include infectious bronchitis virus, avian nephritis virus, and cryptosporidiosis. Noninfectious causes include dehydration, ingestion of feed containing > 3% calcium by nonlaying chickens, vitamin A deficiency, and exposure to myotoxins (eg, oosporein). Other avian species commonly develop visceral deposits secondary to nephrotoxin exposure, most commonly aminoglycoside antibiotics or heavy metals. Articular urate deposition is less common and occurs after longterm increases in serum levels of uric acid. Deposits develop on synovial membranes in the toes and wing joints and incite a chronic granulomatous reaction to urate crystals. Joints are enlarged, and the feet appear deformed. Articular urate deposition may be seen in birds that have hereditary defects in uric acid metabolism or that are fed excessive protein.

Write correct alphabet of the answer in the given bracket

1. Selection of fast growing broilers leads to
   a) Leucosis b) Anemia
   c) Ascites d) All
2. It is a biotin deficiency-related metabolic disease in broiler and layers chicks of ...
   a) 6-8 weeks of age b) 2–3 weeks of age
   c) 12–13 weeks of age d) All
3. Pink disease in birds
   a) Hepatitis b) Fatty liver
   c) Nephitis d) Gastritis
4. To avoid metabolic diseases in birds....
   a) Provision of thermo neutral environment
   b) Growth curve manipulation
   c) Supplementation of Antioxidants
   d) All
5. Which limiting amino acid deficiency in poultry feed causes impaired pigmentation of bronze turkey poultry and results in stunting and retard development in chick?
   a) leucine b) methionine
   c) arginine d) lysine
6. Which limiting amino acid deficiency in poultry feed causes the wing feathers to curl upward giving the chick a distinct ruffled appearance
   a) Leucine b) Methionine
   c) Arginine d) Lysine
7. A large excess protein diet in poultry diet can cause
   a) Hyperuricemia b) Articular goat
   c) A & B d) None
8. Most toxic limiting amino acid for poultry birds when they are feed with excess amount of corn and soya bean diet
   a) Leucine b) Methionine
   c) Lysine d) Cysteine
9. High levels of dietary protein/ methionine in poultry diet causes
   a) Metabolic acidosis b) Bone mineralization
   c) Thinning of egg shell d) All of the above
10. Crazy chick disease in poultry birds is due to which vitamin deficiency
    a) Vitamin E b) Vitamin C
    c) Vitamin D d) Vitamin A

11. Lactose intolerance in chicken which causes severe diarrhoea in birds is use due to
    a) High production of intestine lactose
    b) Low production of intestine lactose
    c) High activity of intestine lactose
    d) Low activity of intestine lactose
12. Fats are important in diet of poultry as concentrated source of energy and source of which essential fatty acids ?
    a) Linoleic acid b) Linolenic acid
    c) Arachidonic acid d) Eicosanopentaenoic acid
13. The most frequent cause of ascites in birds is....
    a) Increased portal pressure
    b) Secondary to right ventricular failure
    c) Liver damage
    d) All
14. Fast growth rate increases the demand for oxygen and hence the workload on the heart predispose broiler for the development of
    a) Pulmonary hypertension syndrome b) CHF
    c) SDS d) DCM
15. ______ is a component of visual pigment in sensory cells of retina which plays an essential role in detection of light
    a) Vitamin a aldehyde b) Retinal
    c) Retinal d) A and B
16. Most dietary vitamin A is in the form of retinol and retinal, which is oxidized by cells to
    a) Retinolic acid b) Retinalic acid
    c) Retinoic acid d) All of the above
17. Flip-Over disease in birds due to
    a) SDS b) DCM
    c) HCM d) All
18. The incidence and severity of blood spots in eggs of chicken and abnormal embryonic development is seen in which vitamin deficiency
    a) Vitamin A b) Vitamin B1
    c) Vitamin B12 d) Vitamin C
19. Valgus-varus deformities is also known as
    a) Toed leg b) Cubbed Leg
    c) Twisted leg d) All
20. Spondylolisthesis also known as
    a) Kinky back b) Twisted back
    c) Goiter d) Gout

21. Which vitamin is required by poultry for proper metabolism of calcium and phosphorus?
    a) Vitamin A b) Vitamin B
    c) Vitamin C d) Vitamin D
22. Which vitamin helps in regulation of calcium metabolism and influences oesteoblast and osteoclast activity?
    a) Vitamin A b) Vitamin B
    c) Vitamin C d) Vitamin D
23. Which vitamin is synthesized from T - dehydrocholestrol in skin under the influence of UV light?
    a) Vitamin A b) Vitamin B
    c) Vitamin C d) Vitamin D
24. The metabolically active form of vit d is formed by how many enzymatic hydroxylation of cholecalciferol (vit d3)
    a) One b) Two
    c) Three d) Four
25. Increase in numbers of thin - shelled and soft shelled eggs in layers is indication off which vitamin deficiency
    a) Vitamin A b) Vitamin B
    c) Vitamin C d) Vitamin D
26. Penguin type squat in poultry bird is seen in which vitamin deficiency
    a) Vitamin A b) Vitamin B
    c) Vitamin C d) Vitamin D
27. Soft and pliable beak , claws & keel bone and bent sternum in poultry birds is seen in which vit deficiency
    a) Vitamin A b) Vitamin B
    c) Vitamin C d) Vitamin D
28. Which vitamin deficiency in chicks and poults causes retard growth and rickets?
    a) Vitamin A b) Vitamin B
    c) Vitamin C d) Vitamin D
29. Which vitamin deficiency in poultry birds causes widening of epiphyseal plate, hypertrophy
    a) Vitamin A b) Vitamin B
    c) Vitamin C d) Vitamin D
30. Which vitamin toxicity results in soft tissue calcification, cellular degeneration and atrophy of parathyroid gland in growing chicks?
    a) Vitamin A b) Vitamin E
    c) Vitamin C d) Vitamin D
31. Tibial dyschondroplasia due to deficiency of ……
    a) Vitamin E b) Vitamin C
    c) Vitamin B d) Vitamin D

32. Death due to spiking mortality syndrome in broiler chickens
    a) Vitamin D
    b) High protein
    c) Hyperglycemia
    d) Hypoglycemia
33. Age of death due to spiking mortality syndrome in broiler chickens
    a) 12-18 Weeks
    b) 2-8 Days
    c) 2-8 Weeks
    d) 12-18 Days
34. Fatty liver haemorrhagic syndrome as excessive accumulation of fat along with haemorrhages in the liver most common in birds with
    a) Vitamin A
    b) High fat ration
    c) Vitamin E
    d) High energy ration
35. Birds with fatty liver haemorrhagic syndrome will have
    a) Cynotic comb
    b) Red comb
    c) Pale comb
    d) A and C
36. Haemorrhages in fatty liver haemorrhagic syndrome in birds due to
    a) Iron deficiency
    b) Oviposition
    c) Copper
    d) All
37. Fatty liver haemorrhagic syndrome in birds noticed more commonly in
    a) Low egg producing birds
    b) High egg producing birds
    c) High body weight birds
    d) Low body weight birds
38. Putty colour liver noticed in birds with
    a) Vitamin D deficiency
    b) Vitamin C deficiency
    c) Vitamin B deficiency
    d) Fatty liver haemorrhagic syndrome
39. Due to deficiency of vitamin E in chicks causes edema of subcutaneous tissue associated with abnormal permeability of capillary walls and this condition is ermed as
    a) Encephalomalacia
    b) Nutritional myopathy
    c) Exudative diathesis
    d) Ascites
40. In high producing female poultry birds increase in production of which hormone is responsible for FLHS condition
    a) Melatonin
    b) Insulin
    c) Progesterone
    d) Estrogen
41. FLHS positive layers have higher levels of which hormones in their blood…
    a) Leptin
    b) Estrogen
    c) Osteocalcin
    d) All
42. In which diseases birds show fat accumulation and liver bleeding in layers
    a) Ascites
    b) Flip Over
    c) Hepatitis
    d) FLHS
43. Feeding poultry birds with rancid fat may results in ….
    a) Fatty liver
    b) Hepatitis
    c) Sudden death
    d) Hepatic bleeding

44. By close monitoring of poultry birds body weight and feed intake on each day can prevent which diseases...
    a) Gout b) Salmonellosis
    c) MD d) FLHS
45. In layers FLHS reduced by feeding with byproduct feeds such as
    a) Distillers grains b) Alfa alfa
    c) Fish meal d) All
46. When layers are fed with chelated trace minerals instead of inorganic minerals have higher prevalence of
    a) Ascites b) Fatty liver
    c) Rickets d) Hepatitis
47. Urate deposits on the visceral organs due to renal failure are semisolid and are which appearance
    a) Blackish b) Chalky white
    c) Greyish d) Brown
48. In addition to visceral organs, urates in renal failure may deposit in synovial fluid of different joints....
    a) Stifle joint b) Fetlock joint
    c) Hack joint d) Carpal joint
49. Urolithiasis in older layers may leads to formation of
    a) Articular gout b) Visceral gout
    c) A and B d) None
50. Atrophy of the affected kidney due to obstruction of uroliths in the urates of poultry birds is observed in ......
    a) Rickets b) Articular gout
    c) Visceral gout d) Ascites
51. Which vitamin acts as cofactor for many enzymes like NAD and NADPH cytochrome reductases and succinic dehydrogenase?
    a) Vitamin B1 b) Vitamin B2
    c) Vitamin B5 d) Vitamin B12
52. Formation of insoluble products like monosodium urates within the kidney and on visceral organs in poultry birds is due to
    a) Liver failure b) Heart failure
    c) Renal failure d) All
53. Ascites in birds may leads to which metabolic disease due to its hypoxic condition
    a) Fatty liver b) Rickets
    c) Gout d) All
54. Renal failure in poultry birds decrease clearance of which metabolic waste product from the blood
    a) Urea b) Ammonia
    c) Uric acid d) Iodine

55. Kidney failure in poultry birds leads to
    a) Visceral gout b) Articular gout
    c) Urolithiasis d) All
56. Gout is also known as
    a) Urea deposition b) Uric acid deposition
    c) Ammonia deposition d) All
57. Which vitamin acts as cofactor in carboxylation and decarboxylation reactions involve fixation of CO2
    a) Vitamin B1 b) Vitamin B5
    c) Vitamin B6 d) Vitamin B7
58. Which among the following mycotoxins are responsible for the visceral gout in poultry birds
    a) Oosporein b) Orchatoxin
    c) Citrinin d) All
59. Acute death syndrome or sudden death syndrome in chicken is by which vitamin deficiency
    a) Vitamin B1 b) Vitamin B5
    c) Vitamin B6 d) Vitamin B7
60. Which among the following metabolic disease causes increased production of uric acid in poultry birds
    a) Rickets b) Gout
    c) SDS d) Ascites
61. Kidney dysfunction can be reduced nutritionally by avoiding overfeeding of nutrients like
    a) Calcium b) Crude protein
    c) Electrolytes d) All
62. High quantities of crude protein diet in poultry birds increase which levels in plasma
    a) Urea b) Potassium
    c) Ammonia d) Uric acid
63. Which vitamin deficiency causes megablastic arrest of erythrocytes which results in macrocytic anaemia in chicks
    a) Vitamin B1 b) Vitamin B6
    c) Vitamin B7 d) Vitamin B9
64. Kidney dysfunction in poultry birds can be reduced nutritionally by avoiding overfeeding of nutrients like
    a) Calcium b) Crude protein
    c) Electrolytes d) All
65. These urates are semisolid and have white chalky appearance should be differentiated form infectious origin of
    a) Synovitis b) Peritonitis
    c) Perihepatitis and pericarditis d) All

66. Laying hens fed with high calcium levels well before sexual maturity may cause which metabolic disease...
   a) Gout b) Urolithiasis
   c) Ascites d) A and B
67. Ascites can be controlled by and also by in the diet
   a) Avoiding lung injury b) Minimizing sodium level
   c) Avoiding liver injury d) All
68. Birds with inherited abnormalities of uric acid metabolism or those fed on excessive protein may develop
   a) Vusceral gout b) Ascites
   c) Articular gout d) Rickets
69. Utilization of calcium and phosphorous depend on presence of an adequate amount of which vitamin in diet
   a) Vitamin D b) Vitamin C
   c) Vitamin E d) Vitamin A
70. Ca and P deficiency in growing broiler chicken causes
   a) Osteomalacia b) Hock enlargement
   c) Rickets d) Chondrodystrophy
71. Which inorganic elements deficiency in laying hens causes eggs production and thin shelled eggs
   a) Copper b) Calcium
   c) Selenium d) Magnesium
72. Cage layers fatigue in layer is due to deficiency of
   a) Copper b) Calcium
   c) Selenium d) Magnesium
73. Visceral gout in chickens is due to excess feeding of ____element
   a) Calcium b) Copper
   c) Magnesium d) Phosphorous
74. Excess sodium in poultry diet causes
   a) Cardiomegaly b) Ascites
   c) Fibrin mass in liver d) All the above
75. Urate deposition on the wing joints and toe synovial membrane in poultry birds is known as
   a) Visceral gout b) Articular gout
   c) Rickets d) All
76. In ascites, affected broilers are
   a) Red b) Cyanotic
   c) White d) Any colour
77. Which trace element is required for HB formation
   a) Iron b) Iodine
   c) Manganese d) Copper

78. Causes of ascites syndrome in birds due to
   a) Vascular damage
   b) Increased vascular hydraulic pressure
   c) Increased tissue oncotic pressure
   d) All
79. The most common cause of liver injury in broiler hens to cause ascites
   a) Obstructive cholangiohepatitis
   b) Iodine b) deficiency
   c) Copper toxicity d) Molybdinum toxicity
80. Pulmonary hypertension can cause in birds
   a) Ascites b) Macrocytic anaemia
   c) Normochromic macrocytic anaemia d) Myocarditis
81. Accumulation of transudate in the abdominal cavity in birds
   a) Hepatitis b) Nephitis
   c) Ascites d) Anasarca
82. Causes of ascites syndrome in birds
   a) Increased sodium intake b) Lung or liver damage
   c) A and B d) Increased water intake
83. What is the end product of nitrogen metabolism in birds
   a) Urea b) Ammonia
   c) Uric acid d) None
84. _____is a condition where uric acid deposits on joints or tissues surface in birds
   a) Gout b) Urate deposition
   c) Osteoporosis d) Both A and B
85. Deposition of uric acid in visceral organs known as
   a) Gout b) Urate deposition
   c) Osteoporosis d) Both A and B
86. Visceral urate deposition in birds is due to
   a) Dehydration b) Vitamin A deficiency
   c) Urolithiasis d) All the above
87. High protein content in poultry feed leads to a condition called as
   a) Articular urate deposition b) Visceral urate deposition
   c) Urotithiasis d) None
88. Factors for SDS in birds in brooding period
   a) Hypoxia b) Low nutrition
   c) Bad hygiene d) All
89. Birds with SDS may show
   a) Ascites b) Anasarca
   c) Pulmonary edema, hydropericardium d) All the above

90. Which vitamin helps in formation of normal skeleton hard beaks and claws in poultry birds
 a) Vitamin B b) Vitamin C
 c) Vitamin D d) Vitamin A
91. Deficiency of Vitamin E in growing chicken leads to
 a) Soft tissue calcification b) Atrophy of parathyroid
 c) A and B d) None of the above
92. Spontaneous cardiomyopathy can affect the birds at
 a) Chick b) Layer
 c) Brooding stage d) None
93. Which may play a role in the pathophysiology of spontaneous cardiomyopathy in turkeys
 a) DCM b) Pericarditis
 c) Ischemia d) None
94. Sudden death syndrome is linked with in birds
 a) Lactic acidosis b) Carbohydrate metabolism
 c) Loss of membrane integrity d) All
95. Death due to sudden death syndrome in birds
 a) Between 2 to 3 days b) Between 21 to 35 days
 c) Between 80 to 95 days d) All the above
96. Sudden death syndrome in birds can cause
 a) Subendocardial purkinje cells b) Cardiomyocytes
 c) A and B d) None
97. Sudden death syndrome in birds prevented by
 a) Exercise b) Nutrition restriction
 c) Brooding time d) All the above
98. Calcium helps in
 a) Egg shell formation b) Clotting of blood
 c) Contraction of muscle d) All the above
99. Rickets in growing broiler chicken is due to
 a) P b) Na
 c) Ca d) A &C
100. Hypochromic microcytic anaemia in chicken is due to _______ element
 a) Fe b) I
 c) Cu d) Ca
101. Which causes sudden mortality of birds in full production
 a) Ascites b) Sudden death syndrome
 c) Fatty liver hemorrhagic syndrome d) None

102. Administering estrogen to layers and even male birds could induce
    a) Ascites b) Sudden death syndrome
    c) FLHS d) None
103. FLHS positive layers have higher levels of ___ in blood
    a) Leptin b) Estrogen
    c) Osterocalcin d) All the above
104. Which of the metabolic disease has liver is friable and " Putty colour"
    a) Ascites b) Sudden death syndrome
    c) FLHS d) None
105. _____ is not a typical postmortem lesion in case of FLHS
    a) Pale yellow colour liver b) Hepatic hemorrhages
    c) Enlarged liver d) None
106. In FLHS affected birds, the liver dry matter is at least
    a) 50% fat b) 40% fat
    c) 20% fat d) 0% fat
107. Among the following _____ is the common side effect of kidney failure
    a) Ascites syndrome b) Gout
    c) Round heart disease d) Sudden death syndrome
108. The urates of gout are semisolid and appear as
    a) White chalky b) Purulent
    c) Fibrinoid d) Serous
109. Asymmetry in size and weight of both parts of kidneys can be used during diagnosis of visceral
    a) Ascites b) FLHS
    c) Gout d) None
110. What are the important infectious causes which intensity the visceral gout condition
    a) Cryptosporidiosis b) Infectious bronchitis virus
    c) Avian nephritis d) All the above
111. Urolithiasis visceral gout is commonly observed in birds, feeding more ____ diet for weeks before sexual maturity.
    a) Calcium b) Sodium
    c) Potassium d) Magnesium
112. ____ olive lops as a result of persistent increase in the uric acid levels in blood and urate deposits in joints, foot
    a) Visceral gout b) Articular gout
    c) Ascites d) None
113. Articular gout occurs in birds who are overfed with
    a) Protein b) K+cl:Na ratio<1
    c) A and B d) None

114. In articular gout, urates deposition occurs mainly on
   a) Wing joints b) Toe synovial membrane
   c) A and B d) None
115. ____ can be used to prevent or cure urolithiasis
   a) Urinary acidification b) Alkalization
   c) Avoid overfeed of calcium d) A and C
116. Accumulation of fluid in the abdomen which is non-inflammatory in nature is known as_______
   a) Peritonitis b) Ascites
   c) Water belly d) B and C
117. The PM lesions of ascites as a result of RVF/PH have an
   a) Increased venous pressure b) Hydro pericardium
   c) Right ventricular dilation d) All the above
118. Based on diagnosis, broilers with ascites as a result of RVF/PH have an
   a) Enlarged heart
   b) Thicker right side of ventricle
   c) Clear fluid in abdomen and pericardial sac
   d) All
119. Which of the metabolic diseases, where young turkeys die suddenly due to cardiac arrest
   a) Ascites b) FLHS
   c) Round heart disease d) None
120. The effected poultry has a substantially enlarged heart due to dilation of both ventricles, congested lungs, enlarged liver in case o f
   a) Round heart disease b) Anasarca
   c) Ascites d) Hydro pericardium
121. Sudden death syndrome in poultry often known as
   a) Flipover b) Heart attack
   c) A and B d) None
122. The etiology of sudden death syndrome is
   a) Cardiac tamponade b) Cardiac arrhythmia
   c) Carbohydrate metabolism d) None
123. On opening of heart, atria contains PM blood clots while ventricles are normally empty with slight hypertrophy in case of
   a) Round heart disease b) Ascites
   c) Sudden death syndrome d) FLHS
124. Heart lesions recognized as white streaks or patches associate with hydro pericardium seen in
   a) Round heart disease b) ascites
   c) Vitamin A def d) Vitamin E and selenium def

125. ______has its greatest effect on rapidly growing broilers in which slight reduction in availability will slow growth
a) Light b) Darkness
c) Temperature d) Hypoxia

126. _____ results in anorexia and could be the reason for failure to eat in these that are in negative energy balance
a) Starvation b) Ketosis
c) Dehydration d) None

127. High______ is stressful for poultry and frequently causes death
a) Starvation b) Temperature
c) Oxygen d) Nutrition

128. The lethal high body temperature for chicks and adult birds is
a) 1160F,1170F b) 1100F,1110F
c) 1170F,1160F d) 1110F,1100F

129. Dead birds are usually found on their breast and intestine may contain fluid content in case of
a) Ascites b) Hyperthermia
c) Hypoxia d) Nutrition def

130. Commercial poultry rarely die from ______
a) Starvation b) Dehydration
c) Hyperthermia d) Hypothermia

131. The lethal low body temperature for chicks and adult birds is
a) 600F,720F b) 720F ,600F
c) 1160F ,1170F d) 1170F ,1160F

132. Hens may become paralyzed or die from acute______while shelling an egg
a) Hyperthermia b) Sudden death syndrome
c) Hypoxia d) Hypocalcaemia

133. "Egg bond" condition occurs in
a) Osteoporosis b) Round heart disease
c) Egg drop syndrome d) Hypocalcaemia

134. Sudden death syndrome of broiler breeders is associated with low dietary_______
a) Na+ b) K+
c) Ca+2 d) Both b and c

135. _____ in laying hens is a condition that involves the progressive loss of bone during laying period
a) Osteoporosis b) Osteopenia
c) Osteomalacia d) Hypocalcaemia

136. Layers in high production and develop osteoporosis due to
a) Inability to metabolise Ca b) Inadequate dietary Ca
c) Vitamin D3 or P d) All

137. Phosphorous deficiency- induced osteoporosis in high producing cage layers …

a) Osteoporosis
b) Cage layer fatigue
c) Osteopenia
d) None

138. To prevent osteoporosis and hypocalcaemia, hens must absorb enough calcium for egg shell formation, it requires

a) 2 g of Ca
b) 1 g of Ca
c) 10 g of Ca
d) no need of Ca

139. In _____ there is damage to spinal cord followed by partial paralysis, lame sit on these tail with their feet extended is

a) Scoliosis
b) Osteochondrosis
c) Spondylolis thesis or kinky back
d) None

140. Which among them causes 50% of the lameness in broiler chickens, where animal protein used in the ration

a) Osteochondrosis
b) Dyschondroplasia
c) Scoliosis
d) Kinky back

141. "Straddle –legged " posture is seen in

a) Kinky back
b) Dyschondroplasia
c) Rotated tibia
(d)None

142. Which is a severe lameness, in which birds are reluctant to rise and walk and spend much of their time squatting

a) Fracture
b) Deep pectoral myopathy
c) Trembling syndrome
d) Shaky leg syndrome

143. Which is an exertional myopathy induced by holding the broilers by its legs and allowing it to flap on wings

a) Deep pectoral myopathy
b) Metabolic myopathy
c) Cardiac myopathy
d) None

144. Myocarditis and ascites have been produced when ______ is fed to poultry

a) Linseed oil
b) Terpentine oil
c) Rapeseed oil
d) None

145. In birds, lesions associated with systemic hypertension, hyperlipemia and hypercholesterolaemia

a) Epicardial fibrosis
b) Atherosclerosis
c) Ruptured aorta
d) Arteriosclerosis

146. Live chicks are found recumbent and uncoordinated, frequently lying on their breasts with legs extended in

a) Fatty liver and kidney syndrome
b) Spiking mortality syndrome
c) FLHS
d) Spleenomegaly syndrome

147. Which is a biotin deficiency related metabolic disease in broiler chicks, resulting in impaired hepatic gluconeogenesis and increased fat deposition.

a) Fatty liver and kidney syndrome
b) Spiking mortality syndrome
c) FLHS
d) Splenomegaly syndrome

148. Which is a degenerative muscle disease that affects the breast tender deep within the breast

a) Ascites
b) Green muscle disease
c) Deep pectoral myopathy
d) B and C

149. Reluctant to move, respiratory distress distended abdomen, combs wattles and sudden death are cyanotic are the clinical signs of

a) Sudden death syndrome
b) Kinky back
c) FLHS
d) Ascites

150. Birds have difficulty in walking and standing with legs for apart in case of

a) Encephalomalacia
b) Exudative diathesis
c) Muscular dystrophy
d) None

Answer Key

1	c	2	b	3	b	4	d	5	d	6	c	7	c
8	b	9	d	10	a	11	d	12	a	13	d	14	a
15	a	16	c	17	a	18	a	19	c	20	a	21	d
22	d	23	d	24	b	25	d	26	d	27	d	28	d
29	d	30	d	31	d	32	d	33	d	34	d	35	c
36	b	37	b	38	d	39	c	40	d	41	d	42	d
43	d	44	d	45	d	46	b	47	b	48	c	49	b
50	c	51	b	52	c	53	c	54	c	55	d	56	d
57	d	58	d	59	d	60	d	61	d	62	d	63	b
64	d	65	d	66	d	67	d	68	c	69	a	70	c
71	b	72	b	73	a	74	d	75	b	76	b	77	a
78	d	79	a	80	a	81	c	82	c	83	c	84	d
85	a	86	d	87	a	88	a	89	d	90	c	91	c
92	c	93	c	94	d	95	b	96	c	97	b	98	d
99	d	100	a	101	c	102	c	103	d	104	c	105	a
106	b	107	b	108	a	109	c	110	d	111	a	112	b
113	c	114	c	115	d	116	d	117	d	118	d	119	c
120	a	121	c	122	b	123	c	124	d	125	d	126	b
127	b	128	a	129	b	130	d	131	a	132	d	133	d
134	d	135	a	136	d	137	b	138	a	139	c	140	b
141	c	142	d	143	a	144	c	145	b	146	b	147	a
148	d	149	d	150	b								

32

Nutritional Disorders

A.K. Singh[1], T. Rana[2] and Shilpi Kerketta[3]

[1]Animal Nutrition, FVAS, Banaras Hindu University, Benaras

[2]Livestock Production and Management, ICAR-IARI, Gauria Karma, Hazaribagh Jharkhand

Nutritional deficiencies can result from a lack of specific nutrients in the diet, adverse interactions between nutrients in seemingly well-balanced diets, or the influence of specific anti-nutrients. The latter two scenarios are particularly challenging to diagnose because dietary analysis may suggest that nutrient levels are adequate. Micronutrients such as vitamins and trace minerals are typically added to diets through standalone micro premixes, making classic signs of individual nutrient deficiencies rare. Instead, the effects are often a combination of various metabolic conditions. Accurate diagnosis often requires comprehensive information about the diet and management practices, clinical signs in affected birds, necropsies, and tissue analyses. However, tissue analysis, especially of the liver and serum, can be misleading. Following the onset of a deficiency, birds may sequester nutrients in the liver, leading to falsely high liver assay values even when the diet is deficient. This effect is particularly significant for minerals such as copper. A diet that appears to contain sufficient levels of certain nutrients based on analysis may actually be deficient in those nutrients to some extent. Stressors such as bacterial, parasitic, or viral infections, as well as extreme temperatures, can interfere with nutrient absorption or increase the nutritional requirements. Toxins or microorganisms may destroy or render unavailable specific nutrients that appear to be present in adequate levels according to conventional chemical or physical assays. Consequently, many trace minerals and vitamins are included in the diet at levels significantly higher than the actual requirements to account for these potential issues.

Poultry do not have a direct protein requirement but need the correct levels and balance of nutritionally essential amino acids, along with sufficient amino nitrogen (from amino acids) to synthesize nonessential amino acids. Traditionally, diets were formulated to contain adequate levels of the first three or four limiting essential amino acids and a minimum level of dietary crude protein, which was generally sufficient for poultry using typical ingredients. However, modern poultry have higher growth rates and different body compositions (meat-type birds) and egg production rates (egg-laying birds). Additionally, there is a growing desire in many regions to reduce dietary crude protein levels to minimize nitrogen excretion by birds, thereby reducing environmental nutrient pollution. Optimal levels of balanced protein intake vary: for growing chicks, it is approximately 18%–23% of the diet; for growing poults and gallinaceous upland game birds, 26%–30%; and for growing ducklings and goslings, 20%–22%. If the protein and amino acid content of the diet falls below these levels, birds tend to grow more slowly. Even when diets meet the recommended protein quantities, optimal growth also requires the proper balance and sufficient quantities of essential amino acids plus sufficient amino nitrogen for synthesizing nonessential amino acids. Few specific signs are associated with deficiencies of individual amino acids, except for a peculiar, cup-shaped appearance of feathers in chickens with arginine deficiency and loss of pigment in some wing feathers in bronze turkeys with lysine deficiency. Deficiencies in any essential amino acids result in retarded growth in growing birds or reduced egg size and egg production in egg-laying birds. If a diet is deficient in crude protein or specific amino acids, birds may initially consume more feed to resolve the deficiency. However, after a few days, this increase in feed intake shifts to reduced feed intake. Consequently, feed efficiency decreases, and birds become fatter due to consuming more energy relative to protein. Commercial breeds of poultry can consume energy according to their requirements regardless of dietary energy concentration, assuming they can physically consume enough feed. An energy deficiency can occur only if the diet is so low in energy concentration that birds cannot compensate by increasing feed consumption. With an energy deficiency, birds will grow slowly or stop ovulating. Amino acids will be deaminated and their carbon skeletons oxidized, and lipids will undergo beta-oxidation. This condition can lead to ketosis, a condition more common in mammals but with similar classic signs in birds.

Deficiencies in essential nutrients can lead to significant health issues in birds:

Calcium or Phosphorus Deficiency: In young birds, this leads to abnormal bone development and lack of skeletal calcification, causing rickets. In laying hens, it results in poor shell quality and osteoporosis.

Sodium Deficiency: This lowers osmotic pressure, disrupts acid-base balance, reduces cardiac output and blood pressure, increases PCV, decreases tissue elasticity, and impairs adrenal function, potentially leading to shock and death. In chicks, it causes retarded growth, soft bones, corneal keratinization, impaired food utilization, and reduced plasma volume. In layers, it reduces egg production, growth, and can lead to cannibalism. Sodium depletion can occur due to diarrhea or renal/adrenal damage.

Selenium Deficiency: In young chickens, it causes exudative diathesis with signs like unthriftiness, ruffled feathers, skin edema, bruising, and scab formation. In laying hens, it reduces egg production, hatchability, and feed conversion efficiency.

Zinc Deficiency: In young chicks, it results in retarded growth, thickened and shortened leg bones, enlarged hock joints, skin scaling, poor feathering, loss of appetite, and mortality. In aging hens, it reduces egg production, and severely affects embryos, leading to weak chicks with respiratory issues, inability to stand, skeletal deformities, and sometimes missing limbs or eyes. Choline, Manganese- Slipped Tendon

List of Deficiency Diseases

Following is a list of major deficiency diseases that occur due to lack of essential minerals and vitamins:

Types of Vitamins	Deficiency Diseases
A (Retinol)	Night blindness
B1 (Thiamine)	Star Gazing Appearance, Polyneuritis
B2 (Riboflavin)	Curled Toe Paralysis
B12 (Cyanocobalamin)	Anaemia
C (Ascorbic acid)	Scurvy
D (Calciferol)	Rickets
K (Phylloquinone)	Excessive bleeding due to injury
Types of Minerals	Deficiency Diseases
Calcium	Brittle bones, excessive bleeding
Phosphorus	Bad teeth and bones
Iron	Anaemia
Iodine	Goitre, enlarged thyroid gland
Copper	Low appetite, retarded growth

1. Which mineral deficiency causes rickets in poultry?
   a) Calcium b) Sodium
   c) Iron d) Copper
2. A deficiency of which mineral leads to poor eggshell quality?
   a) Potassium b) Calcium
   c) Magnesium d) Zinc
3. Iron deficiency in poultry primarily results in:
   a) Goiter b) Anemia
   c) Rickets d) Osteoporosis
4. Which mineral deficiency causes perosis in poultry?
   a) Manganese b) Selenium
   c) Sodium d) Iodine
5. Zinc deficiency in poultry can lead to:
   a) Poor feathering b) Anemia
   c) Weak bones d) Goiter
6. A deficiency of which mineral can cause fatty liver hemorrhagic syndrome?
   a) Iron b) Selenium
   c) Choline d) Iodine
7. Which mineral is essential for preventing goiter in poultry?
   a) Calcium b) Iodine
   c) Magnesium d) Zinc
8. Selenium deficiency in poultry can cause:
   a) Perosis b) Muscular dystrophy
   c) Goiter d) Anemia

9. Which mineral deficiency is associated with weak eggshells?
   a) Iron b) Zinc
   c) Calcium d) Iodine
10. A lack of manganese in poultry diets can lead to:
   a) Rickets b) Anemia
   c) Perosis d) Goiter
11. Copper deficiency in poultry is likely to cause:
   a) Poor growth b) Feather depigmentation
   c) Goiter d) Anemia
12. Which mineral deficiency causes white muscle disease in poultry?
   a) Calcium b) Selenium
   c) Iron d) Iodine
13. A deficiency in sodium can lead to:
   a) Poor feathering b) Muscle cramps
   c) Anemia d) Osteoporosis
14. Which mineral is crucial for preventing anemia in poultry?
   a) Iron b) Iodine
   c) Magnesium d) Calcium
15. Potassium deficiency in poultry may cause:
   a) Weak bones b) Anemia
   c) Muscle weakness d) Goiter
16. Which mineral deficiency is associated with muscular dystrophy in poultry?
   a) Manganese b) Selenium
   c) Zinc d) Iodine
17. Calcium deficiency in poultry can result in:
   a) Goiter b) Anemia
   c) Rickets d) Perosis
18. A deficiency in which mineral can lead to osteomalacia?
   a) Zinc b) Iron
   c) Calcium d) Selenium
19. Iodine deficiency in poultry is most likely to cause:
   a) Anemia b) Goiter
   c) Rickets d) Perosis
20. Which mineral is essential for preventing perosis in poultry?
   a) Magnesium b) Manganese
   c) Zinc d) Calcium
21. A lack of zinc in the diet of poultry can lead to:
   a) Poor feathering b) Rickets
   c) Anemia d) Goiter

22. Copper deficiency in poultry can cause:
    a) Muscle cramps b) Feather depigmentation
    c) Goiter d) Anemia
23. Which mineral deficiency leads to white muscle disease?
    a) Calcium b) Selenium
    c) Iron d) Zinc
24. Sodium deficiency in poultry may result in:
    a) Muscle cramps b) Poor growth
    c) Anemia d) Osteoporosis
25. A deficiency in iron can lead to:
    a) Rickets b) Goiter
    c) Anemia d) Perosis
26. Potassium deficiency affects poultry by causing:
    a) Muscle weakness b) Anemia
    c) Weak bones d) Goiter
27. Which mineral deficiency is linked to muscular dystrophy?
    a) Manganese b) Selenium
    c) Zinc d) Iron
28. Calcium deficiency can lead to:
    a) Anemia b) Rickets
    c) Goiter d) Perosis
29. A lack of which mineral can cause osteomalacia in poultry?
    a) Zinc b) Iron
    c) Calcium d) Selenium
30. Iodine deficiency is associated with:
    a) Anemia b) Goiter
    c) Rickets d) Perosis
31. Manganese deficiency can lead to:
    a) Goiter b) Rickets
    c) Perosis d) Anemia
32. A deficiency of zinc in poultry may cause:
    a) Weak bones b) Poor feathering
    c) Anemia d) Goiter
33. Copper deficiency results in:
    a) Feather depigmentation b) Muscle cramps
    c) Goiter d) Anemia
34. Selenium deficiency can cause:
    a) Anemia b) White muscle disease
    c) Goiter d) Rickets

35. Sodium deficiency in poultry may result in:
    a) Poor feathering   b) Muscle cramps
    c) Anemia   d) Osteoporosis
36 . Iron deficiency leads to:
    a) Rickets   b) Anemia
    c) Goiter   d) Perosis
37. Potassium deficiency can cause:
    a) Muscle weakness   b) Anemia
    c) Weak bones   d) Goiter
38. Which mineral deficiency causes muscular dystrophy?
    a) Manganese   b) Selenium
    c) Zinc   d) Iron
39. Calcium deficiency can result in:
    a) Anemia   b) Rickets
    c) Goiter   d) Perosis
40. A lack of calcium can lead to:
    a) Osteomalacia   b) Anemia
    c) Goiter   d) Perosis
41. Iodine deficiency in poultry is associated with:
    a) Anemia   b) Goiter
    c) Rickets   d) Perosis
42. Manganese deficiency may cause:
    a) Goiter   b) Rickets
    c) Anemia   d) Perosis
43. Zinc deficiency in poultry leads to:
    a) Weak bones   b) Poor feathering
    c) Anemia   d) Goiter
44. Copper deficiency results in:
    a) Muscle cramps   b) Feather depigmentation
    c) Goiter   d) Anemia
45. Selenium deficiency in poultry can cause:
    a) Anemia   b) White muscle disease
    c) Goiter   d) Rickets
46. A lack of sodium can lead to:
    a) Poor feathering   b) Muscle cramps
    c) Anemia   d) Osteoporosis
47. Iron deficiency is likely to result in:
    a) Rickets   b) Anemia
    c) Goiter   d) Perosis

48. Potassium deficiency affects poultry by causing:
    a) Muscle weakness b) Anemia
    c) Weak bones d) Goiter
49. Which mineral deficiency causes muscular dystrophy?
    a) Manganese b) Selenium
    c) Zinc d) Iron
50. Calcium deficiency can lead to:
    a) Anemia b) Rickets
    c) Goiter d) Perosis
51. Which vitamin deficiency causes rickets in poultry?
    a) Vitamin A b) Vitamin D
    c) Vitamin E d) Vitamin K
52 . A deficiency of which vitamin leads to poor feathering in poultry?
    a) Vitamin C b) Vitamin D
    c) Vitamin B6 d) Vitamin B2
53. Vitamin A deficiency in poultry primarily results in:
    a) Anemia b) Poor vision
    c) Rickets d) Perosis
54. Which vitamin deficiency causes encephalomalacia in poultry?
    a) Vitamin A b) Vitamin D
    c) Vitamin E d) Vitamin K
55. Riboflavin (Vitamin B2) deficiency in poultry can lead to:
    a) Curled toe paralysis b) Anemia
    c) Weak bones d) Goiter
56. A deficiency of which vitamin can cause perosis in poultry?
    a) Vitamin B3 b) Vitamin B5
    c) Vitamin B7 d) Vitamin B2
57. Which vitamin is essential for preventing nutritional myopathy in poultry?
    a) Vitamin D b) Vitamin E
    c) Vitamin B1 d) Vitamin K
58. Vitamin K deficiency in poultry can cause:
    a) Poor feathering b) Muscle cramps
    c) Hemorrhage d) Anemia
59. Which vitamin deficiency is associated with exudative diathesis in poultry?
    a) Vitamin A b) Vitamin D
    c) Vitamin E d) Vitamin K
60. A lack of thiamine (Vitamin B1) in poultry diets can lead to:
    a) Rickets b) Anemia
    c) Polyneuritis d) Goiter

61. Vitamin B6 deficiency in poultry is likely to cause:
    a) Poor growth
    b) Feather depigmentation
    c) Goiter
    d) Anemia
62. Which vitamin deficiency causes “crazy chick disease” in poultry?
    a) Vitamin A
    b) Vitamin D
    c) Vitamin E
    d) Vitamin K
63. A deficiency in niacin (Vitamin B3) can lead to:
    a) Poor feathering
    b) Muscle cramps
    c) Black tongue
    d) Osteoporosis
64. Which vitamin is crucial for preventing anemia in poultry?
    a) Vitamin B12
    b) Vitamin A
    c) Vitamin D
    d) Vitamin K
65. Pantothenic acid (Vitamin B5) deficiency in poultry may cause:
    a) Weak bones
    b) Dermatitis
    c) Muscle weakness
    d) Goiter
66. Which vitamin deficiency is associated with curled toe paralysis in poultry?
    a) Vitamin B1
    b) Vitamin B2
    c) Vitamin B6
    d) Vitamin B12
67. Vitamin D deficiency in poultry can result in:
    a) Goiter
    b) Anemia
    c) Rickets
    d) Perosis
68. A deficiency in which vitamin can lead to encephalomalacia?
    a) Vitamin B2
    b) Vitamin B6
    c) Vitamin E
    d) Vitamin K
69. Vitamin A deficiency in poultry is most likely to cause:
    a) Anemia
    b) Poor vision
    c) Rickets
    d) Perosis
70. Which vitamin is essential for preventing perosis in poultry?
    a) Vitamin B2
    b) Vitamin B3
    c) Vitamin B5
    d) Vitamin B6
71. A lack of Vitamin B6 in the diet of poultry can lead to:
    a) Poor growth
    b) Rickets
    c) Anemia
    d) Goiter
72. Vitamin K deficiency in poultry can cause:
    a) Muscle cramps
    b) Feather depigmentation
    c) Goiter
    d) Hemorrhage
73. Which vitamin deficiency leads to “crazy chick disease”?
    a) Vitamin A
    b) Vitamin D
    c) Vitamin E
    d) Vitamin K

74. Thiamine (Vitamin B1) deficiency in poultry may result in:
    a) Muscle cramps b) Polyneuritis
    c) Anemia d) Osteoporosis
75. A deficiency in riboflavin (Vitamin B2) can lead to:
    a) Rickets b) Goiter
    c) Curled toe paralysis d) Perosis
76. Vitamin B12 deficiency leads to:
    a) Rickets b) Anemia
    c) Goiter d) Perosis
77. Niacin (Vitamin B3) deficiency can cause:
    a) Black tongue b) Poor growth
    c) Weak bones d) Goiter
78. Vitamin D deficiency can lead to:
    a) Anemia b) Rickets
    c) Goiter d) Perosis
79. A lack of which vitamin can cause exudative diathesis in poultry?
    a) Vitamin A b) Vitamin D
    c) Vitamin E d) Vitamin K
80. Vitamin A deficiency in poultry is associated with:
    a) Anemia b) Poor vision
    c) Rickets d) Perosis
81. Vitamin B5 deficiency can lead to:
    a) Goiter b) Rickets
    c) Dermatitis d) Anemia
82. A deficiency of Vitamin B2 in poultry may cause:
    a) Poor feathering b) Curled toe paralysis
    c) Anemia d) Goiter
83. Vitamin B12 deficiency results in:
    a) Anemia b) Muscle cramps
    c) Goiter d) Rickets
84. Which vitamin deficiency causes polyneuritis in poultry?
    a) Vitamin B1 b) Vitamin B2
    c) Vitamin B6 d) Vitamin B12
85. Vitamin B3 deficiency can cause:
    a) Anemia b) Black tongue
    c) Goiter d) Rickets
86. A lack of Vitamin E can lead to:
    a) Rickets b) Anemia
    c) Encephalomalacia d) Goiter

87. Vitamin A deficiency primarily affects:
    a) Muscle growth b) Vision
    c) Egg production d) Feathering
88. Vitamin B2 deficiency in poultry is likely to cause:
    a) Weight gain b) Improved egg quality
    c) Curled toe paralysis d) Hyperactivity
89. Which vitamin deficiency leads to black tongue in poultry?
    a) Vitamin B1 b) Vitamin B2
    c) Vitamin B3 d) Vitamin B5
90. Vitamin B6 deficiency affects:
    a) Feathering b) Muscle mass
    c) Growth rate d) Vision
91. Vitamin K deficiency can lead to:
    a) Anemia b) Goiter
    c) Hemorrhage d) Osteomalacia
92. Which vitamin deficiency is associated with dermatitis in poultry?
    a) Vitamin B3 b) Vitamin B5
    c) Vitamin B6 d) Vitamin B12
93. A lack of Vitamin B12 can cause:
    a) Anemia b) Osteoporosis
    c) Polyneuritis d) Dermatitis
94. Vitamin B1 deficiency can result in:
    a) Rickets b) Curled toe paralysis
    c) Polyneuritis d) Anemia
95. Which vitamin is essential for preventing exudative diathesis?
    a) Vitamin D b) Vitamin E
    c) Vitamin B1 d) Vitamin K
96. A deficiency in Vitamin B2 can cause:
    a) Goiter b) Curled toe paralysis
    c) Anemia d) Rickets
97. Vitamin B3 deficiency results in:
    a) Black tongue b) Muscle cramps
    c) Goiter d) Anemia
98. A lack of Vitamin D can lead to:
    a) Anemia b) Rickets
    c) Goiter d) Dermatitis
99. Vitamin A deficiency affects:
    a) Muscle growth b) Vision
    c) Egg production d) Feathering

100. Which vitamin deficiency is associated with poor feathering?
a) Vitamin A b) Vitamin D
c) Vitamin E d) Vitamin B2

101. Which nutrient deficiency causes reduced growth and poor feathering in poultry?
a) Protein b) Carbohydrate
c) Fat d) Water

102. Carbohydrate deficiency in poultry primarily leads to:
a) Anemia b) Energy deficit
c) Rickets d) Perosis

103. A deficiency of fat in poultry diets can result in:
a) Poor vision b) Energy deficit
c) Feather loss d) Anemia

104. Which nutrient deficiency causes fatty liver hemorrhagic syndrome in poultry?
a) Protein b) Carbohydrate
c) Fat d) Water

105. Protein deficiency in poultry can lead to:
a) Curled toe paralysis b) Anemia
c) Poor growth d) Goiter

106. Which condition in poultry is caused by a lack of essential fatty acids?
a) Rickets b) Anemia
c) Poor feathering d) Polyneuritis

107. A deficiency of water in poultry can lead to:
a) Dehydration b) Poor feathering
c) Rickets d) Perosis

108. Which metabolic disorder in poultry is associated with an imbalance of calcium and phosphorus?
a) Goiter b) Fatty liver
c) Rickets d) Anemia

109. Excessive carbohydrate intake in poultry can cause:
a) Rickets b) Obesity
c) Anemia d) Perosis

110. Protein deficiency in poultry diets often results in:
a) Poor growth b) Anemia
c) Rickets d) Goiter

111. Which nutrient deficiency causes ketosis in poultry?
a) Protein b) Carbohydrate
c) Fat d) Water

112. Fat deficiency in poultry is likely to cause:
a) Poor vision b) Muscle cramps
c) Energy deficit d) Anemia

113. Which condition in poultry is caused by a deficiency of methionine?
   a) Goiter b) Poor growth
   c) Rickets d) Anemia
114. A deficiency in carbohydrates can lead to:
   a) Poor feathering b) Energy deficit
   c) Anemia d) Osteoporosis
115. Excessive fat intake in poultry can cause:
   a) Rickets b) Fatty liver
   c) Weak bones d) Goiter
116. Protein deficiency can lead to:
   a) Poor growth b) Rickets
   c) Anemia d) Goiter
117. Which nutrient is essential for preventing dehydration in poultry?
   a) Protein b) Carbohydrate
   c) Fat d) Water
118. A deficiency in lysine can result in:
   a) Poor feathering b) Muscle weakness
   c) Rickets d) Perosis
119. Carbohydrate deficiency is most likely to cause:
   a) Anemia b) Energy deficit
   c) Rickets d) Perosis
120. Fat deficiency in poultry diets may lead to:
   a) Poor growth b) Rickets
   c) Anemia d) Goiter
121. Protein deficiency can cause:
   a) Anemia b) Obesity
   c) Muscle weakness d) Goiter
122. Which nutrient deficiency can cause muscle weakness and poor growth in poultry?
   a) Protein b) Carbohydrate
   c) Fat d) Water
123. Dehydration in poultry is primarily caused by a lack of:
   a) Protein b) Carbohydrate
   c) Fat d) Water
124. Which nutrient is crucial for maintaining proper metabolic functions in poultry?
   a) Protein b) Carbohydrate
   c) Fat d) Water
125. Excessive protein intake in poultry can lead to:
   a) Kidney damage b) Rickets
   c) Anemia d) Obesity

126. A deficiency of carbohydrates can result in:
   a) Energy deficit b) Poor feathering
   c) Muscle weakness d) Goiter
127. Which nutrient deficiency can cause fatty liver syndrome in poultry?
   a) Protein b) Carbohydrate
   c) Fat d) Water
128. A lack of essential amino acids in poultry diet can lead to:
   a) Poor feathering b) Energy deficit
   c) Anemia d) Rickets
129. Which condition in poultry is caused by an imbalance in electrolytes?
   a) Goiter b) Fatty liver
   c) Dehydration d) Anemia
130. Protein deficiency can result in:
   a) Poor vision b) Poor growth
   c) Rickets d) Obesity
131. Carbohydrate deficiency primarily affects:
   a) Feathering b) Egg production
   c) Energy levels d) Bone development
132. Which nutrient is essential for proper feathering in poultry?
   a) Protein b) Carbohydrate
   c) Fat d) Water
133. A lack of fat in the diet can cause:
   a) Poor growth b) Weak bones
   c) Energy deficit d) Goiter
134. Dehydration in poultry can lead to:
   a) Rickets b) Anemia
   c) Kidney damage d) Poor feathering
135. Excessive carbohydrate intake can result in:
   a) Anemia b) Obesity
   c) Rickets d) Perosis
136. Protein deficiency is associated with:
   a) Poor feathering b) Obesity
   c) Energy deficit d) Goiter
137. Which nutrient deficiency can cause reduced egg production in poultry?
   a) Protein b) Carbohydrate
   c) Fat d) Water
138. A deficiency in carbohydrates can result in:
   a) Poor feathering b) Energy deficit
   c) Anemia d) Goiter

139. Fat deficiency in poultry is likely to cause:
a) Poor vision b) Muscle cramps
c) Energy deficit d) Anemia

140. Which nutrient is essential for preventing metabolic disorders in poultry?
a) Protein b) Carbohydrate
c) Fat d) Water

141. Protein deficiency in poultry diets often results in:
a) Anemia b) Poor growth
c) Rickets d) Goiter

142. Excessive water intake in poultry can cause:
a) Dehydration b) Kidney damage
c) Obesity d) Anemia

143. A deficiency of methionine in poultry can lead to:
a) Poor growth b) Rickets
c) Anemia d) Perosis

144. Which nutrient is crucial for maintaining electrolyte balance in poultry?
a) Protein b) Carbohydrate
c) Fat d) Water

145. Carbohydrate deficiency is most likely to cause:
a) Anemia b) Energy deficit
c) Rickets d) Perosis

146. Fat deficiency in poultry diets may lead to:
a) Poor growth b) Rickets
c) Anemia d) Goiter

147. Protein deficiency can cause:
a) Anemia b) Obesity
c) Muscle weakness d) Goiter

148. Which nutrient deficiency can cause muscle weakness and poor growth in poultry?
a) Protein b) Carbohydrate
c) Fat d) Water

149. Dehydration in poultry is primarily caused by a lack of:
a) Protein b) Carbohydrate
c) Fat d) Water

150. Which nutrient is crucial for maintaining proper metabolic functions in poultry?
a) Protein b) Carbohydrate
c) Fat d) Water

Answer Key

1	a	2	b	3	b	4	a	5	a	6	c	7	b
8	b	9	c	10	c	11	b	12	b	13	b	14	a
15	c	16	b	17	c	18	c	19	b	20	b	21	a
22	b	23	b	24	a	25	c	26	a	27	b	28	b
29	c	30	b	31	c	32	b	33	a	34	b	35	b
36	b	37	a	38	b	39	b	40	a	41	b	42	d
43	b	44	b	45	b	46	b	47	b	48	a	49	b
50	b	51	b	52	d	53	b	54	c	55	a	56	d
57	b	58	c	59	c	60	c	61	a	62	c	63	c
64	a	65	b	66	b	67	c	68	c	69	b	70	a
71	a	72	d	73	c	74	b	75	c	76	b	77	a
78	b	79	c	80	b	81	c	82	b	83	a	84	a
85	b	86	c	87	b	88	c	89	c	90	c	91	c
92	b	93	a	94	c	95	b	96	b	97	a	98	b
99	b	100	d	101	a	102	b	103	b	104	c	105	c
106	c	107	a	108	c	109	b	110	a	111	b	112	c
113	b	114	b	115	b	116	a	117	d	118	b	119	b
120	a	121	c	122	a	123	d	124	d	125	a	126	a
127	c	128	a	129	c	130	b	131	c	132	a	133	c
134	c	135	b	136	a	137	a	138	b	139	c	140	d
141	b	142	b	143	a	144	d	145	b	146	a	147	c
148	a	149	d	150	d								

33

Toxicity of Various Minerals Chemicals, Plants, and Gases

Ravi Shankar Kumar Mandal[1], Sonam Bhatt[1], Vivek Joshi[2] and Anil Kumar[1]

[1]*Department of Veterinary Medicine, Bihar Veterinary College, Patna-800014*

[2]*Division of medicine, ICAR-Indian Veterinary Research Institute, Izatnagar*

Paracelsus recognized more than 400 years ago that it is "the dose that makes the poison."Deliberate or inadvertent over dosages may cause illness, and a misplaced decimal in water or feed medication concentrations frequently results in toxicity. A general feature of modern complex poultry rations, feed mill equipment, and feed delivery to poultry farms is that any component included in a ration may at some time be mistakenly included at a higher than desired rate. This may occur through human or mechanical error. For example, sulfaquinoxaline poisoning occurs in meat-type chickens, even at recommended doses, because of high water intake in warm buildings, particularly in hot weather, or because of poor feed mixing.

Poisonous substances are widely distributed in nature. Poisoning occurs more frequently in free-range and backyard flocks and in village poultry where birds forage in neighboring gardens and fields or receive household waste and weeds cut from roadsides and fields. Some of these poisonings are malicious. Contaminated litter on the floor and in nest boxes is an added source of toxins in chickens not raised on wire.

Antimicrobials, Anticoccidials, and Growth Promotants

Most reports of poisoning with chemotherapeutic agents involve inappropriate use or overdose of ionophore anticoccidials or growth promotants. Sulfaquinoxaline and sulfamethazine were most widely used. Chickens with sulfa toxicity are depressed, pale, and frequently underweight. In adults, there is a marked decrease in egg production and shell quality; brown eggs may be depigmented. Ionophores (ion carriers) facilitate movement of some monovalent cations, such as sodium and potassium, and divalent cations, such as calcium and magnesium, across cell membranes. Subchronic monensin toxicity resulted in opaque fibrin plaques on the epicardium, hemorrhage in coronary fat, and decreased liver weight.

Nutrients and Other Feed- and Water-Related Toxicants

Interaction among some amino acids relates to growth, but only methionine is toxic to poultry. A variety of feedstuffs and potential feed stuffs are poorly digestible, contain factors that inhibit digestion (protein inhibitors), depress growth, cause pasting of feces, or increase the incidence of skeletal disorders.

Metals and Metalloids

Arsenic: Inorganic, aliphatic, and trivalent organic arsenicals are used as pesticides, weed and brush killers, and defoliants. Toxic effects include diarrhea, nervous signs, and cyanosis.

Lead: Lead is widespread in the environment, and there are many possible sources for ingested lead when toxicity occurs. Most lead poisoning in birds is chronic. Clinical disease usually is seen as wasting, ataxia, lameness or paralysis, and anemia. In acute cases, anorexia, weakness, prostration, and anemia may be prominent. Basophilic stippling and abnormal erythrocytes may occur in lead-poisoned birds.

Mercury: Residues in chickens given subclinical amounts of methylmercury found highest in liver, least in muscle, and intermediate in kidney. Eggs had 4 times as much mercury in albumin compared with yolk. Wallerian degeneration of peripheral nerves and spinal cord and neuronal damage in the brain may be present. Vasculitis also may be obvious in some vessels, particularly in the brain.

Vanadium: Vanadium can contaminate phosphorus sources and cause reduced egg quality, growth, and hatchability.

Other

Calcium lignosulfonate, a pellet binder, may produce black, sticky cecal contents that adhere to the skin ofprocessed broilers, causing increased condemnation from contamination.

Nitrate and Nitrite: High levels of nitrate cause diarrhea, dyspnea, and death. Lower levels affect growth and egg production. Blood hemoglobin is changed to methemoglobin.

Pen-and Litter-Related Toxicants

Boric acid is used in litter to control darkling beetles and may be consumed by broilers, which results in reduced growth and abnormal feathering.

Ferrous sulfate heptahydrate added to litter to reduce ammonia formation is toxic to broilers.

Pentachlorophenol has been used as a pesticide in industry and agriculture, but its primary use is as a wood preservative. Sawdust and shavings from treated wood frequently have been used as poultry litter; chickens can become contaminated from contact with these shavings.

Disinfectants and Fumigants

Phenol, cresol, creolin, carbolineum, and creosote products cause damage to vascular endothelium, epithelia of respiratory and digestive tracts, and parenchymal organs, such as liver and kidney.

High levels of quaternary ammonia cause epithelial irritation of the mouth, pharynx, and upper respiratory tract, resulting in oral, ocular, and nasal discharges.

Prolonged exposure to high levels of formaldehyde, which dissolves in liquids on mucous membranes to produce formalin, in the hatcher impairs cilial function and causes tracheal epithelial degeneration and sloughing.

Insecticides

Organochloride insecticides often remain longer in the environment than other insecticides. Because they are fat soluble, organochlorides tend to build up in the food chain and be present in yolks of eggs.

Organophosphorus and carbamate insecticides inhibit acetylcholinesterase, causing acetylcholine to accumulate, which results in the overstimulation of parasympathetic nerves and muscles.Delayed neurotoxicity occurs several days to weeks after exposure, causing progressive degeneration of the peripheral nerves and spinal cord, which leads to weak ness and paralysis. Acetyl cholinesterase is not affected.

Rodenticides

Alpha-naphthylthiourea causes depression, anorexia, weakness, prostration, and death. Lesions include pulmonary edema, hydropericardium, fatty change in liver, and myocardial degeneration.

Warfarin, brodifacoum, and diphacinone are anticoagulant rodenticides, inhibit epoxide reductase, which converts vitamin K to its active form. Toxicity causes anemia with fluttering, gasping, and hemorrhages in eyes, mouth, and other tissues

Weakness, diarrhea, opisthotonos, and convulsions occur with zinc phosphide.

Toxic Gases

Ammonia levels should be less than 25 ppm, but in poorly ventilated litter-type houses, ammonia may exceed 100 ppm. Ammonia dissolves in the liquid on mucous membranes and eyes to produce ammonium hydroxide, an irritating alkali causing keratoconjunctivitis.

Carbon monoxide (CO) poisoning may occur in build ings in which defective or unventilated gas-catalytic or open-flame brooders or furnaces are in use, or where poultry are exposed to internal combustion-engine exhaust fumes. Affected chicks or poults show drowsiness, labored breathing, and in-coordination. Spasms and convulsions may occur prior to death. At postmortem, blood is bright red.

Phytotoxins

All or parts of some plants are toxic, or if fed at low levels may only reduce growth rate. Phytotoxin present in some plants are as following: Gossypol in cotton seed meal, cyanide or prussic acid in *Eucalyptus cladocalyx* leaf, conine in hemlock seed, scopolamine and hyoscyamine in *Datura stramonium*, mimosine in *Leucaena leucocephala,* asclepidin in milkweed, belladonna in nightshade (*Solanum nigrum*), taxine in yew.

MCQ

1. I n blood circulation cadmium (C d) is transported after binding with
   a) Metallothionine b) Metallophosphate
   c) Albumin d) Globulin
2. Absorption of Cadmium (CD) in the digestive tract increases deficiencies of minerals such as
   a) Calcium b) Phosphorus
   c) Iron d) Both a and c

3. Ingestion of Cadmium (CD) at a high rate results in areduction in egg production by poultry as a result of
   a) Histopathological damage
   b) Reducing feed intake
   c) Increasing sensitivity to stress
   d) All
4. Arsenic toxicity causes
   a) Block synthesis of acetyl-CoA synthesis
   b) Block synthesis of glutathione (GSH)
   c) Fatty acid oxidation
   d) All of the above
5. Most toxic form of mercury is
   a) Mercuric iodide
   b) Methyl mercury
   c) Mercuric chloride
   d) Mercuric oxide
6. Once absorbed mercury gets distributed throughout the body and is stored mainly in the
   a) Bone
   b) Liver
   c) Kidney
   d) Both b and c
7. "The dose that makes the poison" (All things are poison, and nothing is without poison; the dosage alone makes it so a thing is not a poison) is statement of
   a) Rachel Carson
   b) Paracelsus
   c) W. Eugene Smith
   d) Socrates
8. A chemical substance found within an organism that is not naturally produced or expected to be present within the organism
   a) Probiotic
   b) Prebiotic
   c) Xenobiotic
   d) Symbiotic
9. Sulfaquinoxaline poisoning occurs in meat-type chickens, even at recommended doses, because of
   a) High water intake in warm buildings
   b) Poor feed mixing
   c) Both a and b
   d) None
10. Manifestations of sulfa toxicity are
    a) Hemorrhagic syndrome
    b) Bone marrow depression
    c) Thrombocytopenia
    d) All
11. "Paintbrush" ecchymotic hemorrhages in the myocardium is seen in toxicity of
    a) Ionophores
    b) Sulfonamides
    c) Nicarbazin
    d) Quinolones
12. Lesions in Sulfonamide toxicity is characterized by
    a) Ulcers at the proventricular–ventricular junction.
    b) The entire length of the intestinal tract may be spotted with petechial and ecchymotic hemorrhage.
    c) Hemorrhage may be present in the proventriculus and beneath the ventriculus (gizzard) lining.
    d) All

13. Microscopic lesions associated with sulfa toxicity are
    a) Lymphoid hypoplasia around splenic sheaths
    b) Hemosiderin deposits in necrotic areas.
    c) Degeneration and necrosis of tubular epithelium
    d) All
14. Compounds have both anticoccidial and antibacterial activity, and used extensively in poultry and ruminant feeds
    a) Ionophores
    b) Sulfonamides
    c) Nicarbazin
    d) Quinolones
15. Choose correct statements
    a) Ionophores are coccidiocidal because of their ability to preferentially move ions, usually Na+, into various stages of the parasite.
    b) Toxic levels of ionophores cause potassium to leave and calcium to enter cells, particularly myocytes, resulting in cell death.
    c) Signs of toxicity are related to high extracellular potassium and high intracellular (intramitochondrial) calcium.
    d) All
16. Subchronicmonensin toxicity results in
    a) Opaque fibrin plaques on the epicardium
    b) Hemorrhage in coronary fat
    c) Decreased liver weight
    d) All
17. Signs of Nicarbazin toxicity is
    a) Reduced egg production
    b) Shell depigmentation
    c) Yolk mottling
    d) All
18. The lethal dose 50% (LD50) of tetramisole for chickens is
    a) 2.75 g/kg
    b) 1.75 g/kg
    c) 0.5 g/kg
    d) 0.75 g/kg
19. The following drug has wide margin of safety in birds
    a) Levamisole
    b) Tetramisole
    c) Coumaphos
    d) Ivermectin
20. The amino acid which is toxic to poultry
    a) Alanine
    b) Arginine
    c) Methionine
    d) Leucine
21. Ethinone toxicity in chicks can be relieved by
    a) Alanine
    b) Arginine
    c) Methionine
    d) Leucine
22. Antinutrients that can be found in plants include
    a) Lectins
    b) b-glucans
    c) Pentosans
    d) All

23. Aluminum toxicity causes
    a) Phosphorus retention
    b) Decreased iron absorption
    c) Decreased feed intake
    d) All
24. The condition produced in pullets by feed delivery mistakes in which layer ration is accidentally fed to pullets
    a) Urolithiasis
    b) Nephrosis
    c) Hyperuricemia
    d) All
25. Swollen gunmetalcoloured kidney is observed in toxicity of
    a) Copper
    b) Sulphur
    c) Cadmium
    d) Molybdenum
26. Enlarged spleen with dark, brown-black (blackberry jam) parenchyma is characteristic of toxicity of
    a) Copper
    b) Sulphur
    c) Cadmium
    d) Molybdenum
27. Lead may affect haeme synthesis by interfering enzyme
    a) Amino levulinic acid dehydratase
    b) Haemesynthetase
    c) Coprogen oxidase
    d) All
28. Poor growth and a bizarre syndrome of chicks falling over, lying motionless, getting up,and then repeating falling over, seen in the toxicity of
    a) Copper
    b) Sulphur
    c) Iodine
    d) Molybdenum
29. Sodium toxicity in chicks produces
    a) Heart failure
    b) Edema
    c) Ascites
    d) All
30. Basophilic stippling and abnormal erythrocytes may occur in poisoning of
    a) Copper
    b) Lead
    c) Iodine
    d) Molybdenum
31. The final diagnosis of lead poisoning is based on blood and tissue levels, which includes
    a) Blood lead level greater than 4 ppm
    b) Liver lead level greater than 18 ppm wet weight,
    c) Kidney lead level greater than 20 ppm wet weight
    d) All
32. Acid-fast inclusions in kidney epithelial cells suggest poisoning of
    a) Cadmium
    b) Lead
    c) Mercury
    d) Molybdenum
33. Excess magnesium in diet of poultry causes
    a) Bone abnormalities
    b) Replaces calcium
    c) Affects phosphate utilization
    d) All

34. Excess phosphorus in diet leads to
    a) Affects growth plate development of bones
    b) Hematologic abnormalities
    c) Tibial dyschondroplasia
    d) All
35. Toxic effects of arsenic include
    a) Diarrhea b) Nervous signs
    c) Cyanosis d) All
36. Following antibacterial and antiviral agent used in hatchery impairs cilial function and causes tracheal epithelial degeneration and sloughing
    a) Chlorine b) Formaldehyde
    c) Pentachlorophenol d) KMnO4
37. Sawdust used in poultry litter may cause toxicity of
    a) Chlorine b) Formaldehyde
    c) Pentachlorophenol d) KMnO4
38. Toxicity associated with pentachlorophenol is
    a) Kidney hypertrophy
    b) Decreased humoral immune responses
    c) Musty taste in eggs and broiler meat
    d) All
39. Chlorophenols in litter are metabolized by bacteria and fungi to .... which are responsible for the musty taste in eggs and meat from chickens in contact with contaminated litter
    a) Dioxins b) Chloroanisoles
    c) Both d) None
40. High mortality, ulcerative dermatitis primarily affecting moist areas of the body, irritation of respiratory mucous membranes, and conjunctivitis occurred in chicks due to treatment of building with
    a) Sulfur b) Iron
    c) Pentachlorophenol d) Boric acid
41. Following is added to litter to reduce ammonia formation
    a) Boric acid b) Ferrous sulfate heptahydrate
    c) Pentachlorophenol d) Formaldehyde
42. The following herbicide causes toxicity by converting hemoglobin to methemoglobin
    a) Potassium chlorates b) Sodium chlorates
    c) Nitrate d) All
43. A pellet binder, which may produce black, sticky cecal contents that adhere to the skin of processed broilers, causing increased condemnation from contamination
    a) Calcium lignosulfonate b) Ethoxyquin
    c) Ferrous sulfate heptahydrate d) Uranyl Nitrate

44. Wallerian degeneration of peripheral nerves and spinal cord and neuronal damage in the brain may be due to toxicity of
    a) Methyl mercuric chloride b) Arasan
    c) Captan d) Potassium chlorates
45. Arasan (active ingredient thiram, a dithiocarbamate) has caused poisoning in poultry by
    a) Teratogenic effect b) Soft-shelled eggs
    c) Tibial dyschondroplasia d) All
46. Following dipyridyl herbicides cause toxicity by the inhibition of the glutathione peroxidase system
    a) Paraquat b) Amitrate
    c) 2,4-D d) All
47. The insecticides inhibit acetylcholinesterase, causing acetylcholine to accumulate, which results in the overstimulation of parasympathetic nerves and muscles
    a) Organochlorine b) Carbamates
    c) Lindane d) DDT
48. Sign of toxicity of Dichlorodiphenyltrichloroethane (DDT) and dichlorodiphenyl-trichloroethane (DDE) are:
    a) Tremors b) Lose weight
    c) Eggshell thinning d) All
49. In organophosphorus poisoning following compound is used to reverse clinical signs
    a) Atropine b) Selenium
    c) Diazinon d) Fenthion
50. Toxic effect of Paraquat can be protected by administration of
    a) Atropine b) Selenium
    c) Diazinon d) Fenthion
51. Delayed neurotoxic effects are observed in toxicity of
    a) Organophosphorus b) Carbamates
    c) Malathion d) All
52. Delayed neurotoxicity occurs several days to weeks after exposure due to
    a) Progressive degeneration of the peripheral nerves and spinal cord
    b) Inhibition of acetylcholinesterase
    c) Both a and b
    d) None
53. Signs of delayed neurotoxicity due to Organophosphorus include
    a) Ataxia b) Falling sideways
    c) Lack of leg reflexes d) All

54. Pulmonary edema, hydropericardium, fatty change in liver, and myocardial degeneration are observed in toxicity with

a) Alpha-naphthylThiourea (ANTU) b) Pyrethrum

c) Rotenone d) Lindane

55. Lesions include dark, unclotted blood, pulmonary hemorrhage and edema, clotted bloodin the trachea and air sacs, petechiation, enteritis, and hydropericardium are observed in toxicity of

a) Sodium monofluoroacetate b) Metaldehyde

c) Avitrol d) 2-chloro-4 acetotoluidine (CAT)

56. Toxic effects of strychnine are

a) Tonic spasms

b) Respiratory failure and reproductive failure

c) Increased mortality of progeny from exposed hens

d) All

57. Epoxide reductase inhibitors are

a) Warfarin b) Brodifacoum

c) Diphacinone d) All

58. Anemia with fluttering, gasping, and hemorrhages in eyes, mouth, and other tissues are observed in toxicity of

a) Warfarin b) Brodifacoum

c) Diphacinone d) All

59. A petroleum-like odor from the crop contents is detected in poisoning with

a) Warfarin b) Zinc phosphide

c) Diphacinone d) Brodifacoum

60. Normally in poultry houses ammonia level should not exceed

a) 25 ppm b) 100 ppm

c) 200 ppm d) 300 ppm

61. Ammonia dissolves in the liquid on mucous membranes and eyes to produce ...., an irritating alkali causing keratoconjunctivitis

a) Ammonium sulfate b) Ammonium hydroxide

c) Ammonium chloride d) Ammonium phosphate

62. Signs of ammonia toxicity include

a) Photophobia b) Keratoconjunctivitis

c) Corneal ulcer d) All

63. Poultry are exposed to internal combustion-engine exhaust fumes affected with poisoning of

a) Ammonia b) Polytetrafluoroethylene

c) Carbon monoxide d) Methane

64. Bright red blood at postmortem is observed in poisoning with
   a) Ammonia b) Polytetrafluoroethylene
   c) Carbon monoxide d) Methane
65. Birds frequently are intoxicated from ingesting fermented fruits with
   a) Ethyl alcohol b) Ethylene glycol
   c) Methane d) Hydrogen sulfide
66. Calcium oxalate crystals block renal tubules and cause tubular epithelial necrosis leading to hyperuricemia and urate nephrosis with visceral urate deposits in toxicity with
   a) Ethyl alcohol b) Ethylene glycol
   c) Methane d) Hydrogen sulfide
67. Coccidia oocysts treated with ethylene oxide were toxic to chicks and caused kidney lesions similar to
   a) Ethylene glycol b) Ethyl alcohol
   c) Methane d) Carbon tetrachloride
68. Chick edema factor is
   a) 2,3,7, 8- tetrachl orodibenzodioxin (TCDD)
   b) Polybrominated Biphenyl (PBB)
   c) Polychlorinated Biphenyl (PCB)
   d) All
69. Chick edema disease develops due to addition of contaminants tallow with
   a) 2,3,7, 8-tetrachl orodibenzodioxin (TCDD)
   b) Polybrominated Biphenyl (PBB)
   c) Polychlorinated Biphenyl (PCB)
   d) All
70. Poisonous substances produced by living organisms are
   a) Biotoxins b) Endotoxins
   c) Exotoxins d) Phytotoxins
71. A chemical substance found within an organism that is not naturally produced or expected to be present within the organism is
   a) Biotoxin b) Phytotoxin
   c) Xenobiotic d) Endotoxin
72. Clinical signs after ingestion of Rose chafers (Macrodactylussubspinosus) include
   a) Weakness b) Prostration
   c) Convulsions d) All
73. Ricin poisoning is seen with ingestion of
   a) Carolina Jessamine b) Castor Bean
   c) Theobroma cacao d) Corn Cockle

74. Gossypol toxicity is seen with ingestion of
  a) Castor Bean
  b) Theobroma cacao
  c) Cotton Seed Meal
  d) Corn Cockle
75. Cyanide or Prussic Acid toxicity is observed with ingestion of
  a) *Eucalyptus cladocalyx*
  b) *Conium maculatum*
  c) *Daturastramonium*
  d) Death Camas
76. Conine toxicity is associated with
  a) *Zygadenus*spp
  b) Hemlock seed
  c) *Leucaenaleucocephala*
  d) *Convallariamajalis*
77. Mimosine toxicity is associated with
  a) *Zygadenus*spp
  b) Hemlock seed
  c) *Leucaenaleucocephala*
  d) *Convallariamajalis*
78. Asclepidin toxicity is associated with
  a) Milkweed
  b) Hemlock seed
  c) Cotton seed
  d) *Convallariamajalis*
79. Belladonna toxicity is associated with
  a) Milkweed
  b) Hemlock seed
  c) Cotton seed
  d) Nightshade
80. Osteolathyrism is associated with
  a) Sweet Pea
  b) *Lathyrus odoratus*
  c) *Allium ascalonicum*
  d) Both a and b
81. Neurologic disease, neurolathyrism is associated with
  a) *Lathyrus sativa*
  b) *Lathyrus odoratus*
  c) *Allium ascalonicum*
  d) Both a and b
82. Sudden death with epicardial hemorrhage and pallor, hydropericardium, and hepatosplenomegaly and hemosiderin in hepatocytes, Kupffer cells, and renal tubules are observed in
  a) Allium ascalonicum
  b) Onion poisoning
  c) Oxalate poisoning
  d) Both a and b
83. Ergot alkaloids cause
  a) Vasoconstriction
  b) Uterine contraction
  c) Adrenergic blockade
  d) All
84. Acute ergotism is
  a) Nervous ergotism
  b) Convulsive ergotism
  c) Gangrenous ergotism
  d) Both a and b
85. Nephrotoxic mycotoxins are
  a) Ocharotoxin
  b) Citrinin
  c) Oosporein
  d) All

86. Yellow rice toxin is due to
   a) Citreovirdin
   b) Penitrem A
   c) Trichothecenes
   d) Vomitoxin
87. Mechanism of toxicity of T-2 toxin (Trichothecenes) is
   a) Interaction with 60 S subunit of ribosomes
   b) Inhibits synthesis of DNA
   c) Inhibition of peptidyl transferase
   d) All
88. T-2 toxin is produced by
   a) *Fusarium tricinctium*
   b) *Penicillium citreoviride*
   c) *Penicillium citrinum*
   d) *Pithomyces chartarum*
89. Competitive ANTU antagonist is
   a) 1-ethyl-1-phenyl thiourea
   b) Warfarin
   c) Fluoroacetate
   d) Zinc phosphide
90. Fluoroacetate as such is non-toxic but becomes highly toxic after its metabolic conversion (lethal synthesis) in the body to
   a) Phosphine
   b) Fluorocitrate
   c) Glycerol monoacetate
   d) Fluorosulfate
91. Fluorocitrate has affinity for
   a) Aconitase
   b) 60 S subunit of ribosomes
   c) 30 S subunit of ribosomes
   d) Acetylcholinesterase
92. Toxicity of zinc phophide is due to
   a) Zinc
   b) Phosphorus
   c) Phosphine
   d) All
93. One of the safest rodentiicde is
   a) Red squill
   b) Fluoroacetate
   c) Warfarin
   d) ANTU
94. Type –I pyretroids induced trmors are referred as
   a) CS- syndrome
   b) T-syndrome
   c) Both a and b
   d) Delayed neuropathy
95. Type –II pyretroids cause burrowing behavious, clonic seizure, writhing and profuse salivation which is also referred as
   a) CS- syndrome
   b) T-syndrome
   c) Both a and b
   d) Delayed neuropathy
96. Which statement is correct
   a) AChE inhibition by carbamates is irreversible but that by OPI's is reversible.
   b) OPI's can detach from AChE much more easily and rapidly than Carbamates.
   c) Decarbamylation of carbamates is easier than dephosphorylation of OPI's.
   d) OPI's can bind both at anionic as well esteratic site of AChE whereas carbamates can bind only at esteratic site.

97. The chlorinated hydrocarbons are neuro-poisons and produce toxicity by
    a) Inhibiting Na^{+}-K^{+} and Ca^{2+}-Mg^{2+} ATPase
    b) Inhibit acetylcholinesterase (AChE)
    c) Inhibition of aconitase
    d) All
98. Cytotoxic anoxia is associated with
    a) *Nerium oleander*
    b) *Sorghum vulgare*
    c) *Zea mays*
    d) All
99. Taxine toxicity is associated with
    a) Yew
    b) Tobacco
    c) Velvetweed
    d) Onions
100. Photosensitization is associated with
    a) Phenothiazine
    b) Acridine
    c) Rose Bengal
    d) All

Answer Key

1	a	2	d	3	d	4	d	5	b	6	d	7	b
8	c	9	c	10	d	11	b	12	d	13	d	14	a
15	d	16	d	17	d	18	a	19	d	20	c	21	c
22	d	23	d	24	d	25	a	26	a	27	d	28	c
29	d	30	b	31	d	32	b	33	d	34	d	35	d
36	b	37	c	38	d	39	b	40	a	41	b	42	d
43	a	44	a	45	d	46	a	47	b	48	d	49	a
50	b	51	d	52	a	53	d	54	a	55	a	56	d
57	d	58	d	59	b	60	a	61	b	62	d	63	c
64	c	65	a	66	b	67	a	68	d	69	d	70	a
71	c	72	d	73	b	74	c	75	a	76	b	77	c
78	a	79	d	80	d	81	d	82	d	83	d	84	d
85	d	86	a	87	d	88	a	89	a	90	b	91	a
92	c	93	a	94	b	95	a	96	c	97	a	98	d
99	a	100	d										

34

Field and Laboratory Investigation for Disease Diagnosis

Sirigireddy Sivajothi, Bhavanam Sudhakara Reddy, Dadireddy Narmada Raghavi and Devupalli Satyanarayana Murthy

College of Veterinary Science - Proddatur, Sri Venkateswara Veterinary University Andhra Pradesh, India

All infectious agents, toxins, and nutritional imbalances have an impact on the performance of the farm and consequently on the local poultry industry. Additionally, poultry can be infected with common diseases like endoparasites, ectoparasites, infectious bronchitis, Marek's disease, fowl cholera, salmonellosis, infectious coryza, fowl pox, avian encephalomyelitis, etc.

Controlling infectious diseases is vital for poultry health and diagnostic methods are an indispensable feature to resolve disease etiologies and the impact of infectious agents on the host. Although the basic principles of disease diagnostics have not changed, the spectrum of poultry diseases constantly expanded, with the identification of new pathogens and improved knowledge on epidemiology and disease pathogenesis. In parallel, new technologies have been devised to identify and characterize infectious agents, but classical methods remain crucial, especially the isolation of pathogens and their further characterization in functional assays and studies.

In poultry medicine, the diagnostic process originally shifted from the traditional veterinarian approach centered on individual animals to the health assessment of entire flocks. Flocks are commonly classified as "healthy" if they perform according to their genetic potential and are considered free from clinical disease. On-farm, diagnostic activities comprise routine sampling and investigations in line with health control programs; nationally and/or internationally adopted control programs for certain *Mycoplasma* and *Salmonella* species represent examples of paramount importance. Samples may be investigated immediately on site (e.g., rapid antigen test for avian influenza) or sent for further processing to a laboratory (e.g., ELISA and PCR). Field veterinarians further implement diagnostic surveillance in order to provide epidemiological data for flock management purposes. The periodical collection of samples (e.g., feces, serum samples, and swabs from mucosal surfaces) is primarily used to confirm the infection (free) status of a flock or to monitor vaccine response. Altogether, generated data facilitate objective judgment and decision making in order to optimize flock health and production.

In the field, diagnostic procedures are initiated as soon as flock health is compromised, using morbidity and/or mortality as initial indicators. In such a scenario, investigations start with the compilation of a case history pertaining to relevant flock, management and infection/ disease characteristics (e.g., bird type and origin, age, routine medications, vaccination program, previous diseases, husbandry system, standard operation procedures such as feeding and watering systems, ventilation, lighting program, hygiene and biosecurity processes, production parameters, morbidity and mortality data, duration of signs/problems and epidemiological links to other production sites). On the farm, diagnostics starts with the clinical examination of flocks, individual birds in various stages of the disease and their products (e.g., feces and eggs) by experienced poultry workers and veterinarians thoroughly familiar with the appearance of a healthy flock and the environment. Clinical examinations are time consuming and labor intensive and can regrettably fail to detect diseases; especially subclinical diseases can be challenging to be accurately diagnosed) The manifestation of an infectious disease can vary from subclinical to severe clinical illness, depending on various etiological factors and influences such as the causative agent, host and/or environment altogether complicating diagnosis. Clinical signs comprise non-specific, general signs (e.g., apathy, ruffled feathers, and inappetence), which can be associated with a wide range of diseases, often together with more specific signs indicative of a certain disorder (e.g., enteric, respiratory, and neurologic) or even pathognomonic for a specific disease (e.g., histomonosis). Diagnostic procedures continue with post mortem investigations, on farm or in the laboratory, which serve to identify gross pathological changes in organs and tissues in order to further specify a tentative cause of impaired performance and clinical signs. Altogether, a comprehensive case history together with the accurate assessment of clinical signs and thorough post mortem investigations narrows the range of presumptive diagnoses. This provides the basis to select appropriate laboratory methods.

Write correct alphabet of the answer in the given bracket

1. Typical star-grazing posture is characteristic symptoms of which vitamin deficiency

   a) Vitamin A b) Thiamine

   c) Riboflavin d) Vitamin D

2. Sudden death without any clinical signs, accompanied by marked reddish discoloration of comb, wattle and toes is seen in which disease of poultry

   a) Bird flu b) Marek's disease

   c) Ascites d) Candidiasis

3. Paralysis of leg and wing in birds with 6 weeks age

   a) Marek's disease b) Gumboro disease

   c) Coccidiosis d) Bird flu

4. A bird with nasal discharges, facial oedema, conjunctivitis and open-mouth breathing is characteristic symptom of

   a) Marek's disease b) Infectious coryza

   c) Ascites d) Candidiasis

5. Falling forward with leg outstand behind and lying paralyzed for several minutes is characteristic of which deficiency

   a) Chloride deficiency b) Choline deficiency

   c) Riboflavin deficiency d) All of the above

6. A poultry species laying thin shelled eggs, rough and rebound eggs are symptoms of which disease

a) Infectious bronchitis b) Gumboro disease
c) Egg drop syndrome d) Bird flu

7. A healthy fast-growing broilers dying on their back suddenly, flap wings intensely and have convulsions

a) Sudden death syndrome b) Gumboro disease
c) Egg drop syndrome d) Bird flu

8. On post mortem examination of chicken bird, abscess is found in the foot pad is characteristic of which disease

a) Rickets b) Bumble foot
c) Egg drop syndrome d) Egg peritonitis

9. Subcutaneous cellulitis of head is highly suggestive of which disease

a) Swollen head syndrome b) Salmonellosis
c) Pasteurellosis d) Bird flu

10. Swollen head syndrome in poultry is differentially diagnosed with which bacterial disease

a) Brucellosis b) Salmonellosis
c) Pasteurellosis d) Bumble foot

11. Symble pharon condition is associated with which of the following

a) Swollen head syndrome b) Salmonellosis
c) E. coli infection d) Mycoplasmosis

12. A bird with enlarged yolk sac, typical omphalitis in 3 day old chick is seen is diagnosed as

a) Swollen head syndrome b) Salmonellosis
c) E. coli infection d) Mycoplasmosis

13. Reserved carriers from pullorum disease can be identified using which laboratory test

a) PCR
b) Tube Agglutination test
c) Rapid whole blood plate agglutination test
d) Hemagglutination tset

14. Enrichment medium for identification of Salmonella pullorum

a) Tetrathionate broth b) SSDA
c) Both d) Blood agar

15. Birds showing copious white diarrhea with faecal matter adherent to plumage surrounding vent

a) Pullorum b) Pasteurellosis
c) Salmonellosis d) All

16. Panopthamitis in turkey poultry is characteristic of
    a) Salmonella pullorum b) Salmonella Arizona
    c) Pasteurella multocida d) All
17. Characteristic bipolar organisms observed in Giemsa stained smear is seen in which disease
    a) Pasteurellosis b) Salmonellosis
    c) Mycoplasmosis d) Coccidiosis
18. In which of the following disease torticollis is seen commonly
    a) Pasteurellosis b) E.coli infections
    c) Newcastle disease d) All of the above
19. A bird with caseous cellulitis of wattles and sero-purulent arthritis may be diagnosed as
    a) Pasteurellosis b) E.coli infections
    c) Newcastle disease d) Spirochetosis
20. Enlarged spleen with mottling due to subscapular hemorrhages is predominant lesion of which disease
    a) Pasteurellosis b) E.coli infections
    c) Newcastle disease d) Spirochetosis
21. Avian encephalomyelitis is differentiated with which of the following
    a) Encephalomalacia b) E.coli infections
    c) Newcastle disease d) Spirochetosis
22. The major site of blood collection in poultry is
    a) Jugular vein b) Wing vein
    c) Comb d) Both b & c
23. A bird presented with perivascular cuffing and degeneration of neuron are characteristic symptom seen in which of the following
    a) Influenza b) Avian pox
    c) Epidemic tremor d) Pullorum
24. Lenticular opacity (cataract) in poultry birds is seen after recovery from which disease.
    a) Influenza b) Avian pox
    c) Epidemic tremor d) Pullorum
25. Cofal test is gold standard test for which disease
    a) Lymphoid Leucosis b) Ranikhet Disease
    c) Salmonellosis d) Anthrax
26. Incoordination and lateral recumbency in chicken between 7-14 day old is associated with
    a) Spiking Mortality Syndrome b) Ranikhet Disease
    c) Mycoplasmosis d) Lymphoid Leucosis

27. Intra nuclear inclusion bodies shown on histopathological examination of infected liver associated with which infective disease
    a) Adenovirus infection b) Salmonellosis
    c) Herpes virus infection d) Mycoplasmosis
28. A bird with sudden drop in egg production with no specific clinical abnormalities is characteristic of ______
    a) Salmonellosis b) Mycoplasmosis
    c) Egg drop syndrome d) Fowl typhoid
29. Characteristic hydropericardium condition is associated with which disease
    a) Angara disease b) Salmonellosis
    c) E. coli infection d) Pullorum
30. For histopathology of birds tissue sample are collected from
    a) Live animals b) dead
    c) Both d) None
31. For histopathology of birds size of tissue should not be more than
    a) 10 cm b) 5 cm
    c) 3 cm d) 1 cm
32. Double pored tape worm of poultry is
    a) Dipylidium caninum b) Moniezia expansa
    c) Cotugnia digonopora d) All of the above
33. Trichomonas gallinae predilection site
    a) Pharynx b) Oesophagus
    c) Crop d) All of the above
34. In which disease yellow buttons are characteristics in liver and lungs of birds
    a) Ascardia galli b) Trichomonas gallinae
    c) Histomonas meleagridis d) Tetrameres spp.
35. For which parasite earth worms will act as transport host in poultry
    a) Ascardia galli b) Trichomonas gallinae
    c) Histomonas meleagridis d) Tetrameres spp.
36. Hemorrhagic enteritis with ulceration and necrosis seen in
    a) Histomonas meleagridis b) Tetrameres spp.
    c) Ornithostrogylus quadriradiatus d) All
37. Intermediate host for Raillietina tetragona
    a) Ants b) Snails
    c) Earthworms d) Slugs
38. Caecal worm of poultry
    a) Ascardia galli b) Syngamus trachea
    c) Histomonas meleagridis d) Heterakis spp.

39. Gapeworm of poultry
    a) Ascardia galli
    b) Syngamus trachea
    c) Histomonas meleagridis
    d) Heterakis spp.
40. Coccidia positive material cab be preserved in
    a) 2.5% k2Cr2O7
    b) 70% Alcohol
    c) Formalin
    d) NS
41. Air sac mite in birds
    a) Sternostoma tracheacolum
    b) Demodex spp.
    c) Sarcoptes spp
    d) Psoroptes spp.
42. In postmortem examination, white spots on the surface at air sacs and pulmonary edema can be seen due to
    a) Sternostoma tracheacolum
    b) Demodex spp.
    c) Sarcoptes spp
    d) Psoroptes spp.
43. A bird is presented with history of blood stained dropping and pallor comb and wattles is associated with
    a) Coccidiosis
    b) Pullorum
    c) Avian influenza
    d) Angora disease
44. Osteopenia and proximal epiphysis of femur fracture is seen in which disease Condition
    a) Coccidiosis
    b) Renting Syndrome
    c) Avian influenza
    d) Angora disease
45. Haemorrhagic typhilitis is caused by which species of coccidian
    a) Eimeria mivati
    b) Eimeria brunette
    c) Eimeria tenella
    d) Eimeria necatrix
46. On postmortem examination Hemorrhages are seen on duodenum and ceaca in which of the following disease.
    a) Angora disease
    b) Renting Syndrome
    c) Avian influenza
    d) Coccidiosis
47. Ladder like lesions in intestine is due to
    a) Eimeria acervulina
    b) Eimeria brunetti
    c) Eimeria tenella
    d) Eimeria necatrix
48. salt and pepper appearance of intestine is due to
    a) Eimeria acervulina
    b) Eimeria brunette
    c) Eimeria tenella
    d) Eimeria necatrix
49. Principle pathogen responsible for necrotic enteritis in poultry is
    a) Clostridium perfringes
    b) Salmonella typhimurium
    c) Eimeria tenella
    d) Eimeria necatrix
50. Stiffness and death within one hour in poultry farm is associated with which disease
    a) Nectrotic enteritis
    b) Salmonellosis
    c) Botulism
    d) Coccidiosis

51. Samples meant for virological examination transported at
    a) 40C b) -200C
    c) -1960C d) 00C
52. Bipolar plugs and unsegmented embryonic mass inside eggs is seen in
    a) Capillarisis b) Ascariasis
    c) Coccidiosis d) Schistosomosis
53. Cestode of jejunum resulting in nodular granulomas and catarrhal enteritis
    a) Davainea proglottina b) Raillietina echinobothrida
    c) Choanotaenia infundibulum d) Cotugnia dignophora
54. Curled toe paralysis in poultry is seen in deficiency of
    a) Vit.D b) Vit. B2
    c) Vit.B1 d) Vit. A
55. Recumbency and paralysis with hyperextension of vent is due deficiency of
    a) Vit.D b) Vit. B2
    c) Vit.B1 d) Vit. A
56. Displacement of gastrocnemius tendon is due to deficiency of
    a) Vit.D b) Vit. B2
    c) Vit.B1 d) Pyridoxine
57. Enlargement of hock joint with reduction of length of leg bones is due to deficiency of
    a) Magnesium b) Manganese
    c) Selenium d) None of the above
58. Bending of tibio-tarsus and distortion of ribs on postmortem examination is due to deficiency of
    a) Vit.D b) Vit. B2
    c) Vit.B1 d) Pyridoxine
59. Hock sitting posture of bird is seen in which of the following disease
    a) Rickets b) Both a and b
    c) Mycoplasmic arthritis d) None of the above
60. Serous arthritis and enlargement of hock joint is characteristic of
    a) Reoviral arthritis b) Mycoplasmic arthritis
    c) Both a and b d) None of the above
61. In Staphylococcus aureus, which type of arthritis is more common
    a) Purulent arthritis b) Serous arthritis
    c) Catarrhal arthritis d) All of the above
62. Bollinger's bodies in infected tracheal mucosa is seen in which disease
    a) Avian pox b) Rabies
    c) Avian flu d) Salmonellosis

63. In which form of avian pox, presence of nodular hyperplasia of mucosa of pharynx and trachea is seen in
    a) Cutaneous form b) Diphtheritic form
    c) Both a and b d) None of the above
64. In Diphtheritic form of avian pox, death of bird is due to
    a) Anorexia b) Asphyxiation
    c) Oedema d) Abscess
65. A bird with focal lesion on comb and wattle is seen in which of the following poultry disease
    a) Avian pox b) Rabies
    c) Avian flu d) Salmonellosis
66. The lice infestation which are observed as spherical white structures adherent to shaft of the feathers
    a) Nits b) Festoons
    c) Both a & b d) None of the above
67. Subcutaneous hemorrhages on de-feathered carcass due to nocturnal feeding of
    a) Argas persicus b) Dermacentor variabilis
    c) Ornithonyssus spp. d) Dermanyssus gallinae
68. Gray scaly appearance of comb and wattles and non-feathered areas of the head is characterized by
    a) Influenza b) Dermacentor variabilis
    c) Ornithonyssus spp. d) Dermatomycosis
69. Enlargement of bursa fabricius and haemorrhages are seen in which form of IBD
    a) Chronic b) Acute
    c) Subacute d) Mild
70. Sulfur yellow colour droppings are most commonly seen in which disease of poultry
    a) Newcastle disease b) Histomonosis
    c) Coccidiosis d) Ascariasis
71. Symptoms such as greenish diarrhea, paralysis and cyanotic comb and wattle are associated with which poultry disease
    a) Newcastle disease b) Histomonosis
    c) Coccidiosis d) Ascariasis
72. Lesions such as petechial hemorrhages in pro ventriculus and necrotic caecal tonsil are seen in postmortem of which poultry disease
    a) Gumbor b) Histomonosis
    c) RD d) Influenza
73. Diagnostic test used for confirmation of RD is
    a) Hemagglutination test b) Hemagglutination inhibition test
    c) ELISA d) PCR

74. On Postmortem examination, haemorrhages at the junction of proventriculus and gizzard and pectoral leg muscle are typical lesion of

a) Gumboro b) Histomonosis
c) RD d) Influenza

75. Tracheal congestion, pale, swollen kidney and atrophied oviduct are macroscopic lesion seen in postmortem of which poultry disease

a) Gumboro b) Infectious Bronchitis
c) RD d) Infectious Laryngio tracheitis

76. On microscopic examination of trachea showing formation of intra nuclear inclusion bodies in mucosal epithelium in which disease

a) Gumboro b) Infectious Bronchitis
c) RD d) Infectious Laryngio tracheitis

77. Signs such as nasal discharge, head shaking, obstruction of trachea with mucosal plug and conjunctivitis are seen in which disease

a) Avian Pox b) Infectious Bronchitis
c) RD d) Infectious Laryngotracheitis

78. Yellow cheesy, necrotic pseudo diphtheritic membrane is seen in postmortem of which poultry disease

a) Avian Pox b) Infectious Bronchitis
c) RD d) Infectious Laryngotracheitis

79. Diagnostic test used for confirmation of Avian Influenza is

a) Hemagglutination test b) Hemagglutination inhibition test
c) ELISA d) PCR

80. Oedema and discoloration of shank and feet due to subcutaneous ecchymotic haemorrhages

a) Avian Influenza b) Infectious Bronchitis
c) RD d) Infectious Laryngotracheitis

81. Characteristic posture observed in the farm affected with Marek's disease

a) Nodules on comb and wattles b) Conjunctivitis
c) Unilateral Paralysis d) None of the above

82. Skin Leucosis noticed in broiler after de-feathering during processing is observed in which disease condition

a) Influenza b) Infectious Bronchitis
c) RD d) Marek's disease

83. On postmortem examination of dead bird diffuse nodular lymphoid tumor may be seen in liver and other organs

a) Influenza b) Infectious Bronchitis
c) RD d) Marek's disease

84. Marek's Disease in poultry develops at which age group and that is different from lymphoid Leucosis

a) > 14 weeks b) >10 weeks
c) 3 weeks d) 5 weeks

85. Diffuse or nodular lymphoid tumors are common in the liver, spleen, and bursa are characteristic lesions of

a) Influenza b) Infectious Bronchitis
c) Lymphoid Leucosis d) Marek's disease

86. which is a neoplastic disease of poultry

a) Influenza b) Infectious Bronchitis
c) Lymphoid Leucosis d) Marek's disease

87. Chick showing ataxia and inclination to sit on their hocks and falling a side are more pronounced in which disease

a) Avian Encephalomyelitis b) Marek's disease
c) Influenza d) Lymphoid Leucosis

88. Demonstration of intra nuclear inclusion body in Hematoxylin and Eosin stain in hepatocytes of chicken

a) Inclusion body hepatitis b) Avian Pox
c) Avian Encephalomyelitis d) Lymphoid Leucosis

89. On postmortem examination pericardial sac is filled with straw coloured fluid is seen in which condition

a) Avian Encephalomyelitis b) Hydropericardium syndrome
c) Lymphoid Leucosis d) All of the above

90. In Hydropericardium syndrome heart may be appeared as

a) Congested b) Balsam
c) Litchi d) Gauva

91. Haemorrhages in proventriculus, subcutaneous and muscular hemorrhages associated with aneamia seen in

a) Avian Encephalomyelitis b) Hydropericardium syndrome
c) Lymphoid Leucosis d) Chicken Infectious Anaemia

92. On microscopic examination of aneamic which characterized by panmyelophthitis and lymphoid atrophy

a) Avian Encephalomyelitis b) Hydropericardium syndrome
c) Lymphoid Leucosis d) Chicken Infectious Anaemia

93. Anaemia is characterized by watery blood, clotting time increased and paler plasma with aplasia of bone marrow is characteristic of

a) Avian EncephalomyelitisT b) Hydropericardium syndrome
c) Lymphoid Leucosis d) Chicken Infectious Anaemia

94. EDS can be distinguished from which of the following

a) Influenza b) Infectious Bronchitis
c) Lymphoid Leucosis d) Marek's disease

95. Indications for Bone marrow biopsy
    a) Non regenerative anaemia
    b) Neoplastic diseases of bone marrow
    c) Both a &b
    d) None
96. Materials for laboratory investigation of disease is collected from
    a) Living (Ante mortem) b) Dead (Post-mortem)
    c) Both d) None
97. In a poultry form birds are walking with stiffed joints. This is a classical sign of
    a) Viral arthritis b) Infectious Bronchitis
    c) Lymphoid Leucosis d) Marek's disease
98. Swollen abdomen and congestion of abdominal skin is characteristic symptom of
    a) Viral arthritis b) Ascites
    c) Lymphoid Leucosis d) Coccidiosis
99. On postmortem examination of dead poultry birds revealed that ovaries are inactive and decreased in size of oviduct. What may be the cause of the disease
    a) Thrush b) Egg Drop Syndrome
    c) Lymphoid Leucosis d) Coccidiosis
100. A layer of white cheesy material present in the crop region of bird is indicative of which disease
    a) Thrush b) Aflatoxicosis
    c) Rickets d) Coccidiosis
101. Pedunculated, irregular, cystic and discoloured ova are seen in which of the following disease
    a) Fowl Cholera b) Pullorum disease
    c) Salmonellosis d) Coccidiosis
102. Autolysed samples are not fit for
    a) Blood test b) Histopathological
    c) Serum test d) Microscopy
103. Preferable size of tissue for histopathology studies
    a) 5-7 mm b) 7-12 mm
    c) 12- 17 mm d) 17-25 mm
104. What is the volume of phosphate-buffered 10% formalin to ensure adequate fixation for histopathology
    a) 20 times b) 10 times
    c) 2times d) Equal
105. On post mortem examination dark, enlarged, friable liver than often has a coppery bronze tinge is seen in which disease
    a) Fowl Cholera b) Pullorum disease
    c) Tuberculosis d) Fowl Typhoid

106. Irregular greyish yellow nodules in liver, spleen, intestine and bone marrow are the characteristic post mortem findings of
   a) Fowl Cholera b) Pullorum disease
   c) Tuberculosis d) Mycoplasmosis
107. On postmortem, cheese like inflammatory material in air sacs and some degree of pneumonia is seen in which disease
   a) Fowl Cholera b) Pullorum disease
   c) Tuberculosis d) Mycoplasmosis
108. In aflatoxicosis which organ in poultry is primarily affected
   a) Kidney b) Liver
   c) Heart d) Spleen
109. Parasites present in the proventriculus of birds
   a) Tetrameres spp. b) Prosthagonimus ovatus
   c) Certophyllus gallinae d) Echidnophaga gallinacea
110. Which disease is popularly known as fowl plague
   a) Fowl Cholera b) Bird flu
   c) Pullorum disease d) All
111. The following disease is caused by fungal infection
   a) Pullorum disease b) Aspergillosis
   c) Enteritis d) Psittacosis
112. Avian Nephritis is also called as
   a) Cutaneous gout b) Visceral Gout
   c) Both a and b d) None
113. Clinical materials for diagnosis of aspergillosis
   a) Lung tissue b) Skin tissue
   c) A and B d) None
114. Sample required in dermatophytosis
   a) Infected hair b) Scab from edges of skin lesions
   c) A and B d) None
115. Scattered piece of yolk, thickened yolk, cheesy semi solid material and milky fluid in abdominal cavity is seen in
   a) Egg Peritonitis b) Salmonellosis
   c) Egg Drop Syndrome d) Pullorum
116. On post mortem examination of dead bird, egg is bound and lodged in the abdominal cavity
   a) Egg Peritonitis b) Egg Bound Condition
   c) Egg Drop Syndrome d) Pullorum
117. Carcass markedly dehydrated and congested, breast muscle is pale to white cooked meat appearance is seen in
   a) Heat Stress b) Cage layer fatigue
   c) Egg Drop Syndrome d) Rickets

118. A bird with soft bones and beak, keel bone is bend, ribs are leaded and legs are bowed. These are characteristic of

a) Heat Stress b) Cage layer fatigue
c) Egg Drop Syndrome d) Rickets

119. An acute respiratory disease of chickens characterized by decreased activity, nasal discharge, sneezing, a serous nasal discharge and occasionally slight facial swelling. With increased severity extreme swelling of one or both infraorbital sinuses

a) Infectious Coryza b) Fowl Cholera
c) Fowl Typhoid d) None

120. White, firm masses of various sizes in the liver, spleen, and bone marrow. The intestinal wall is thickened and pale, and there may be serosal masses is seen in which disease

a) Fowl Cholera b) Pullorum disease
c) Tuberculosis d) Mycoplasmosis

121. In the candidiasis infected birds, which part of body is used for identification

a) Crop b) Liver
c) Kidney d) Trachea

122. Haemorrhages and Oedema accompanied by atrophy of spleen, bursa of fabricius are characteristic lesion of

a) Fowl Cholera b) Blue wing disease
c) Pullorum disease d) Mycoplasmosis

123. The condition in poultry where birds in flock attack their pen mates and eat their Flesh

a) Cannibalism b) Vent picking
c) Blue wing disease d) Head picking

124. Chondrodystrophy is differentiated from which metabolic disease

a) Rickets b) Vit. D deficiency
c) Osteomalacia d) Perosis

125. Long bones are short, thick and usually deformed and enlargement of hock joint is seen in which condition

a) Rickets b) Osteomalacia
c) Perosis d) Both b and c

126. In a poultry farm where sudden death of healthy birds mostly males are due to

a) Cage Layer Fatigue b) Sudden Death Syndrome
c) Perosis d) All

127. On postmortem examination, liver is enlarged, fatty and greyish to yellow colour and showing Hemorrhages is suggestive of

a) Sudden Death Syndrome b) Cage Layer Fatigue
c) Fatty Liver d) A and B

128. On postmortem examination, kidneys are markedly reduced in size and center dilated
   a) Hypercalcaemia b) Fever of unknown origin
   c) Urolithiasis d) Cage Layer Fatigue
129. Oviduct fluke of poultry
   a) Prosthagonimus ovatus b) Fasciola gigantica
   c) Dicrocoelium dendriticum d) Paragonimus westermanii
130. Largest poultry tape worm
   a) Raillietina tetragona b) Raillietina echinobothrida
   c) Davainea proglottina d) Cotugnia dignopora
131. Double pored tapeworm of poultry
   a) Raillietina tetragona b) Raillietina echinobothrida
   c) Davainea proglottina d) Cotugnia dignopora
132. Dwarf tape worm of poultry
   a) Raillietina tetragona b) Raillietina echinobothrida
   c) Davainea proglottina d) Cotugnia diagnophora
133. Most pathogenic poultry tape worm
   a) Raillietina tetragona b) Raillietina echinobothrida
   c) Davainea proglottina d) Cotugnia diagnophora
134. Nodular taeniosis in poultry is caused by
   a) Raillietina tetragona b) Raillietina echinobothrida
   c) Davainea proglottina d) Cotugnia diagnophora
135. Most pathogenic trematode in poultry
   a) Prosthagonimus ovatus b) Fasciola gigantica
   c) Dicrocoelium dendriticum d) Paragonimus westermanii
136. Birds with clinical signs of abnormal eggs production, discharge of albumen from cloaca and gluing of feathers are indicative of which disease
   a) Prosthagonimus ovatus b) Fasciola gigantica
   c) Dicrocoelium dendriticum d) Paragonimus westermanii
137. Penguin like moments of pregnant women posture in poultry is a characteristic feature of which disease condition in poultry
   a) Prosthagonimus ovatus b) Fasciola gigantica
   c) Dicrocoelium dendriticum d) Paragonimus westermanii
138. Synonym for histomoniosis in poultry
   a) Infectious Entero-Hepatitis b) Black Head disease
   c) Both a and b d) None of the above
139. Stick tight flea of fowl
   a) Certophyllus gallinae b) Echidnophaga gallinacea
   c) Xenopssylla chepis d) Ctenocephalides canis

140. Common flea of domestic poultry and responsible for irritation and anaemia is
   a) Certophyllus gallinae b) Echidnophaga gallinacea
   c) Xenopssylla chepis d) Ctenocephalides canis
141. Tularemia caused by Fracisella tularensis, mechanically transmitted by
   a) Certophyllus gallinae b) Echidnophaga gallinacea
   c) Xenopssylla chepis d) Ctenocephalides canis
142. Menopon gallinae is commonly known as
   a) Wing louse of poultry b) Body louse of poultry
   c) Shaft louse of poultry d) Tropical Bird louse
143. Menacanthus stramineus is commonly known as
   a) Wing louse of poultry b) Body louse of poultry
   c) Shaft louse of poultry d) Tropical Bird louse
144. Heavy lice infestation in birds is known as
   a) Puritis b) Pediculosis
   c) Lousiness d) All
145. Fowl tick/ Tampan
   a) Argas persicus b) Boophilus microplus
   c) Ornithodoros moubata d) Otobius megnini
146. Following tick acts as vector for Borrelia ansarina which causes fowl Spirochetosis
   a) Argas persicus b) Boophilus microplus
   c) Ornithodoros moubata d) Otobius megnini
147. Common name of Lipeurus caponis
   a) Wing louse of poultry b) Body louse of poultry
   c) Shaft louse of poultry d) Tropical Bird louse
148. Identified the flea that associated with formation of nodules
   a) Certophyllus gallinae b) Echidnophaga gallinacea
   c) Xenopssylla chepis d) Ctenocephalides canis
149. The following lice is considered as destructive louse of poultry, causes severe irritation and scab covered skin
   a) Menacnthus stramineus b) Menopan gallinae
   c) Lipeurus caponis d) Echidnophaga gallinacea
150. Tracheal rail sounds in poultry is caused by
   a) Ascardia galli b) Heterakis gallinarum
   c) Syngamus Trachea d) Trichomonas gallinae

Answer Key

1	b	2	a	3	a	4	b	5	a	6	a	7	a
8	b	9	a	10	c	11	a	12	c	13	c	14	a
15	a	16	b	17	a	18	d	19	a	20	d	21	c
22	d	23	c	24	c	25	a	26	a	27	a	28	c
29	a	30	c	31	d	32	c	33	a	34	c	35	a
36	c	37	a	38	d	39	b	40	a	41	a	42	a
43	a	44	b	45	c	46	d	47	a	48	d	49	a
50	a	51	b	52	a	53	b	54	b	55	c	56	d
57	b	58	a	59	c	60	c	61	a	62	a	63	b
64	b	65	a	66	a	67	b	68	d	69	b	70	b
71	a	72	c	73	b	74	a	75	a	76	d	77	d
78	a	79	a	80	a	81	c	82	d	83	d	84	c
85	c	86	c	87	a	88	a	89	b	90	c	91	d
92	d	93	d	94	b	95	c	96	c	97	a	98	b
99	b	100	a	101	b	102	b	103	a	104	b	105	d
106	c	107	d	108	b	109	a	110	b	111	b	112	b
113	a	114	c	115	a	116	b	117	c	118	d	119	a
120	c	121	a	122	b	123	a	124	d	125	d	126	b
127	c	128	c	129	a	130	a	131	d	132	c	133	b
134	b	135	a	136	a	137	a	138	c	139	b	140	a
141	b	142	c	143	b	144	c	145	a	146	a	147	a
148	b	149	a	150	c								

35

Clinical Pathology

Sushma Kajal[1], Vikas Nehra[1], Deepika Lather[1] and Surbhi Gupta[2]

[1]Department of Veterinary Pathology

[2]Department of Veterinary Physiology & Biochemistry, Lala Lajpat Rai University of Veterinary and Animal Sciences, Hisar-125004, India

In avian medicine, because clinical signs in birds can be vague, veterinarians must rely on additional clinical tests to accurately diagnose and treat conditions. These tests, including hematology, urine analysis and others, are essential for understanding diseases early and tailoring effective treatments. Clinical hematology is qualitative and quantitative assessment of blood and other blood component for the treatment of clinical patient. In comparison to mammals, bird's erythrocytes are oval and nucleated cells, nucleated thrombocytes, heterophiles instead of neutrophils. RBCs of birds have relatively short life span and regenerate more quickly than mammals. The preferred vein for blood collection in birds varies with the species. In most species the wing veins is preferred site. Both EDTA and heparin have been used in avian clinical haematology as anticoagulant. The average blood volume of most birds is approximately 10% body weight. Avian plasma samples frequently are yellow due to carotenoid pigments, not bilirubin. Uric acid is the major nitrogenous waste product of birds it is relatively inert and substantially less toxic than ammonia or urea. Both BUN and creatinine levels are normally low in birds and may be below the minimum detectable limit of the assays in the laboratory. It may be useful to evaluate BUN and uric acid together to differentiate among dehydration, postprandial effects and renal pathology.

Urinalysis is indicated when there is azotemia, uratemia, polyuria/polydipsia, abnormal urates. Avian urine is generally collected from a voided sample by removal of cage paper and thorough cleaning of the cage surface. Specific gravity in normal birds reported as 1.005-1.020 and avian urine is usually acidic. Normal urine sediment is composed of uric acid precipitates and crystals and sloughed epithelial cells. Majority of uric acid in avian urine exists as urates made up of uric acid, sodium and/or potassium and protein. Urine specific gravity tends to be lower in birds and reptiles than in mammals.

The common parasitic infections occur in poultry include gastrointestinal helminthes (cestodes, nematodes) and *Eimmeria* species that cause considerable damage and great economic losses to the poultry industry due to malnutrition, decreased feed conversion ratio, weight loss, lowered egg production and death in young birds.

1. Sero-mucus exudates in trachea is due to degeneration of cilia by viropexin enzyme produced by

   a) IBV b) NCDV

   c) IBDV d) AIV

2. Pink or red plasma is usually indicative of which condition in poultry
   a) Bilirubinemia b) Hemolysis
   c) Lipidemi d) Urobilinogen
3. Avian plasma samples frequently are yellow due towhich pigments
   a) Bilirubin b) Urochrome
   c) Biliverdin d) Carotenoids
4. Due to active renal tubular secretion, blood levels of which are not notably affected by dehydration until GFR is significantly decreased which may occur in severe dehydration
   a) Calcium b) ALT
   c) Uric acid d) AST
5. Biliverdinuria is not a normal finding in poultry due to
   a) Lack of bilirubin reductase b) Excess of bilirubin reductase
   c) Lack of bilirubin oxidase d) Excess of bilirubin reductase
6. Liver damage is associated with elevations in the enzymes
   a) Glutamate dehydrogenase, LDH, and AST
   b) CK, AST
   c) BUN, creatinine
   d) Lipase, amylase
7. Hypercalcemia, hypeglobulinemia, and an elevation in alkaline phosphatase may be seen in the
   a) Broiler breeder b) Chicks
   c) Layer hen d) All of the above
8. Avian red cells are
   a) Nucleated round b) Nucleated oval
   c) Non nucleated round d) Non nucleated oval
9. Muscle damage, which may include intramuscular injections, can cause elevations in the enzymes
   a) Glutamate dehydrogenase, LDH, AST b) ALT, Uric acid
   c) BUN, creatinine d) Creatine kinase, AST, LDH
10. Which side jugular vein is often sampled in most avian species as it is larger than the other side
   a) Right jugular vein b) Sub clavian vein
   c) Left jugular vein d) Brachiocephalic vein
11. Which anaemia can be seen as a consequence of chronic inflammatory or infectious disease and bone marrow pathology in avian spp
   a) Regenerative anaemia b) Hemorrhagicanemia
   c) Non-regenerative anaemia d) Hemolyticanemia

12. Regenerative anaemia in poultry may occur as a result of
    a) Haemorrhage
    b) haemoparasites such as Plasmodium
    c) Toxicosis from lead or zinc poisoning
    d) All of the above
13. Dehydration can cause what type changein PCV/HCT
    a) Relative increase b) Relative decrease
    c) Absolute increase d) Absolute decrease
14. Chronic infectious diseases such as include aspergillosis, avian tuberculosis and Chlamydia psittaci infectionscommonly leads to
    a) Neutrophilia b) Monocytosis
    c) Lymphocytosis d) All the cells
15. Enzyme which can increase due to cholestasis but lacks sensitivity
    a) GGT b) ALT
    c) AST d) CK
16. The major bile pigment in birds, which is not metabolised
    Cholebilirubin Biliverdin
    Bilirubin Hemobilirubin
17. Elevated alpha and beta globulins usually indicate acute inflammation or infection, whereas
    a) Acute inflammation or infection
    b) All of the above
    c) Chronic inflammatory or infectious process
    d) None of the above
18. High mortalityin a turkey flock coinciding with sulfur-colored droppings paired with necropsy as a result oftyphlitis and hepatitis indicates an infection with
    a) Histomonas meleagridis b) Salmonella spp.
    c) Escherichia coli d) Eimeria spp.
19. Elevated gamma globulins can indicate a more
    a) Acute inflammation or infection
    b) All of the above
    c) Chronic inflammatory or infectious process
    d) None of the above
20. Avian erythrocytes are typically nucleated; however, a small proportion of anucleated erythrocytes are seen which are termed as termed erythroplastids
    a) Kinetoplastids b) Erythroleucoblasts
    c) Erythroplastids d) Erythroblasts

21. Biliverdinuria is not a normal finding and is most birds commonly caused by liver compromise resulting in toxicinsult due to
    a) Bilestasis due to inflammation, infection and neoplasia
    b) Haemolytic anemia
    c) Lipidosis
    d) All of the above
22. Increase in AST in poultry birds may be caused by
    a) Hepatocellular damage b) Vit E/Selenium deficiency
    c) Muscle damage d) All of the above
23. Which is the primary and reliable indicator(s) of renal function in birds
    a) Blood uric acid level b) Electrolytes
    c) AST &ALT levels d) CK-MB
24. Elevated serum phosphorus is frequently observed in
    a) Advanced liver failure b) Advanced renal failure
    c) Early renal failure d) Early liver failure
25. Hypoglycemia is extremely rare in birds and the primary cause of hypoglycemia in farm birds is
    a) Insulin deficiency b) Diabetes insipidius
    c) Septicemia d) Diabetes mellitus
26. An elevated AST without a concurrent elevation in CK is highly suggestive of
    a) Hepatocellular disruption b) Cardiac failure
    c) Renal dysfunction d) Shock condition
27. Impaired liver functionis suggested in case when there is
    a) Elevation of bile acids in the portal circulation
    b) Elevation of bile acids in the general circulation
    c) Decrease in bile acids in the portal circulation
    d) Decrease in bile acids in the general circulation
28. Feather tips have been validated for use in the detection of viral antigen for molecular detection of which avian disease
    a) Marek's disease b) Avian Influenza
    c) Lymhoid leucosis d) Avian encephalomyelitis
29. Uric acid (an oxidized form of hypoxanthine) is synthesized predominantly in which organ frompurine metabolism
    a) Liver b) Lymph node
    c) Kidney d) Intestine
30. Specific gravity in most clinically normalbirds has been reported as
    a) <1.000 b) 1.005-1.020
    c) 1.000-1.001 d) >1.020

31. A measure of the degree of size variation inerythrocytes (anisocytosis) and is expressed as a percentage
    a) PT b) PCV
    c) MCV d) RDW
32. Iron deficiency can cause
    a) Hypochromia b) Increased MCHC
    c) Hyperchromasia d) Increased MCV
33. Which avain leucocyte has prominent small, round cytoplasmic granules that vary in color from bright red to pink depending on the species
    a) Heterophil b) Eosinophil
    c) Basophil d) Neutrophil
34. Most predominant leukocyte in avian species with lobulated, condensed nucleus and a cytoplasm that is filled with elongate, rod- to spindle-shaped, orange to brick-red granules
    a) Eosinophil b) Heterophil
    c) Basophil d) Neutrophil
35. Natt and Herrick's method allows the direct measurement of total
    a) Leucocytes, Erythrocytes b) Erythrocytes only
    c) Leucocytes only d) Thrombocytes
36. Elevated levels of cholesterol can be seen in birds in which condition
    a) low-fat diets b) Hpothyroisism
    c) Emaciation d) All of the above
37. Low levels of cholesterol can be seen in birds with
    a) Liver and kidney disease b) Pancreatic disease
    c) Bone disease d) Both a and c
38. Normal serum glucose for most birds ranges between
    a) 50-100 mg% b) 500-700 mg%
    c) 200 and 450 mg% d) 700-1000 mg%
39. Hypoglycemia (low blood sugar) in birds occurs with
    a) Malnutrition b) Fasting
    c) Liver disease d) All of the above
40. Hyperglycemia (high blood sugar) may occur during
    a) Pancreatitis b) Egg yolk peritonitis
    c) Stress d) All of the above
41. Elevated levels of amylase, as high as three times the upper limit of the normal range, may be seen with
    a) Acute gastritis b) Acute pancreatitis
    c) Acute hepatitis d) Acute cholecystitis
42. In healthy birds, albumin is the largest protein fraction, constituting up to
    a) 40% of total serum protein b) 60% of total serum protein
    c) 50% of total serum protein d) 70% of total serum protein

43. Causes of decrease in the A/G ratio in birds include
    a) Egg yolk peritonitis
    b) Both a and b
    c) Chronic diseseas
    d) None of the above
44. An inflammatory process in birds will result in increase in total protein due to
    a) Elevation of alpha-, beta-globulin fractions
    b) Both a and b
    c) Elevation of gammaglobulin fractions
    d) Increase in albumin
45. Decrease in serum albumin level in birds can develop due to
    a) Chronic liver/ renal disease
    b) Over hydration
    c) Parasitism
    d) All of the above
46. An increase in gammaglobulins in birds, which are composed primarily of immunoglobulins are seen in
    a) Chronic active hepatitis
    b) Nephrotic syndrome
    c) Severe active hepatitis
    d) Systemic mycotic infections
47. An increase in alpha- and betaglobulins can result in birds is seen in
    a) Vaccinations
    b) Immune-mediated disorders
    c) Severe active hepatitis
    d) Chronic active hepatitis
48. Ovulating birds have
    a) Elevated calcium levels
    b) Normal calcium levels
    c) Decreased calcium levels
    d) None of the above
49. Oversupplementation with _____________ will increase serum calcium and lead to renal mineralization
    a) Vitamin A
    b) Vitamin C
    c) Vitamin D3
    d) Vitamin B2
50. Elevated values of protein are found in
    a) Dehydration
    b) Hemolysis and lipemia
    c) Shock or infection
    d) All of the above
51. The ___________ of most bird species has a cytoplasm that is filled with elongate, rod- to spindle-shaped,orange to brick-red granules
    a) Eosinophils
    b) Basophils
    c) Heterophils
    d) Lymphocytes
52. The__________ has prominent small, round cytoplasmic granules that vary in color from bright red to pink depending on the species
    a) Eosinophils
    b) Basophils
    c) Heterophils
    d) Lymphocytes
53. The ______________ has prominent small, round, deep-magenta to purple cytoplasmic granules
    a) Eosinophils
    b) Basophils
    c) Heterophils
    d) Lymphocyte

54. _____________ lack the prominent cytoplasmic granules of the granulocytes but maycontain fine, dustlike, pink granulation and small, clear vacuoles

a) Monocytes
b) Basophils
c) Heterophils
d) Lymphocytes

55. The eosinophil Unopette 5877 system is used to quantify the numbers of__________________, but estimation is necessary to determine total number of leukocytes

a) Basophils and Eosinophils
b) Heterophils and Eosinophils
c) Monocytes and Eosinophils
d) Lymphocytes and Eosinophils

56. __________frequently results in transient heterophilia accompanied by normal or increased lymphocyte counts. It is often seen in young birds and birds notaccustomed to handling

a) Physiologic leukocytosis
b) Inflammation
c) Corticosteroid release or administration
d) Chronic myelogenous leukemia

57. __________ is characterized by transient heterophilia accompanied by lymphopenia in poultry

a) Physiologic leukocytosis
b) Inflammation
c) Corticosteroid release or administration
d) Chronic myelogenous leukemia

58. Stress leukogram is the term associated with _________in birds

a) Physiologic leukocytosis
b) Corticosteroid release or administration
c) Inflammation
d) Chronic myelogenous leukemia

59. Physiologic leukocytosis, corticosteroids, and inflammation result in heterophilia by

a) Heterophil redistribution
b) Decreased hematopoietic production
c) Increased egress from the circulation to tissues
d) Lymphocytes redistribution

60. ______________ may result in heteropenia with left shift and heterophil toxicity

a) Mild inflammation
b) Severe inflammation
b) Moderate inflammation
d) Both Mild and Moderate inflammation

61. _______________results in heterophil redistribution
   a) Adverse pharmacologic effects of cyclophosphamide
   b) Leukemia
   c) Multicentriclymphosarcoma
   d) Endotoxemia
62. Birds with leukemia, myelosuppressive therapy, or idiosyncratic drug reactions may have_________
   a) Lymphocytopenias   b) Pancytopenias
   c) Monocytopenias   d) Eosinopenias
63. Lymphocytosis due to _____________is rarely seen in birds especially pet birds
   a) Physiologic leukocytosis   Lymphoproliferative disease
   c) Chronic antigenic stimulation   Pathological leukocytosis
64. _______________ is the predominant cause of monocytosis in pet birds
   a) Inflammatory disease (acute or chronic) b) Phamacological drug toxicity
   c) Chronic antigenic stimulation   d) Multicentriclymphosarcoma
65. The most common reported cause of thrombocytopenia in birds is _____________
   a) Viral infections
   b) Phamacological drug toxicity
   c) Disseminated intravascularcoagulopathy (DIC)
   d) Bacterial septicemia
66. Which of the following is not a characteristic feature ofavian erythrocyte
   a) Nucleated, elliptic cell with orange-pink cytoplasm
   b) Nucleus is elliptic, condensed, and centrally positioned
   c) Generally smaller than mammalian erythrocytes
   d) Slight anisocytosis and poikilocytosis may be normally seen in healthy birds
67. What is the most common erythrocyte abnormality in pet bird
   a) Hyperchromasia   b) Anaemia
   c) Microcystosis   d) Polycythemia
68. Which of the following is not a feature in Conure bleeding syndrome affecting birds
   a) Birds have episodic bleeding
   b) Has high numbers of polychromatophils and immature erythrocytes
   c) Microscopic analysis shows amarked regenerative response
   d) Has high numbers of mature erythrocytes
69. Microcytosis in pet birds isnot seen in
   a) Iron deficiency either nutritional orresulting from chronic blood loss
   b) Chicks infected with Salmonella Gallinarum
   c) Chicks experimentally treated with cyclophosphomide
   d) Chicks infected with viral diseases

70. Hypochromasiain poultry birds is not seen in
    a) Iron deficiency (nutritional, chronic blood loss)
    b) Inflammatory diseases
    c) Cases of arsenic intoxication
    d) During regenerative responses (due to presence of polychromatophils)

71. __________ is characterized by increased numbers of erythrocytes with high intracytoplasmic Hb concentrations and measured by increased MCHC, is an artifact caused by in vitroor in vivo hemolysis
    a) Hyperchromasia   b) Polychromasia
    c) Microcytosis   d) Macrocystosis

72. Birds in general tolerate acute blood loss well. Under experimental conditions, loss of ____________ of blood volume in chickens and pigeons, respectively, does not produce hemorrhagicshock, and PCV values return to normal in 3 to 7 days
    a) 10% to 20%   b) 20% to 30%
    c) 30% to 60%   d) 30% to 40%

73. Which of the following is not a cause of hemolysis in birds
    a) Parasites: Plasmodium and Aegyptianella spp.
    b) Viral septicaemia
    c) Bacterial septicemia
    d) Toxins: aflatoxin, petroleum products, heavy metals

74. Increased reticulocytosis or polychromasia (>5%-10% of erythrocytes) indicates an
    a) Myleoid regenerative response to anemia
    b) Erythroid regenerative response to polycythemia
    c) Erythroid regenerative response to anemia
    d) Myleoid regenerative response to polycythemia

75. Which of the following is false related to infectious agents that cause blood parasitic diseases in birds
    a) Plasmodium spp.: gametocytes and multicellular schizonts generally found within
    b) Leucocytozoon spp.: gametocytes found within erythrocytes and leucocytes
    c) Erythrocytes but also in other blood cells
    d) Atoxoplasma spp.: sporozoites found within mononuclear leukocytes only

76. Which of the following is not the cause of decreased erythrocyte production
    a) Inflammatory disease: acute or chronic, infectious or noninfectious
    b) Adverse pharmacologic effects: fenbendazole in storks
    c) Myelosuppressive therapy: radiation
    d) Hyperthyroidism

77. Birds has _____blood volume as compared to mammalian counterparts
    a) Smaller   b) Milder
    c) Larger   d) Very milder

78. Which of the following is not the reported patterns of anemia seen in birds

a) Microcytic b) Macrocytic

c) Normocytic c) Normocytic

79. Which ectoparasite commonly affects poultry by causing small reddish brown flecks around breast, tail and vent?

a) Eimeria tenella *b) Ornithonyssus sylviarum*

c) Syngamus trachea *d) Cotugnia digonophora*

80. Which parasite is responsible for causing scaly leg in poultry?

The recommended level of EDTA for avian blood

a) *Ascaridia galli* *b) Echidnophaga gallinacea*

c) Ornithonyssus sylviarum *d) Knemidocoptes mutans*

81. Which parasite is commonly found in the respiratory tract of poultry?

a) *Ornithonyssus sylviarum* *b) Syngamus trachea*

c) Roundworm *d) Knemidocoptes mutans*

82. Which ectoparasite can lead to decreased egg production and weight loss in poultry?

a) *Eimeria necatrix* *b) Menopon gallinae*

c) Raillietina echinobothrida *d) Prosthogonimus ovatus*

83. Which parasite is commonly found in the intestines of poultry and can lead to haemorrhagic diarrhea, decreased growth rates and heavy mortality?

a) *Raillietina tetragona* *b) Eimeria tenella*

c) Ornithonyssus sylviarum *d) Ascaridia galli*

84. Which parasite is found in proventriculus of desi chicken?

a) *Tetrameres mohtedai* *b) Ascaridia galli*

c) Syngamus trachea *d) Eimeria tenella*

85. Which ectoparasite is responsible for anaemia in poultry birds?

a) Tapeworm b) Gapeworm

c) Roundworm d) Fowl tick

86. Which parasite is responsible for causing blackhead disease leading to cyanosis of comb and wattles in poultry?

a) Histomonas meleagridis b) Roundworm

c) Heterakis gallinarum d) Both a and b

87. Which nocturnal ectoparasite is commonly known as the "chicken mite" and is responsible for feather loss, irritiation and anaemia?

a) Knemidocoptes mutans b) Ornithonyssus sylviarum

c) Dermanyssus gallinae d) Argas persicus

88. Which parasite can cause neurological symptoms such as head shaking and circling in poultry?

a) Lice b) Roundworm

c) Fleas d) Gapeworm

89. Which parasite can lead to anemia and pale combs in poultry?
a) Tetramere b) Coccidia
c) Gapeworm d) Northern fowl mite

90. Which parasite is responsible for poor food absorption in poultry?
a) Railletina tetragona b) Railletina cesticillus
c) Railletina echinobothrida d) Hymenolepis carioca

91. Which parasite is responsible for blindness in young poultry?
a) Menopon gallinae b) Goniodes gigas
c) Menacanthus stramineus d) Echidnophaga gallinaceae

92. Which parasite can cause intestinal obstruction and catarrhal enteritis in poultry?
a) Ascaridia galli b) Gapeworm
c) Tetrameres mohtedai d) Coccidia

93. Which parasite is responsible for sulphur yellow droppings in poultry?
a) Histomonas meleagridis b) Trypanosoma sp.
c) Trichomonas avium d) Prosthogonimus sp.

94. Which parasite can be controlled using urea solution in poultry farm?
a) Fleas b) Lice
c) Coccidia d) Tapeworm

95. Which parasite is commonly spread through arthopods containing cysticercoid?
a) Tapeworm b) Gapeworm
c) Roundworm d) Northern fowl mite

96. Which parasite is mainly responsible for ladder like appearance in duodenum of poultryt?
a) Eimeria acervulina b) Eimeria tenella
c) Eimeria necatrix d) Eimeria brunetti

97. Which parasite is responsible for nodular taeniasis in poultry?
a) Railletina echinobothrida b) Railletina cesticillus
c) Railletina tetragona d) Cotugnia digonophora

98. Which parasite can be controlled through the use of acaricides and prevent blood loss in poultry?
a) Dermanyssus gallinae b) Argas persicus
c) Ornithonyssus sylviarum d) All of the above

99. Which parasite can cause decreased egg production and direct yolk release from vent in poultry chicks?
a) Prosthogonimus sp. b) Eimeria leukarti
c) Histomonas meleagridis d) Ascaridia galli

100. Which parasite is commonly found in the digestive tract of poultry and can cause nutritional deficiencies?
a) Tapeworm b) Northern fowl mite
c) Roundworm d) Both a and b

101. Which ectoparasite is known for causing severe itching and irritation around the vent area of poultry?
   a) Gapeworm b) Lice
   c) Fleas d) Northern fowl mite

102. Which parasite is responsible for severe anemia and paleness of comb in affected poultry birds?
   a) Dermanyssus gallinae b) Cnemidocoptes mutans
   c) Argas persicus d) Both a and b

103. Which roundworm is commonly found in the ceca of poultry?
   a) Gapeworm b) Echinostomum sp.
   c) Heterakis gallinarum d) Northern fowl mite

104. Which dwarf tapeworm is diagnosed in mucus collected from duodenal bumps and is responsible for heavy mortality in poultry?
   a) Davainea proglottina b) Cotugnia
   c) Raillietina d) Hymenolepis carioca

105. Which fluke is responsible for the formation of subcutaneous cysts in poultry birds?
   a) Postharmostomum commutatum b) Philopthalmus gralli
   c) Collyriclum faba d) Prosthogonimus macrorchis

106. Which parasite is claimed as eyeworm of poultry?
   a) Postharmostomum commutatum b) Philopthalmus gralli
   c) Collyriclum faba d) Prosthogonimus macrorchis

107. Which parasite is commonly spread through contact with contaminated bedding and litter?
   a) Northern fowl mite b) Gapeworm
   c) Tapeworm d) Lice

108. What is the primary function of hemoglobin in poultry blood?
   a) Oxygen transport b) pH regulation
   c) Nutrient absorption d) Waste removal

109. Which blood parameter is an indicator of the oxygen-carrying capacity of poultry blood?
   a) Hemoglobin concentration b) White blood cell count
   c) Platelet count d) Red blood cell count

110. Which blood parameter is responsible for clotting and preventing excessive bleeding in poultry?
   a) Hemoglobin b) Platelet count
   c) Hematocrit d) Red blood cell count

111. What is the primary function of erythrocytes (red blood cells) in poultry blood?
   a) Fighting infections b) Transporting oxygen
   c) Clotting d) Removing toxins

112. Which blood parameter indicates the volume percentage of red blood cells in the total blood volume?
a) Hemoglobin concentration
b) Platelet count
c) Hematocrit
d) Red blood cell count

113. What is the average lifespan of a chicken's red blood cell?
a) 28-35 days
b) 45-55 days
c) 65-90 days
d) 95-98 days

114. Which blood parameter is indicative of the body's ability to fight infections in poultry?
a) Hemoglobin concentration
b) White blood cell count
c) Hematocrit
d) Red blood cell count

115. What is the main function of leukocytes (white blood cells) in poultry blood?
a) Transporting oxygen
b) Clotting
c) Fighting infections
d) Nutrient absorption

116. Which blood parameter indicates the number of white blood cells per unit volume of blood?
a) Hemoglobin concentration
b) Platelet count
c) Hematocrit
d) White blood cell count

117. What is the normal range for hematocrit levels in poultry?
a) 20-30%
b) 40-50%
c) 30-40%
d) 50-60%

118. What is the role of thrombocytes in poultry blood?
a) Transporting oxygen
b) Fighting infections
c) Clotting
d) Removing toxins

119. Which of the following serum biochemical parameters is a measure of liver function in poultry?
a) Uric acid
b) Alanine aminotransferase (ALT)
c) Creatinine
d) Glucose

120. Which serum biochemical parameter is indicative of muscle damage in poultry?
a) Creatine kinase (CK)
b) Total protein
c) Cholesterol
d) Sodium

121. Elevated levels of which serum biochemical parameter may indicate dehydration in poultry?
a) Potassium
b) Chloride
c) Magnesium
d) Sodium

122. Which serum biochemical parameter is often used to assess lipid metabolism in poultry?
a) Cholesterol
b) Bilirubin
c) Iron
d) Total protein

123. High levels of which serum biochemical parameter can indicate egg yolk coagulation in poultry?
   a) Calcium
   b) Uric acid
   c) Phosphorus
   d) Total protein
124. Which serum biochemical parameter can indicate inflammation or infection in poultry?
   a) Albumin
   b) Potassium
   c) C-reactive protein (CRP)
   d) Iron
125. Which serum biochemical parameter is essential for bone health in poultry?
   a) Sodium
   b) Calcium
   c) Magnesium
   d) Bilirubin
126. End product of nitrogen metabolism in birds is
   a) Uric acid
   b) Bile pigments
   c) Urea
   d) Bile salts
127. Hemosiderin is
   a) Iron containing pigment
   b) Zinc containing pigment
   c) Copper containing pigment
   d) Sulphur containing pigment
128. The best site for collection of blood from avian species is
   a) Wing vein
   b) Heart
   c) Jugular vein
   d) None of the above
129. The best anticoagulant for routine haematological tests which preserves cellular elements is
   a) Heparin
   b) EDTA
   c) Oxalates
   d) All of the above
130. The recommended level of EDTA for avian blood
   a) 1 mg EDTA/ml of blood
   b) 2 mg EDTA/ml of blood
   c) 2 mg EDTA/ml of blood
   d) 2 mg EDTA/10ml of blood
131. Excess of EDTA in avian blood can cause
   a) Shrinkage of erythrocytes
   b) Low packed cell volume
   c) Low mean corpuscular volume
   d) All of the above
132. The recommended level of heparin for avian blood is
   a) 1 IU/ml of blood
   b) 5 IU/ml of blood
   c) 10 IU/ml of blood
   d) 15 IU/ml of blood
133. The recommended level of Heller and Paul oxalate for avian blood
   a) 0.1 ml of the mixture/ml of blood
   b) 0.2 ml of the mixture/ml of blood
   c) 0.5 ml of the mixture/ml of blood
   d) 1 ml of the mixture/ml of blood
134. Hyperlipemia can the ESR value in birds
   a) Increase
   b) Decrease
   c) No effect
   d) None of the above

135. Mean ESR ranging from mm/hr
a) 0.0 to 0.2 b) 0.5 to 9
c) 10 to 20 d) 20 to 30

136. Normal erythrocytes (millions/μl) value for chicken is
a) 1.18-1.50 b) 2.18-4.12
c) 5.18-9.12 d) 10.18-14.12

137. Normal haemoglobin (g/dl) value for chicken is
a) 2-4 b) 4-5
c) 7-13 d) 14-15

138. Anaemia usually associated with the following condition
a) Copper deficiency b) Iron deficiency
c) Both a and b d) None of the above

139. Polycythemia is usually associated with starvation
a) Starvation b) Hypoxia
c) Both a and b d) None of the above

140. Leukocytosis is usually associated with
a) Inflammatory diseases b) Avian leucosis
c) Mild type marek's disease d) All of the above

141. Lymphocytosis is usually associated with
a) Lymphocytic leukemia b) Adrenocortical insufficiency
c) Both a and b d) None of the above

142. Lymphopenia is usually associated with
a) X-ray irradiation b) Infectious bursal disease
c) Both a and b d) None of the above

143. Which haematological parameter is not affected by age and sex in birds?
a) MCHC b) MCH
c) MCV d) None of the above

144. Which of the following condition present in parasitic infection in poultry?
a) Eosinophilia b) Monocytosis
c) Lymphocytosis d) Heterophilia

145. Name the main nitrogenous excretory product in case of poultry?
a) Urea b) Uric acid
c) Ammonia None of the above

146. Which of poultry disease is known as acquired immunodeficiency syndrome
a) Infectios Bronchitis b) Infectious bursal disease
c) Pox d) Inclusionbody hepatitis

147. A metabolic disorder results in abnormal accumulation of urates in birds is :
a) Nephrosis b) Gout
c) Flipover disease d) Ascites

148. Coccidiosis in poultry diagnosed in faecal sample by:

a) Flotation b) Both a and b

c) Sedimentation d) None of the above

149. Avian urine is usually :

a) Acidic b) Neutral

c) Basic d) None of the above

150. Normal uric acid level in poultry :

a) 5-7mg /100ml b) 2-3mg/100ml

c) 7-9mg/100ml d) None of the above

Answer Key

1	a	2	b	3	d	4	c	5	a	6	a	7	c
8	b	9	d	10	a	11	c	12	d	13	a	14	b
15	a	16	b	17	a	18	a	19	c	20	c	21	d
22	d	23	a	24	b	25	c	26	a	27	b	28	a
29	a	30	a	31	b	32	a	33	b	34	b	35	a
36	b	37	a	38	c	39	d	40	d	41	b	42	a
43	b	44	b	45	d	46	a	47	c	48	a	49	c
50	d	51	c	52	a	53	b	54	a	55	b	56	a
57	c	58	b	59	a	60	b	61	d	62	b	63	b
64	a	65	d	66	c	67	b	68	d	69	d	70	c
71	a	72	c	73	b	74	c	75	b	76	d	77	c
78	c	79	b	80	d	81	b	82	b	83	b	84	a
85	d	86	d	87	c	88	a	89	a	90	c	91	d
92	a	93	a	94	c	95	a	96	a	97	a	98	d
99	a	100	d	101	b	102	d	103	c	104	a	105	c
106	b	107	d	108	a	109	a	110	b	111	b	112	c
113	a	114	b	115	c	116	d	117	b	118	c	119	b
120	d	121	a	122	a	123	d	124	c	125	b	126	a
127	a	128	a	129	b	130	c	131	d	132	d	133	a
134	a	135	b	136	b	137	c	138	c	139	c	140	d
141	c	142	c	143	a	144	a	145	b	146	b	147	b
148	a	149	a	150	a								

36

Therapeutic Applications of Drugs and Management

Sindhu K.

Department of AHVS, Govt. of Karnataka, Karnataka

Introduction

Poultry is one of the most widespread food industries worldwide. Chicken is the most common type of poultry in the world. The term broiler is applied to chickens that have especially been bred for meat; they grow rapidly. Broiler strains are based on hybrid crosses between Cornish White, New Hampshire and White Plymouth Rock. In broiler production there are two main production phases – keeping of parent stock and production of day-old-chicken (DOC); and growing and finishing of broilers.

The primary purpose of any enterprise is to maximize return on investment over the long-term. It is therefore necessary to market poultry, meat products, and eggs at a price which allows farmers or integrators to maintain profitability in a competitive market. Cost-effective programs of biosecurity and vaccination are required to prevent or limit the impact of disease. It is emphasized that the incremental return in the form of enhanced egg production, hatchability, liveability, growth rate, and feed conversion efficiency must exceed capital and operating expenditures on disease prevention.

Antibiotics are naturally occurring, semi-synthetic, or synthetic compounds with antimicrobial activity and are most widely used drugs in the poultry industry. They are administered parenterally or intravenously, topically, and orally. Antibiotic drugs are typically used to serve three purposes in poultry,(1) therapeutic use where animals (either individually or in small groups) are administered with high doses of antibiotics for relatively shorter periods, (2) prophylactic use that involves exposure of animals with moderate doses of antimicrobials for longer time durations, and (3) growth promotion where antibiotics in subtherapeutic doses, Wide range of antibiotic are used in poultry industry such as beta lactums, tetracyclines, fluoroquinolones, aminoglycosides along with many multivitamins and trace mineral supplements etc

A surge in the development and spread of antibiotic resistance has become a major cause for concern. Over the past few decades, no major new types of antibiotics have been produced and almost all known antibiotics are increasingly losing their activity against pathogenic microorganisms. Poultry products are among the highest consumed products worldwide but a lot of essential antibiotics are employed during poultry production in several countries; threatening the safety of such products (through antimicrobial residues) and the increased possibility of development and spread of microbial resistance in poultry settings. Therefore strict guidelines and regulations to control the indiscriminate use of antibiotics and growth supplements should be incorporated.

Multiple Choice Questions

1. Hyperpnea (panting) occurs in mature chickens exposed to temperatures exceeding.
   a) 40°C b) 30°C
   c) 35°C d) 45°C
2. Costs relating to live bird production can be classified into
   a) stable and recurring components b) movable and statice components
   c) fixed and variable components d) none of the above
3. Productivity and profitability in poultry can be enhanced by
   a) sound principles of biosecurity b) regular vaccination
   c) scientific management d) all of the above
4. The 3 levels of biosecurity components comprise of
   a) Operational Biosecurity b) Structural Biosecurity
   c) Conceptual Biosecurity d) all of the above
5. The net present value (NPV) of an investment in biosecurity can be calculated from the annual cash flows, discounted by an appropriate interest factor.
   a) true statement b) wrong prediction
   c) maybe d) irrelevant
6. Breeder farms should be operated on an ____________ preferably with absolute separation of rearing and laying flocks.
   a) few in few out basis b) all in system
   c) all out system d) all-in-all-out basis
7. Strategies to prevent infection are based on the purchase of breeding stock free of
   a) vertically-transmitted disease b) horizontally-transmitted disease
   c) both of the above d) none of the above
8. The severity of viral respiratory diseases such as bronchitis/ laryngotracheitis is influenced by
   a) housing b) environmental and clinical stress
   c) host factors d) none of the above
9. Which among the following are examples of Poultry emerging diseases affecting flocks in Asia, Africa, and Latin Americ a)
   a) Angara disease b) Virulent infectious bursal disease
   c) Reoviral stunting syndrome d) All of the above
10. The effect of intercurrent low-grade conditions such as pasteurellosis, mycoplasmosis or coccidiosis may be exacerbated by
    a) increasing vaccination strategies b) increased biodensity
    c) both a & b d) only a

11. The velogenic Newcastle disease (vvND) or highly pathogenic avian influenza (HPAI) can be effectively controlled by
    a) effective regular vaccination
    b) monitoring horizontal transmission
    c) monitoring vertical transmission
    d) genetic engineering
12. Pododermatitis (Bumble foot) resulting from
    a) excess potassium b) lack of calcium
    c) dry litter d) Wet litter
13. Keratitis (inflammation of the cornea) and conjunctivitis following exposure to high levels of
    a) atmospheric ammonia b) high amount of carbon di oxide
    c) high amount of carbon mono oxide d) all of the above
14. Vent peck and disembowelment in cage housed hens can be avoided by
    a) isolating individual stocks b) precision beak trimming
    c) trimming of the feathers d) none of the above
15. Following are the mechanisms of disease transmission
    a) Biological transmission b) Mechanical transmission
    c) both a & b d) none of the above
16. The ability of an organism to resist the killing effects of an antibiotic to which it was normally susceptible
    a) Antibiotic Resistance b) Antibiotic Susceptibility
    c) Antimicrobial Sensitivity d) none of the above
17. Contact between susceptible flocks and clinically affected or asymptomatic reservoirs of disease will result in infection
    a) Transmission on the egg shell b) Transovarian transmission
    c) Indirect transmission d) Direct transmission
18. Pathogens may be transmitted by the vertical route from hen to progeny via the egg is ______
    a) Transmission on the egg shell b) Transovarian transmission
    c) Indirect transmission d) Direct transmission
19. ___________ may be introduced into brooding and rearing units by contaminated egg-shells.
    a) Coryza b) Laryngotracheitis
    c) Mycoplasmosis d) Omphalitis and Salmonellosis
20. Pathogens including infectious bursal disease virus (IBDV) and Salmonella spp which can infect successive placements are classical examples of____________
    a) Transmission on the egg shell b) Transovarian transmission
    c) Indirect transmission d) Direct transmission

21. The disease transmitted by mosquitoes (Vector borne diseases) to poultry are
    a) Pox virus
    b) West Nile virus
    c) Highland J arbovirus
    d) All of the above
22. Argasid ticks transmits which of the following poultry disease
    a) Spirochetosis
    b) Marek's disease
    c) IBD
    d) Salmonellosis
23. House flies transmits which of the following poultry disease
    a) Spirochetosis
    b) Marek's disease
    c) IBD
    d) Campylobacteriosis
24. Rodents are major vectors and reservoirs of poultry and zoonotic pathogens like
    a) Pasteurella multocida
    b) Salmonella typhimurium
    c) Salmonella enteritidis
    d) All of the above
25. Free-living migratory and resident birds serve as reservoirs and disseminators of numerous infections of commercial poultry like ________
    a) Newcastle disease
    b) Avian influenza
    c) Duck viral enteritis
    d) All of the above
26. Epidemic tremor in poultry is seen in
    a) Avian encephalomyelitis
    b) Infectious bursal disease
    c) Egg drop syndrome
    d) Infectious laryngotracheitis
27. Linoleic and linolenic acid deficiency leads to condition
    a) poor skin quality
    b) deformed feathers
    c) gout
    d) fatty liver syndrome
28. Xerophthalmia ("dry eye") is due to deficiency of
    a) Vitamin D3
    b) Vitamin C
    c) Vitamin A
    d) none
29. Visceral gout; urate deposit on the viscera in the advanced cases seen during PM examination is due to deficiency of
    a) Avitaminosis A
    b) Thiamine Deficiency
    c) Cholecalciferol Deficiency
    d) Riboflavin Deficiency
30. ____________ can be confirmed by histological examination of the proximal end plate of the tibia and parathyroid gland tissue.
    a) Fatty liver syndrome
    b) Rickets
    c) Chronic purulent conjunctivitis
    d) Metabolic gout
31. Transudative diathesis in chicks causes degeneration of the endothelium can be corrected by supplementing
    a) Vitamin D3
    b) Vitamin C
    c) Vitamin A
    d) Vitamin E
32. Star gazing in 10-to-20-day old chicks is due to
    a) Avitaminosis A
    b) Thiamine Deficiency
    c) Cholecalciferol Deficiency
    d) Riboflavin Deficiency

33. Curled toe paralysis characterized by rotation of the legs in chicks aged 10 - 30 days is due to
    a) Avitaminosis A b) Thiamine Deficiency
    c) Cholecalciferol Deficiency d) Riboflavin Deficiency
34. The displacement of the gastrocnemius tendon occurs as perosis /slipped tendon is due to
    a) Calcium deficiency b) Manganese deficiency
    c) Magnesium deficiency d) Zinc deficiency
35. Young chicks showing tail picking and cannibalism is due to
    a) Sodium & Chloride deficiency b) Manganese deficiency
    c) Magnesium deficiency d) Zinc deficiency
36. Hyperkeratosis (thickening of the skin) of the plantar surface of the feet associated with
    a) Pantothenic acid deficiency b) Thiamine Deficiency
    c) Cholecalciferol Deficiency d) Riboflavin Deficiency
37. Which among these are Immunosuppressive diseases in poultry birds
    a) Marek's disease b) Infectious bursal disease
    c) Infectious anemia d) All of the above
38. The diseases of poultry which affects the respiratory system
    a) Newcastle disease b) Mycoplasmosis
    c) Infectious coryza d) All of the above
39. Adenovirus infections in poultry includes
    a) Inclusion body hepatitis b) Angara disease
    c) Egg drop syndrome d) All of the above
40. Bacillary White Diarrhea condition is otherwise known as
    a) Pullorum disease b) Fowl typhoid
    c) Paratyphoid d) None of the above
41. Fowl Cholera is also known as
    a) Pullorum disease b) Fowl typhoid
    c) Paratyphoid d) Pasteurellosis
42. Hydropericardium-Hepatitis Syndrome (HHS) in chickens is caused due to
    a) Type 1 adenovirus b) Type 2 adenovirus
    c) Type 3 adenovirus d) all of the above
43. Hemorrhagic enteritis of turkeys is caused due to
    a) Type 1 adenovirus b) Type 2 adenovirus
    c) Type 3 adenoviru d) All of the above
44. Type 3 adenovirus infections lead to
    a) Hydropericardium-Hepatitis Syndrome (HHS) in chickens
    b) Hemorrhagic enteritis of turkeys
    c) Egg drop syndrome in chickens
    d) None of the above

45. Hydropericardium-Hepatitis syndrome in India is known as
    a) Lychee disease b) Angara disease
    c) both a & b d) Moist rales
46. Which among these is known as "helicopter disease" in chickens
    a) Runting syndrome b) Rickets-like syndrome
    c) Infectious Stunting Syndrome d) All of the above
47. hemorrhagic typhlitis (inflammation of the cecum) is caused by
    a) E. necatrix b) E. tenella
    c) E. brunetti d) E. necatrix
48. The diagnosis and identification of Eimeria sp. Is done using intestine from a sacrificed, affected bird preserved in ___________ for culture
    a) 1% potassium dichromate b) 2% potassium dichromate
    c) 4% potassium dichromate d) 5% potassium dichromate
49. Coccidiosis can be treated by adding ______ in drinking water for 5 days
    a) Amprolium solution b) Sulfonamides
    c) both a & b d) cephalosporins
50. The principal pathogen responsible for necrotic enteritis (NE)
    a) *Clostridium perfringens* b) *Clostridium botulinum*
    c) both a & b d) none of the above
51. The nematode typically occurring in the jejunum is_______
    a) *Ascaridia galli* b) *Cheilospirura hamulosa*
    c) *Oxyspirum mansoni* d) *Heterakis gallinarum*
52. The nematode typically present beneath the nictitating membrane of the eye.
    a) *Ascaridia galli* b) *Cheilospirura hamulosa*
    c) *Oxyspirum mansoni* d) *Heterakis gallinarum*
53. The cestodes of the jejunum resulting in nodular granulomas and catarrhal enteritis.
    a) *Davainea proglottina* b) *Choanotaenia infundibulum*
    c) *Raillietina tetragona* d) *Raillietina echinobothridia*
54. Mycoplasma responsible for serous arthritis and teno-synovitis in chickens is
    a) *Mycoplasma bovis* b) *Mycoplasma synoviae*
    c) *Mycoplasma gallinarium* d) None of the above
55. Characteristic Hock sitting posture of broiler is due to
    a) *Mycoplasma bovis* b) *Mycoplasma synoviae*
    c) *Mycoplasma gallinarium* d) None of the above
56. Valgus (x-legged) and Varus (bow-legged) deformities occur in rapidly growing broilers
    a) bacterial origin b) viral origin
    c) deficiency disorder d) genetic in origin

57. The presence of intracytoplasmic inclusions (Bollinger bodies) in the respiratory mucosa and skin is characteristic in which disease

a) leucocytozoonosis b) scaly leg mites' infestation
c) avian pox d) dermatomycosis

58. _________are effective in the treatment of sinusitis and chronic respiratory disease in poultry.

a) Penicillin b) Tetracyclines
c) Aminoglycosides d) All of the above

59. _______ is often the treatment of last resort for methicillin-resistant Staphylococcus aureus (MRSA) infections

a) Amoxicillin b) Oxytetracycline
c) Gentamicin d) Vancomycin

60. The feed additives used in the control of coccidiosis, primarily when raising broilers, broiler breeders and replacement pullets is

a) Glycopeptides b) Lincosamides
c) Ionophores d) Macrolides

61. All supplementary fats and animal byproducts should be stabilized with ________ ethoxyquin compound.

a) 100-300 ppm b) 300-600 ppm
c) 600-900 ppm d) 1000 ppm

62. The vitamin E supplementation as per NRC levels for stressed flocks

a) 20 IU/kg b) 30 IU/kg
c) 40 IU/kg d) 40IU/kg

63. The process of physically removing biological and inorganic material from the surfaces of a building or equipment is termed as ____________

a) Fumigation b) Sterilization
c) Decontamination d) Disinfection

64. Compounds used to disinfectants the poultry buildings and soil is __________

a) Cresols b) Organic phenols
c) Quaternary ammonium compounds d) Chlorine compounds

65. __________ used in hatcheries to decontaminate hatcheries equipment.

a) Cresols b) Organic phenols
c) Quaternary ammonium compounds d) Chlorine compounds

66. ___________ are widely used in processing plants and to purify water on poultry farms.

a) Cresols b) Organic phenols
c) Quaternary ammonium compounds d) Chlorine compounds

67. Compound suitable to fumigate eggs in purpose-designed cabinets is______

a) Organic phenols b) QAT
c) Formalin d) Hypochlorite

68. The surface of the litter and the lower side walls should be sprayed with ________ for effective disinfection.

a) 1% carbamate insecticide b) 2% carbamate insecticide

c) 3% carbamate insecticide d) 4% carbamate insecticide

69. Maximum Acceptable Level of Coliform bacteria in the water supplied for poultry is______

a) 10 CFU/ml b) 50 CFU/ml

c) 100 CFU/ml d) 500 CFU/ml

70. ________is stimulated in breeding stock in response to exposure to pathogens or Vaccination

a) Maternal Antibody (MAB's) b) Maternal Antigens

c) T-cell mediated immunity d) all of the above

71. *In ovo* vaccination using the patented Embrex InovoJect® system at ____ days of incubation

a) 0th day of incubation b) 10th day of incubation

c) 18th day of incubation d) 30th day of incubation

72. Eradication of vectors and dusting birds can be done using

a) 5% carbamate b) 10% carbamate

c) 15% carbamate d) 20% carbamate

73. Antibiotic indicated for growth proportion in poultry

a) Amoxicillin b) Oxytetracycline

c) Virginiamycin d) Vancomycin

74. An alkaloid derivative used as feed additive for prevention and control of coccidiosis

a) Halofuginone b) Vancomycin

c) Vincristine d) Hypochlorite

75. used as a premix for the prevention of coccidiosis in broiler chicken

a) Duramicin 2% b) Vancomycin 5%

c) Maduramicin 1% premix d) None of the above

76. Apramicin sulphate is approved by CDSCO to treat the following poultry diseases

a) Bacterial enteritis b) Cellibacillosis

c) Salmonellosis d) All of the above

77. ___________is a type of avian cancer were tumors in nerves cause lameness and paralysis in poultry

a) Marek's disease b) Aspergillosis

c) Mycoplasma synoviae d) NCD

78. Condition in which affected chicks shows external navel infection, large unabsorbed yolk sacs, peritonitis with foetid odour, exudates adhering to the navel and oedema of the skin.

a) Avian Encephalomyelitis b) Infectious Bursal Disease

c) Omphalitis d) Egg Drop Syndrome

79. Avian Metapneumovirus disease is also known as
   a) Turkey Rhinotracheitis (TRT)   b) Rhinotracheitis (RT)
   c) Swollen Head Syndrome (SHS)   d) All of the above
80. The diagnosis of Turkey Rhinotracheitis can be done after infection several serological methods can be used to detect antibodies.
   a) VN   b) ELISA
   c) IFT   d) All of the above
81. Infectious Coryza treatment can be done with following antibiotics
   a) erythromycin   b) tetracycline
   c) both a & b   d) none
82. Laboratory confirmation with histopathology showing intranuclear inclusion bodies in tracheal epithelial cells is characteristic of which disease
   a) Infectious Coryza
   b) Infectious Laryngotracheitis (ILT)
   c) Swollen Head Syndrome
   d) None of the above
83. Vertical transmission of disease in poultry means
   a) Agents gets transmitted through the egg to their offspring/ parent to progeny
   b) Agents gets transmitted by contact or by airborne dust or droplets
   c) Agents gets transmitted by birds to birds directly
   d) Agents gets transmitted indirectly through feed supplements
84. Horizontal transmission of disease in poultry means
   a) Agents gets transmitted through the egg to their offspring/ parent to progeny
   b) Agents gets transmitted by contact or by airborne dust or droplets
   c) Agents gets transmitted by birds to birds directly
   d) Agents gets transmitted indirectly through feed supplements
85. The Newcastle disease strains used for live vaccines are mainly
   a) Lentogenic   b) Mesogenic
   c) Velogenic   d) All of the above
86. Histological examination showing intranuclear inclusion bodies of liver is diagnostic feature of _____ disease
   a) Inclusion Body Hepatitis
   b) Hydropericardium-Hepatitis Syndrome (HHS)
   c) both a & b
   d) Egg drop syndrome
87. The malabsorption syndrome (MAS) is also known as
   a) Femoral head necrosis/ brittle bone disease,
   b) Infectious proventriculitis,
   c) Runting and stunting syndrome
   d) All of the above

88. The most widely used vaccines live attenuated virus vaccines which can be administered to birds by techniques such as
    a) Drinking water,
    b) Spray application,
    c) Eye drop or by injection
    d) All of the above
89. Ingestion of tissues and organs (meat, offals, eggs, etc.) containing drug remnants above safe maximum residual levels (MRLs) leads to
    a) directly as initiation of hypersensitive or allergic reactions
    b) indirectly as carcinogens, teratogens,
    c) development of Antibiotic resistance often leads to drug toxicity.
    d) All of the above
90. first drug of choice for colibacillosis include
    a) ormethoprim-sulfadimethoxine
    b) trimethoprim-sulfadiazine
    c) both a & b
    d) lincosamides
91. Bacteria counteract the actions of antibiotics by the following mechanisms such as
    a) alteration in target binding sites
    b) enzyme modification
    c) decreased permeability of bacterial membrane
    d) All of the above
92. ______ is usually the drug of choice for the treatment of Campylobacter infections
    a) Erythromycin
    b) Amoxicillin
    c) trimethoprim
    d) Levamisole
93. According to OECD, the estimated global average annual consumption of antimicrobials to produce one kilogram of chicken meat is
    a) 100mg
    b) 126mg
    c) 148mg
    d) 174mg
94. The ____________introduced a new norm that specifies the withdrawal period, or the timeframe for poultry, livestock and marine products to be kept off antibiotics before they enter the food chain.
    a) Central Drugs Standard Control Organization
    b) AMR control bureau
    c) MOEF & CC
    d) FSSAI
95. According to the Food Safety and Standards (Contaminants, Toxins and Residues) Amendment Regulation 2017; the tolerance limit of antibiotics and pharmacology active substances in food of animal origin will be
    a) 1 mg/kg
    b) 0.5 mg/kg
    c) 0.1 mg/kg
    d) 0.01mg/kg
96. Administered in-water (Prescription) FDA approved medications for poultry.
    a) Penicillium G
    b) Neomycin
    c) both a & b
    d) none of the above

97. Aminoglycoside class of antimicrobials approved for use in poultry by FDA
    a) Streptomycin
    b) Gentamicin
    c) Neomycin
    d) All of the above
98. Tetracycline class of antimicrobials approved for use in poultry by FDA
    a) Tetracycline Hcl
    b) Chlortertracycline
    c) Oxytetracycline
    d) All of the above
99. _________lay down science-based standards for articles of food and to regulate their manufacture, storage, distribution, sale and import to ensure availability of safe and wholesome food for human consumption.
    a) CFTRI
    b) CDSCO
    c) DAHD&F
    d) FSSAI
100. ______ is the inoculation of specific biological substance (antigen) to stimulate resistance or immunity to the birds against diseases.
    a) Vaccination
    b) Antibiotic treatment
    c) Supplementation
    d) All of the above

Answer Key

1	b	2	c	3	d	4	d	5	a	6	d	7	a
8	b	9	d	10	b	11	a	12	d	13	a	14	b
15	c	16	a	17	d	18	b	19	d	20	c	21	d
22	a	23	d	24	d	25	d	26	a	27	d	28	c
29	a	30	b	31	d	32	b	33	d	34	b	35	a
36	a	37	d	38	d	39	d	40	a	41	d	42	a
43	b	44	c	45	a	46	d	47	b	48	d	49	c
50	a	51	a	52	c	53	d	54	b	55	b	56	d
57	c	58	a	59	d	60	c	61	b	62	a	63	c
64	a	65	b	66	d	67	c	68	b	69	a	70	b
71	c	72	a	73	c	74	a	75	c	76	d	77	a
78	c	79	d	80	d	81	c	82	b	83	a	84	b
85	a	86	c	87	d	88	d	89	d	90	c	91	d
92	a	93	c	94	a	95	d	96	c	97	d	98	d
99	d	100	a										

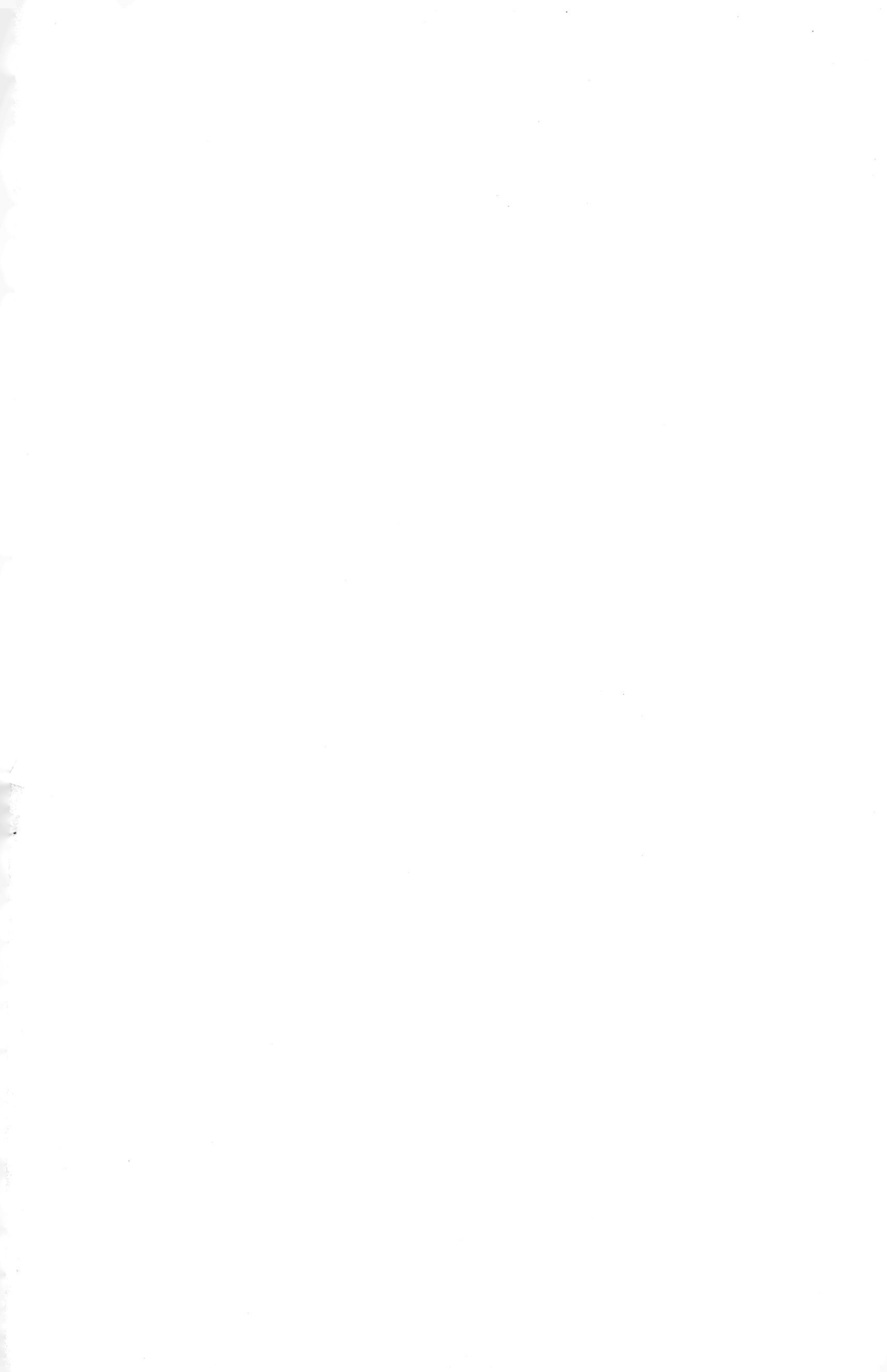